Drugs in Sport

Drugs in Sport is the most comprehensive and accurate text on the emotive, complex and critical subject of doping and illegal performance enhancement in sport. Thoroughly updated in light of the latest World Anti-Doping Code and taking into account the latest regulations, methods and landmark cases, this seventh edition explores the science behind drug-use in sport, as well as its ethical, social, political and administrative context.

Introducing an increased focus on inadvertent doping, athlete-support personnel as key stakeholders in the doping process, societal drug-use, and the role of national governing bodies and anti-doping organisations, the book covers key topics including:

- an assessment of the prevalence of drug-taking in sport
- the latest doping control regulations stipulated by the World Anti-Doping Agency (WADA)
- the science and side effects of each major class of drug used in sport
- cutting-edge issues such as gene doping and biological passports
- issues surrounding legal substances and ergogenic aids in supplements
- medical and pharmaceutical services at major sporting events

Accessibly written, and supported throughout with illustrative case studies and data, *Drugs in Sport* provides a crucial and objective resource for students and researchers, athletes, sports scientists, coaches and athlete-support staff, journalists, sports administrators and policymakers, alike.

David R. Mottram is Emeritus Professor of Pharmacy at Liverpool John Moores University, UK. He was a member of the organising committee for pharmacy services for the London 2012 Olympic and Paralympic Games, and part of the medical services team at the Polyclinic in the Athlete Village during the Rio 2016 Olympic Games. David is currently providing education and training programmes on medicines management in sport for the International Olympic Committee (IOC), the World Anti-Doping Agency (WADA) and UK Anti-Doping (UKAD).

Neil Chester is Senior Lecturer in Sport and Exercise Sciences at Liverpool John Moores University, UK. His teaching commitments are in exercise physiology with a particular focus in sports nutrition, supplementation, drug use and anti-doping in addition to research ethics and ethics in sport and professional practice. Neil works closely with UK Anti-Doping in a research, education and testing capacity and is a committee member of the British Association for Sport and Exercise Sciences Clean Sport Interest Group.

Drugs in Sport

Seventh Edition

Edited by David R. Mottram
and Neil Chester

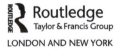

Routledge
Taylor & Francis Group

LONDON AND NEW YORK

Seventh edition published 2018
by Routledge
2 Park Square, Milton Park, Abingdon, Oxon, OX14 4RN

and by Routledge
711 Third Avenue, New York, NY 10017

Routledge is an imprint of the Taylor & Francis Group, an informa business

First edition published by Human Kinetics 1988
Sixth edition published by Routledge 2015

British Library Cataloguing-in-Publication Data
A catalogue record for this book is available from the British Library

Library of Congress Cataloging-in-Publication Data
Names: Mottram, D. R. (David R.), 1944- editor. | Chester, Neil, editor.
Title: Drugs in sport / [edited by] David R. Mottram and Neil Chester.
Description: Seventh edition. | Milton Park, Abingdon ; New York, NY :
    Routledge, 2018. | Includes bibliographical references and index.
Identifiers: LCCN 2017042157 (print) | LCCN 2017043366 (ebook) |
    ISBN 9781315222790 (Master eBook) | ISBN 9780415789394 (hbk) |
    ISBN 9780415789417 (pbk) | ISBN 9781315222790 (ebk)
Subjects: LCSH: Doping in sports. | Sports medicine. | Substance abuse.
Classification: LCC RC1230 (ebook) | LCC RC1230 .D783 2018 (print) |
    DDC 617.1/027—dc23
LC record available at https://lccn.loc.gov/2017042157

ISBN: 978-0-415-78939-4 (hbk)
ISBN: 978-0-415-78941-7 (pbk)
ISBN: 978-1-315-22279-0 (ebk)

Typeset in Goudy
by Swales & Willis Ltd, Exeter, Devon, UK

Contents

Figures

Tables

Boxes

Contributors

Susan H. Backhouse is Director of Research and Professor of Psychology and Behavioural Nutrition in the Carnegie School of Sport at Leeds Beckett University, UK.

Kelsey Erickson is a Research Fellow in the Carnegie School of Sport at Leeds Beckett University, UK.

Neil King is Senior Lecturer in Sport in the Sport Studies and Sports Development Department at Edge Hill University, UK.

Jim McVeigh is Director of the Public Health Institute at Liverpool John Moores University, UK.

Yorck Olaf Schumacher is Sports Medicine Physician at Aspetar Sports Medicine Hospital, Qatar.

Mark Stuart is Clinical Lead for Pharmacy, Nursing and Allied Healthcare at the British Medical Journal, UK.

Dominic J. Wells is Professor in Translational Medicine at the Department of Comparative Biomedical Sciences, Royal Veterinary College, UK.

Nick Wojek is Head of Science and Medicine at UK Anti-Doping.

The use, misuse and regulation of drugs in sport

Chapter 1

Drugs and their use in sport

David R. Mottram

1.1 Introduction

In this chapter we will review what is meant by the term "drug". Having established how drugs exert their effects and side effects within the body, we will reflect on the various circumstances by which athletes may take drugs. Finally, we will consider why drugs are used by athletes for the purpose of performance enhancement.

1.2 What is a drug?

Definition of a drug

The branch of science investigating drug action is known as pharmacology. Drugs are chemical substances which, by interaction with biological targets, can alter the biochemical systems of the body. For example, drugs such as ephedrine can lead to an increase in the force and rate of beating of the heart; amphetamines can produce changes in mood and behaviour; drugs such as insulin interact with metabolic processes in the treatment of disorders such as diabetes.

Banned drugs in sport

In this chapter, frequent reference is made to drugs that appear on the World Anti-Doping Agency (WADA) Prohibited List (http://list.wada-ama.org). The 2017 list is presented in Table 1.1.

Mazzoni et al. (2011) have provided a comprehensive description of the structure, review and update processes for the WADA Prohibited List. Each class of drug is described in detail in Section 2 of this book.

Classification and description of drug names

Drugs are variously classified and described by their:

- generic name (International Non-proprietary Name: INN)
- proprietary name (manufacturer's name)
- mechanism of action

The generic name (INN) is the internationally recognised name of the drug and should normally be used when describing the drug. However, when a pharmaceutical company first

Table 1.1 WADA Prohibited List: January 2017

Substances and methods prohibited at all times (in- and out-of-competition)
Prohibited substances
S.0 Non-approved substances
S.1 Anabolic agents
S.2 Peptide hormones, growth factors, related substances and mimetics
S.3 Beta-2 agonists
S.4 Hormone and metabolic modulators
S.5 Diuretics and masking agents
Prohibited methods
M.1 Manipulation of blood and blood components
M.2 Chemical and physical manipulation
M.3 Gene doping
Substances and methods prohibited in-competition
Categories S.0 to S.5 and M.1 to M.3 plus:
S.6 Stimulants
S.7 Narcotics
S.8 Cannabinoids
S.9 Glucocorticoids
Substances prohibited in particular sports
P.1 Alcohol
P.2 Beta blockers

Source http://list.wada-ama.org/

develops a new drug, it patents the drug under a proprietary name. When the patent expires, other pharmaceutical companies may produce the same drug under their own proprietary name. Some examples of the classification and names of drugs which appear on the WADA Prohibited List are presented in Table 1.2.

Drugs may be classified by their mechanism of action (pharmacology) or by the therapeutic use for which the drug is designed. Examples are given in Table 1.3.

Development of new drugs

Over the centuries, herbalists and apothecaries have extracted drugs from plant and animal sources. For example, morphine is extracted from the opium poppy and digoxin from the

Table 1.2 Examples of the classification and description of drugs by their names

Class of drug	Generic name	Proprietary name
Anabolic androgenic steroids	Nandrolone	Deca-Durabolin
Diuretics	Furosamide	Lasix
Beta-2 agonists	Terbutaline	Bricanyl
Narcotics	Morphine	Sevredol
Beta blockers	Atenolol	Tenormin
Human growth hormone	Somatropin	Humotrope

Table 1.3 Examples of the classification of drugs by their mechanism of action and use

Class of drug	Pharmacological action	Therapeutic use in:
Diuretics	Prevention of re-absorption of water from the kidneys	Heart failure; Hypertension
Beta-2 agonists	Bronchodilation through stimulation of beta-2 adrenoreceptors	Asthma; Chronic obstructive pulmonary disease
Morphine	Agonist on opioid μ receptors	Severe pain
Beta blockers	Antagonists on beta adrenoreceptors	Angina; Hypertension; Cardiac arrhythmias; Anxiety

foxglove plant. However, the majority of drugs are produced by pharmaceutical companies through chemical synthesis. Current research into gene technology is revolutionising the development of new drugs.

Drug development is monitored by government agencies who evaluate the activity and safety of new drugs before awarding a Product Licence which states the therapeutic purpose(s) for which the drug may be used. The development of new drugs can take between 10 and 12 years and have a cost of several hundred million dollars. The WADA Prohibited List includes a class S.0, Non-approved Substances, which includes drugs that are still under development. The pharmaceutical industry is ideally placed to identify the doping potential of new medicines and to support early development of detection methods (Elliott and Leishman, 2012).

Dosage forms for drug delivery to the body

There are many different dosage forms through which drugs can be administered to the body. Some examples for drugs that are subject to restrictions in sport are presented in Table 1.4.

Table 1.4 Examples of dosage forms for drugs used in sport

Generic drug name	Dosage forms
Testosterone (anabolic androgenic steroid)	Oral capsules
	Intramuscular injection
	Transdermal patches
Terbutaline (beta-2 agonist)	Aerosol inhaler
	Oral tablets
	Syrup
	Injection
Hydrocortisone (glucocorticoid)	Oral tablets
	Injection
	Ear/eye drops
	Cream/ointment
Pethidine (narcotic analgesic)	Oral tablets
	Injection

The absorption, distribution, metabolism and elimination of drugs

For a drug to exert its effect it must reach its site of action. This will involve its passage from the site of administration to the cells of the target tissue or organ. The principal factors which can influence this process are absorption, distribution, metabolism and elimination, known as the *pharmacokinetics* of drug action.

Absorption

The absorption of a drug is, in part, dependent upon its route of administration. Most drugs must enter the bloodstream in order to reach their site of action and the most common route of administration for this purpose is orally, in either liquid or tablet form.

Where a drug is required to act more rapidly, or is susceptible to breakdown in the gastrointestinal tract, the preferred route of administration is by injection. The main routes of injection are subcutaneous (under the skin), intramuscular (into a muscle) and intravenous (directly into the blood stream via a vein).

Some drugs can be applied topically for a localised response. This may take the form of applying a cream, ointment or lotion to an area of skin for treatment of abrasions, lesions, infections or other such dermatological conditions. Topical applications may also involve applying drops to the eye, the ear or the nose. Drugs administered by a topical route are not normally absorbed into the body to the same extent as drugs administered orally. Consequently, the WADA regulations regarding some prohibited drugs take into account the route of administration.

Distribution

Apart from topical administration, a significant proportion of a drug will reach the blood stream. Most drugs are then dissolved in the water phase of the blood plasma. Within this phase some of the drug molecules may be bound to proteins and thus may not be freely diffusible out of the plasma. This will affect the amount of drug reaching its target receptors.

An additional obstruction to the passage of drugs occurs at the "blood–brain barrier" which comprises a layer of cells which covers the capillary walls of the vessels supplying the brain. This barrier effectively excludes molecules which are poorly lipid soluble. The blood–brain barrier is an important factor to be considered in drug design since a drug's ability to cross this barrier can influence its potential for centrally-mediated side effects.

Metabolism

The body has a very efficient system for transforming chemicals into safer molecules which can then be excreted by the various routes of elimination. This process is known as metabolism and many drugs which enter the body undergo metabolic change.

There are several enzyme systems which are responsible for producing metabolic transformations. These enzymes are principally located in the cells of the liver but may also be found in other cells. They produce simple chemical alteration of the drug molecules by processes such as oxidation, reduction, hydrolysis, acetylation and alkylation.

The consequences of drug metabolism may be seen in a number of ways:

1   An active drug is changed into an inactive compound. This is the most common means for the termination of the activity of a drug.
2   An active drug can be metabolised into another active compound. The metabolite may have the same pharmacological action as the parent drug or it may differ in terms of higher or lower potency or a different pharmacological effect.
3   An active drug can be changed into a toxic metabolite.
4   An inactive drug can be converted into pharmacologically active metabolites. This mechanism can be used for beneficial purposes where a drug is susceptible to rapid metabolism before it reaches its site of action. In this case a "prodrug" can be designed which is metabolised to an active drug on arrival at its target tissue.

Generally speaking, the metabolism of drugs results in the conversion of lipid soluble drugs into more water-soluble metabolites. This change affects distribution, in that less lipid-soluble compounds are unable to penetrate cell membranes. The kidneys are able to excrete water-soluble compounds more readily than lipid-soluble molecules since the latter can be reabsorbed in the kidney tubules and therefore re-enter the plasma.

Metabolism is a very important factor in determining a drug's activity since it can alter its intrinsic activity, its ability to reach its site of action, and its rate of elimination from the body.

Many drugs are completely metabolised before being excreted in the urine. The WADA testing procedures in doping control detect both the parent drug and its metabolite(s), where appropriate.

Elimination

There are many routes through which drugs can be eliminated from the body:

*   Kidneys (urine)
*   Salivary glands (saliva)
*   Sweat glands (sweat)
*   Pulmonary epithelium (exhaled gases)
*   Mammary glands (mammary milk)
*   Rectum (faeces)

The most important route for drug excretion is through the kidneys into the urine. *Urine sampling is therefore the principal method used in dope testing.* The methods available for detecting drugs and their metabolites are extremely sensitive and capable of determining both the nature and the concentration of the drug and/or metabolite present.

Pharmacological means have been used in an attempt to mask illegal drug taking. Diuretics have also been used to mask drug taking by accelerating urine excretion.

Effect of exercise on pharmacokinetics

Under most circumstances exercise does not affect the pharmacokinetics of drug action. During severe or prolonged exercise, blood flow within the body will be altered, with a decrease in blood supply to the gastrointestinal tract and to the kidneys. However, there is little documentary evidence to suggest that such changes significantly affect the pharma-cokinetics of the majority of drugs.

Drugs and their targets

Ideally, a drug should interact with a single target to produce the desired effect within the body. However, all drugs possess varying degrees of side effects, largely dependent on the extent to which they interact with sites other than their primary target. During a drug's development, pharmaceutical companies ensure that it undergoes a rigorous evaluation in order to maximise therapeutic effects and minimise side effects. "Designer" drugs, produced by "back-street" laboratories to supply the illicit sport market, will not have undergone such rigorous testing for safety.

The sites through which most drug molecules interact are known as receptors, which are normally specific areas of cell membranes. Receptors are present within cells to enable naturally occurring substances, such as neurotransmitters, to induce their biochemical and physiological functions within the body. We exploit the fact that receptors exist, by design-ing drugs to stimulate (agonists) or block (antagonists) these receptors and thereby intensify or reduce biochemical processes within the body.

The interaction between a drug (ligand) and a receptor is the first step in a series of events which eventually leads to a biological effect. The drug–receptor interaction can therefore be thought of as a trigger mechanism.

There are many different receptor sites within the body, each of which possesses its own spe-cific arrangement of recognition sites. The more closely a drug can fit into its recognition site the greater the triggering response and therefore the greater the potency of the drug on that tissue.

Agonists and antagonists

A drug which mimics the action of an endogenous biochemical substance (i.e. one which occurs naturally in the body) is said to be an agonist. The potency of agonists depends on two parameters:

- *Affinity* – The ability to bind to receptors.
- *Efficacy* – The ability, once bound to the receptor, to initiate changes which lead to effects.

Antagonists have the ability to interact with receptor sites (affinity) but, unlike agonists, do not trigger the series of events leading to a response. The pharmacological effect of antago-nists is produced by preventing the body's own biochemical agents from interacting with the receptors and therefore inhibiting particular physiological processes.

A typical example of this can be seen with beta blockers. They exert their pharmacologi-cal effect by occupying beta receptors without stimulating a response, but prevent the neuro-transmitter, noradrenaline (norepinephrine), and the hormone, adrenaline (epinephrine), from interacting with these receptors. Beta blockers therefore reduce heart rate under stress conditions or in exercise.

Many receptor classes can be sub-classified. This can be illustrated by looking at how adrenaline (epinephrine) interacts with adrenergic receptors. We know that there are at least five subclasses of adrenergic receptors, known as alpha-1 (α_1), alpha-2 (α_2), beta-1 (β_1), beta-2 (β_2) and beta-3 (β_3). Adrenaline can interact with all of these receptors, producing

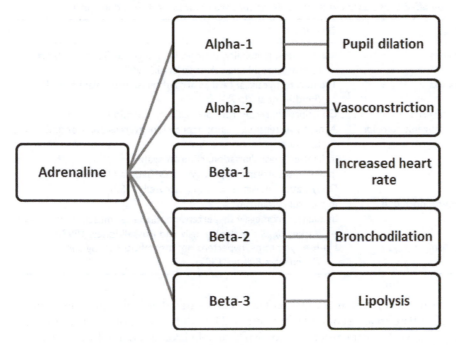

Figure 1.1 Some physiological effects of adrenaline mediated through the five principal classes of adrenergic receptors

a variety of physiological effects, examples of which are shown in Figure 1.1. Some drugs have selectivity for particular sub-classes of receptors. For example, the drug Salbutamol was developed to have a selective effect on beta-2 receptors. It therefore produces bronchodilation, without the other effects associated with adrenaline. As such it is a first-line drug in the treatment of asthma. The selective nature of Salbutamol, Salmeterol and Formoterol is recognised by the WADA who permit their use in sport, subject to certain specific restrictions, whilst other less selective sympathomimetics are totally banned.

Side effects of drugs

All drugs produce side effects. Some of these side effects occur at normal, therapeutic dose levels whilst other side effects are experienced only at higher doses. In many instances, where athletes misuse drugs for doping, they take doses far in excess of those required for therapeutic purposes and in so doing increase the risk of toxic side effects. Predictable side effects associated with some of the drugs that are commonly misused in sport are shown in Table 1.5.

Non-predictable toxicity can occur following the administration of therapeutic or even sub-therapeutic doses of drugs. An example of this is *idiosyncrasy* where a drug produces an unusual reaction, normally genetically determined and often due to a biochemical deficiency. This over-reaction to the drug may be due to an inability to metabolise the drug.

A second type of non-predictable toxicity is *drug allergy*. Patients will only exhibit allergic reactions after previous exposure to the drug or a closely related chemical which sensitises the patient. The drug combines with a protein within the body to produce an antigen, which,

Table 1.5 Side effects associated with some drugs that are commonly misused in sport

Class of drugs	Side effects
Amphetamines	Restlessness; irritability; tremor; insomnia; cardiac arrhythmias; aggression; addiction (Knopp et al., 1997)
Beta-2 agonists	Tremor; tachycardia; cardiac arrhythmias; insomnia; headache (Prather et al., 1995)
Narcotic analgesics	Constipation; respiratory depression; addiction
Anabolic androgenic steroids	Acne; hypertension; mania; depression; aggression; liver and kidney tumours
	In females: masculinisation; cliteromegaly
	In males: testicular atrophy; gynaecomastasia (Tucker, 1997)
Diuretics	Dehydration; muscular cramp (Caldwell, 1987)
Human growth hormone	In children: gigantism
	In adults: acromegaly (hypertension; diabetes; muscular weakness; thickening of the skin) (Healy and Russell-Jones, 1997)
Erythropoietin	Flu-like symptoms; hypertension; thromboses (*Drug and Therapeutics Bulletin*, 1992)

in turn, leads to the formation of other proteins called antibodies. Subsequent exposure to the drug will initiate an antigen-antibody reaction. This allergic reaction can manifest itself in a variety of ways. An acute reaction is known as anaphylaxis and normally occurs within one hour of taking the drug. This response frequently involves the respiratory and cardiovascular systems and is often fatal. Sub-acute allergic reactions usually occur between one and twenty-four hours after the drug is taken and the most common manifestations involve skin reactions, blood dyscrasias, fever and dysfunctions of the respiratory, kidney, liver and cardiovascular systems. Examples of drugs known to produce such allergic responses are aspirin and some antibiotics including penicillins and cephalosporins.

Complex drug reactions

Complex reactions may occur during long-term usage of a drug or where more than one drug is being taken simultaneously.

If the frequency of administration exceeds the elimination rate of a drug, then *drug cumulation* occurs thereby increasing the likelihood of toxicity reactions. The reason for a slow elimination may be related to a slow metabolism, a strong tendency to plasma protein binding or an inhibition of excretion such as occurs in patients with kidney disease.

The opposite response to cumulation is seen in patients with *drug resistance*, which may be genetically inherited or acquired. Inherited resistance is not common in humans, though it is an increasing problem in antibacterial therapy where pathogenic microbes can develop genetic changes in their structure or biochemistry which renders them resistant to antibiotic drugs. Acquired resistance to drugs, also known as *tolerance*, can develop with repeated administration of a drug. Where tolerance occurs, more drug is needed to produce the same pharmacological response. A very rapidly developing tolerance is known as *tachyphylaxis*. This is usually caused by a slow rate of detachment of the drug from its receptor sites, so that subsequent doses of the drug are unable to form the drug-receptor complexes which are required to produce an effect.

A number of drugs acting on the central nervous system, particularly narcotic analgesics, produce tolerance which is accompanied by *physical dependence*. This is a state in which an abrupt termination of the administration of the drug produces a series of unpleasant symptoms known as the abstinence syndrome. These symptoms are rapidly reversed after the readministration of the drug. A further manifestation of this problem involves psychogenic dependence in which the drug taker experiences an irreversible craving, or compulsion, to take the drug for pleasure or for relief of discomfort.

Where more than one drug is being taken there is a possibility for a *drug interaction* to occur. Less commonly, drugs may interact with certain foodstuffs, particularly milk products in which the calcium can bind to certain drugs and limit their absorption. The effects of interactions can range from minor toxicity to fatality.

Drugs and the law

The manufacture and supply of drugs is subject to legal control. This legislation may vary from country to country but the principles are the same.

The definition of a medicinal product

Medicinal product means any substance which is manufactured, sold, supplied, imported or exported for use in either or both of the following ways:

(a) Administered to human beings or animals for medicinal purposes
(b) As an ingredient in the preparation of substances administered to human beings or animals for medicinal purposes

"Medicinal purpose" means any one or more of the following:

(a) Treating or preventing disease
(b) Diagnosing of disease or physiological condition
(c) Contraception
(d) Inducing anaesthesia
(e) Otherwise preventing or interfering with the normal operation of physiological function

Classes of medicinal products

In many countries, there are three classes of medicinal products:

(1) General sale list medicines (GSL)
(2) Pharmacy medicines (P)
(3) Prescription-only medicines (POM)

The law of the country dictates which medicines may be purchased and which can only be obtained through a prescription. In general these laws are similar from country to country but exceptions do occur. Regrettably, most drugs can be obtained legally or illegally, without professional advice, through internet sources.

Patients can obtain prescription-only medicines (POMs) from medical practitioners in a hospital, clinic or community practice. Prescriptions are then dispensed by a pharmacist or, in some cases, by a dispensing doctor. Once the prescription has been dispensed, the medicine becomes the property of the patient.

Over-the-counter (OTC) medicines are available for purchase, without a prescription. These medicines are normally only available from a pharmacy (P medicines) although some medicines, such as aspirin and other analgesics, may be obtained in small pack sizes from other retail outlets (GSL medicines). OTC drugs pose particular problems for athletes, since a number of drugs subject to WADA regulations are available in OTC preparations.

Controlled drugs (CDs), normally those drugs with addictive properties, are subject to more extensive legal restrictions. In most countries CDs include:

- Hallucinogenic drugs (e.g. LSD and marijuana)
- Opiates (narcotic analgesics e.g. morphine, heroin)
- Amphetamines
- Cocaine

For these drugs, the law states that it is illegal to possess such drugs, except where the user is a registered addict and has obtained their drug legally on prescription.

In some countries anabolic androgenic steroids, clenbuterol and some polypeptide hormones are classed as CDs as a further deterrent to their misuse in sport and in body building.

1.3 Why might athletes take drugs?

There are many reasons why sportsmen and women may take drugs. These can be broadly categorised as:

- Legitimate therapeutic use for the treatment of medical conditions (prescription drugs or self-medication)
- Social or "recreational" use (legal and illegal)
- Performance enhancement

Within each of the above categories there are drugs which appear in the WADA Prohibited List (see Table 1.1). Both the deliberate and inadvertent use of prohibited drugs carries significant consequences for athletes. Athletes should always carefully consider the specific need for taking a drug and the full implications of their action.

Therapeutic use of drugs for the treatment of medical conditions

Like any other person, an athlete is liable to suffer from a major or minor illness that requires treatment with drugs. A typical example might involve a bacterial or fungal infection necessitating the use of an antibiotic or antifungal agent. Apart from side effects such treatment would be unlikely to affect an athlete's ability to compete and most drugs are not subject to WADA restrictions. However, there are a number of medical conditions for which athletes may require drug treatment, involving drugs that appear on the WADA Prohibited List. Examples of these conditions are shown in Table 1.6.

For each condition, the more commonly used classes of drugs are listed, with those classes of drugs subject to WADA regulations highlighted.

Table 1.6 Medical conditions for which athletes may require drug treatment involving drugs that appear on the WADA Prohibited List

Type of medical condition	Medical condition	Drug classes commonly used
Long-term chronic conditions	Asthma	Beta-2 agonists +
		Glucocorticoids +
		Leukotriene antagonists
	Diabetes mellitus (Type 1)	Insulin +
	Hypertension	ACE inhibitors
		Beta blockers +
		Calcium channel blockers
		Diuretics +
		Angiotensin II receptor antagonists
Short-term acute conditions	Viral cough and cold	Antitussives
		Decongestant stimulants +
		Non-narcotic analgesics
Sports injuries	Musculo-skeletal damage and inflammation	Non-steroidal anti-inflammatories
		Non-narcotic analgesics
		Narcotic analgesics +
		Glucocorticoids +

Drugs marked with + are subject to WADA Prohibited List (2017) regulations

For minor illnesses, such as coughs, colds, gastrointestinal upsets and hay fever, there is a wide range of preparations available which can be purchased from a pharmacy without a prescription. Athletes should carefully scrutinise the label on such medication to check that banned substances such as ephedrine, methylephedrine, pseudoephedrine or cathine are not included in the medicine.

Athletes frequently experience injuries involving muscles, ligaments and tendons for which they commonly take palliative treatment in the form of analgesic and anti-inflammatory drugs. This enables the athlete to continue to train and even compete during the period of recovery from the injury. The wisdom of such action is open to question but the use of analgesics under these circumstances is unlikely to confer an unfair advantage. However, the doping regulations restrict the type of analgesics which can be used, with narcotic analgesics being prohibited. Regulations also control the routes of administration for anti-inflammatory drugs such as glucocorticoids.

It is in the athlete's interest, in the event of visiting a medical practitioner, to discuss the nature of any drug treatment, to avoid the prescribing of prohibited substances wherever possible.

The WADA regulations relating to the drugs listed in Table 1.6 are described within the respective chapters of this book.

Therapeutic Use Exemption

On the occasions when an athlete needs to be prescribed a drug that appears on the WADA Prohibited List, the athlete and their medical practitioner must obtain a Therapeutic Use Exemption (TUE) (http://www.wada-ama.org/en/Science-Medicine/TUE/), in order to avoid an adverse analytical finding (AAF) during anti-doping testing.

The broad criteria for granting a TUE are:

- The athlete would experience significant health problems without taking the prohibited substance or method.
- The therapeutic use of the substance would not produce significant enhancement of performance.
- There is no reasonable therapeutic alternative to the use of the otherwise prohibited substance or method.
- Requirement to use that substance or method is not due to the prior use of the substance or method without a TUE which was prohibited at the time of use.

TUEs are normally granted to athletes by International Federations or National Anti-Doping Organisations. Requests are dealt with by a panel of independent physicians (Therapeutic Use Exemption Committee). Professor Ken Fitch, as Chair of the IOC Therapeutic Use Exemption Committee, provided an interesting insight into the medical indications and pitfalls in the TUE process (Fitch, 2012).

How to identify if a medicine contains a prohibited substance

Clearly, it is in the athlete's interest to ensure that accurate identification of those medicines that contain prohibited substances is undertaken on each occasion that a medicine is taken. The website Global DRO (http://www.globaldro.com) provides an up-to-date reference source for athletes and healthcare professionals to identify whether or not a medicine contains a prohibited substance. Global DRO was developed through a partnership between UK Anti-Doping (UKAD), the Canadian Centre for Ethics in Sport (CCES) and the United States Anti-Doping Agency (USADA). The Japanese, Australian and Swiss anti-doping authorities are now partners.

Visitors to the site can search for specific information on products sold in the partner countries. The website asks the user to provide information on:

- User type (athlete, coach, health professional etc.)
- The user's sport
- The country in which the medicine was obtained
- The name of the medicine

From this information, Global DRO provides details on the active ingredients of the medicine and their permitted or prohibited status, in-competition or out-of-competition, relative to the country of purchase and sport within which the medicine is to be used.

Social or "recreational" use of drugs

Many cultures, throughout the ages, have used drugs for social and recreational purposes. These drugs include caffeine, a constituent of beverages; drugs that are variably tolerated, such as nicotine, alcohol and cannabinoids; and addictive drugs such as the narcotic analgesics related to heroin and morphine or psychomotor stimulants such as cocaine. Although these drugs may be taken in a social or recreational setting, they can all influence sporting performance, hence many are subject to WADA regulations. The social/recreational drugs that are subject to WADA regulations are shown in Figure 1.2, with an indication of their

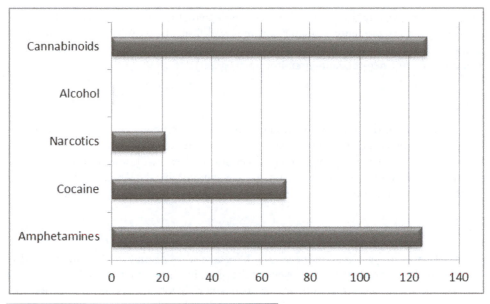

Drug	WADA regulation
Amphetamines	Prohibited class S6 (stimulants)
Cocaine	Prohibited class S6 (stimulants)
Narcotics	Prohibited class S7
Alcohol	Prohibited in particular sports class P1
Cannabinoids	Prohibited class S8

Figure 1.2 **Drugs used socially or recreationally that are subject to WADA regulations and the number of adverse analytical findings, for each class of drug, reported by WADA laboratories in 2015**

extent of use by athletes, as indicated by the number of positive test results for each class of drug reported by WADA laboratories in 2015.

Amphetamines

Amphetamines are used socially to produce alertness and energy. However, they also impair judgement and mental concentration, with excessive use leading to depression and anxiety. There is a risk of addiction with regular use of amphetamine (Knopp et al., 1997).

Cocaine

Cocaine is a powerful stimulant. It is usually inhaled as a powder but a crystalline ("crack") form of cocaine is smoked as a vapour that increases the absorption and effect of the drug. The complex pharmacology of cocaine leads to a wide spectrum of adverse effects, including a negative effect on glycogenolysis, paranoid psychosis, seizures, hypertension and myocardial toxicity, which could lead to ischaemia, arrhythmias and sudden death, especially following intense exercise (Conlee, 1991; Eichner, 1993). After regular use, addictive cravings for cocaine can persist for a period of months.

Caffeine

Perhaps the most widely used social drug is caffeine, which is present in many of the beverages that we consume daily. Caffeine was removed from the WADA Prohibited List in January 2004. However, it remains on the WADA Monitoring List (https://www.wada-ama.org/en/resources/science-medicine/monitoring-program).

Narcotics

Narcotics are potent drugs whose effects are primarily on the central nervous system. The discovery of opiate receptors within the brain has helped in the understanding of the mode of action of morphine, heroin and other related narcotic analgesics. They appear to be mimicking the effect of certain endogenous opiates, known as endorphins and enkephalin. Narcotics are renowned for their ability to cause tolerance and dependence in the regular user.

Alcohol

Though taken for recreational purposes, the effects of alcohol may well be manifested in the field of sport. Some sporting events even take place in an environment where alcohol is freely available both to the spectator and the performer. Alcohol suppresses inhibitions but also impairs judgement and reflexes. Alcohol is prohibited in particular sports.

Cannabinoids

The precise mode of action of cannabinoids is not fully understood but the effects produced are principally euphoria and elation accompanied by a loss of perception of time and space. Although unlikely to be used as a performance-enhancing substance in sport, events in recent years have shown that marijuana is used as part of the lifestyle of many athletes. Cannabinoids are prohibited, by WADA, within competition, in all sports.

1.4 The use of drugs for performance enhancement

What are the factors that influence athletic performance?

In addition to an athlete's innate ability and their commitment to training, many external factors influence an athlete's attempt to reach the peak within his or her chosen sport. These include:

- Coaches
- Sponsorship deals
- Resources and equipment
- Sports nutritionists
- Sports psychologists
- Physiotherapists
- Sports physicians

Inevitably, there are many athletes who achieve excellence in their sport but who consider they have not reached their ultimate goal. It is these athletes, as well as those who seek a short-cut to glory, who may be tempted to experiment with performance enhancement through pharmacological means. This culture within sport of using substances to enhance performance dates back over two thousand years to the ancient Olympic Games.

What is performance enhancement?

The performance-enhancing effects of substances are for the most part directly related to (Barroso et al., 2008):

- Ergogenic effects (enhanced strength, higher energy production, improved recovery)
- Anabolic potential (increased protein synthesis)
- Stimulating properties (improved attention, decreased anxiety)

How can we classify performance-enhancing substances?

Substances that are used in an attempt to enhance performance can be broadly divided into two types:

- Legal supplements
- Illegal performance-enhancing drugs

Legal supplements

Evidence suggests that the majority of today's athletes, regardless of their level of sporting achievement, use supplements (Outram and Stewart, 2015; Knapik et al., 2016). However, a study by Backhouse et al. (2013) concluded that illegal doping behaviour is three-and-a-half times more prevalent in nutritional supplement users than in non-users. The authors suggested that their results offered support for the gateway hypothesis, whereby athletes who engage in legal performance enhancement practices appear to embody an "at risk" group for transition toward doping.

ARE SUPPLEMENTS SAFE TO USE?

The landmark study by Geyer et al. (2004) showed that of 634 non-hormonal nutritional supplements, purchased in 13 countries, 14.8 per cent contained anabolic androgenic steroids, which were not declared on the label. Other studies have indicated that 10–15 per cent of supplements may contain prohibited substances (Krug et al., 2014; Outram and Stewart, 2015). Athletes are therefore vulnerable to the inadvertent use of prohibited substances. There have been many cases reported in recent years involving athletes recording adverse analytical findings following supplement use.

ADVICE REGARDING SUPPLEMENT USE

WADA advise extreme caution: "The use of dietary supplements by athletes is a concern because in many countries the manufacturing and labelling of supplements may not follow strict rules. This may lead to a supplement containing an undeclared substance that is prohibited under anti-doping regulations. A significant number of positive tests have been attributed to the misuse of supplements and taking a poorly labelled dietary supplement is not an adequate defense in a doping hearing" (http://www.wada-ama.org/en/Resources/Q-and-A/Dietary-and-Nutritional-Supplements/).

CHECKING SUPPLEMENTS

Informed-Sport (http://www.informed-sport.com/) is an organisation which provides a risk-minimisation programme for sports nutrition products. The programme certifies that speci-fied batches of nutritional supplements and/or ingredients that bear the Informed-Sport logo have been tested for banned substances in their laboratory. However, this still does not guarantee a supplement is completely free from prohibited substances as there can even be differences in ingredients within the one batch.

Organisations within other countries, such as Cologne List (http://www.koelnerliste.com/en/cologne-list.html) and NZVT (http://www.dopingautoriteit.nl/nzvt/disclaimer) provide similar advice on supplements.

Illegal performance-enhancing drugs

Prohibited performance-enhancing substances can be of two origins: exogenous substances, which are produced synthetically and are not normally produced by the body; and endog-enous substances, which are produced, naturally, in the body. Anti-doping detection meth-ods for exogenous substances are clear cut, whereas for endogenous substances the proof of substance use is more problematical.

The criteria for including substances and methods on the WADA Prohibited List are specified in the World Anti-Doping Code and can be summarised as:

A substance or method shall be considered for inclusion on the Prohibited List if WADA determines that the substance or method meets any two of the following three criteria:

1   the substance or method, alone or in combination with other substances or meth-ods, has the potential to enhance or enhances sport performance;
2   the use of the substance or method represents an actual or potential health risk to the athlete;
3   WADA's determination that the use of the substance or method violates the spirit of sport

The WADA Prohibited List is subject to annual review with revised lists coming into force each January.

Why do athletes use prohibited performance-enhancing substances?

The reasons why athletes use drugs that appear on the WADA Prohibited List are manifold, complex and vary from athlete to athlete and from sport to sport.

In a review of 33 studies, published between 2000 and 2011, Morente-Sánchez and Zabala (2013) reported that the initial reasons given by elite athletes for using banned substances included:

- Achievement of athletic success by improved performance
- Financial gain

- Improving recovery
- Prevention of nutritional deficiencies
- The idea that others use them

In addition, this study found that there is a belief by athletes about the inefficiency of anti-doping programmes and athletes criticise the way tests are carried out.

Some compounding factors that encourage the use of prohibited substances are:

MEDIA COVERAGE

The media tend to give extensive coverage to doping scandals within sport which gives athletes a misleading impression of the extent to which performance-enhancing drugs are used in sport.

PEER PRESSURE

Athletes may directly observe or may hear of the practices of fellow athletes who use per-formance-enhancing drugs and may be offered performance-enhancing drugs by their fellow competitors or team members.

SUPPORT TEAM PRESSURE

Athlete Support Personnel, including family members, coaches, healthcare professionals may instil additional pressure on athletes to improve performance by whatever means are available, including drug use.

AVAILABILITY OF SUBSTANCES

Athletes can obtain virtually any product they wish through the internet.

MISLEADING INFORMATION

The labelling of some supplements may not be complete or accurate and some, apparently, safe supplements may be contaminated with traces of prohibited substances.

LACK OF UNDERSTANDING

Athletes are not pharmacologists and the plethora of information that appears on medicinal products can be confusing to the untrained eye.

Clearly, drug use in sport is a complex picture. The remaining chapters of this book provide a detailed analysis of the substances and methods that are used for performance enhancement in sport and the rules and regulations for doping control.

1.5 Summary

- Drugs are potent substances that are used widely in modern society.
- The mechanisms by which drugs are taken and interact within the body are complex. All drugs produce side effects whose severity largely depends on dose and frequency of use.

- There are many reasons why athletes may take drugs, ranging from accepted social use, therapeutic use for the treatment of medical conditions and the use of supplements through to the illegal use of drugs for performance enhancement.
- The prescribing of drugs that appear on the WADA Prohibited List, when used in athletes for legitimate medical conditions, requires Therapeutic Use Exemption procedures.
- The factors that may influence athletes to take illegal performance-enhancing drugs are complex and vary from athlete to athlete and from sport to sport.

1.6 References

Backhouse, S.H., Whitaker, L. and Petróczi, A. (2013) Gateway to doping? Supplement use in the context of preferred competitive situations, doping, attitude, beliefs and norms. *Scandinavian Journal of Medical Science in Sports* 23: 244–252.

Barroso, O., Mazzoni, I. and Rabin, O. (2008) Hormone abuse in sports: The antidoping perspective. *Asian Journal of Andrology* 10(3): 391–402.

Caldwell, J.E. (1987). Diuretic therapy and exercise performance. *Sports Medicine* 4: 290–304.

Conlee, R.K. (1991) Amphetamine, caffeine and cocaine. In *Perspectives in Exercise Science and Sports Medicine*. New York, Brown and Benchmark, 285–328.

Drug and Therapeutics Bulletin (1992) Epoetin: An important advance. *Drug and Therapeutics Bulletin* 30(8): 29–32.

Eichner, E.R. (1993) Ergolytic drugs in medicine and sports. *American Journal of Medicine* 94: 205–211.

Elliott, S. and Leishman, B. (2012) Abuse of medicines for performance enhancement in sport: Why is this a problem for the pharmaceutical industry? *Bioanalysis* 4(13): 1681–1690.

Fitch K. (2012) Proscribed drugs at the Olympic Games: Permitted use and misuse (doping) by athletes. *Clinical Medicine* 12(3): 257–260.

Geyer, H., Parr, M.K., Mareck, U. et al. (2004) Analysis of non-hormonal nutritional supplements for anabolic-androgenic steroids: Results of an international study. *International Journal of Sports Medicine* 25: 124–129.

Healy, M.-L. and Russell-Jones, D. (1997) Growth hormone and sport: Abuse, potential benefits, and difficulties in detection. *British Journal of Sports Medicine* 31: 267–268.

Knapik, J.J., Steelman, R.A., Hoedebecke, S.S. et al. (2016) Prevalence of dietary supplement use by athletes: Systemic review and meta analysis. *Sports Medicine* 46: 103–123

Knopp, W.D., Wang, T.W. and Bacch, B.R., Jr. (1997) Ergogenic drugs in sports. *Clinics in Sports Medicine* 16: 375–392.

Krug, O., Thomas, A., Walpurgis, K. et al. (2014) Identification of black market products and potential doping agents in Germany 2010–2013. *European Journal of Clinical Pharmacology* 70(11): 1303–1311.

Mazzoni, I., Barroso, O. and Rabin, O. (2011) The list of prohibited substances and methods in sport: Structure and review process by the World Anti-Doping Agency. *Journal of Analytical Toxicology* 35: 608–612.

Morente-Sánchez, J. and Zabala, M. (2013) Doping in sport: A review of elite athletes' attitudes, beliefs and knowledge. *Sports Medicine* 43: 395–411.

Outram, S. and Stewart, B. (2015) Doping through supplement use: A review of the available empirical data. *International Journal of Sport Nutrition and Exercise Metabolism* 25: 54–59.

Prather, I.D., Brown, D.E., North P. et al. (1995) Clenbuterol: A substitute of anabolic steroids? *Medicine and Scence in Sports and Exercise* 27: 1118–1121.

Tucker, R. (1997) Abuse of anabolic-androgenic steroids by athletes and body builders: A review. *Pharmaceutical Journal* 259: 171–179.

Chapter 2

The evolution of doping and anti-doping in sport

David R. Mottram

2.1 Introduction

Organised sport has a history dating back to ancient Greece. By the seventh century BC, religion, culture and sport were all an integral part of Greek society and this tradition continued through to the Roman era. There is little documented evidence for organised sport between the fall of the Roman Empire and the mid-nineteenth century. At this time, sport comprised recreational activities associated with religious, cultural and seasonal events. By the end of the nineteenth century, urbanisation and industrialisation had transformed sport into a more organised activity with associated rules and the formation of sporting clubs and institutions. As the twentieth century progressed, participation in sport increased. More people became spectators and commercial interests in sport developed.

In the 1950s, international pharmaceutical companies expanded the armoury of medicines available to tackle ill-health. Drugs that had hitherto been derived principally from plant and animal sources were now manufactured in the laboratory. Some athletes turned to these new, potent drugs to enhance performance.

Attempts to control substance misuse in sport began around the 1950s. However, ignorance of the extent of the problem, a lack of sophistication of testing procedures and uncoordinated systems for legislating against doping meant that those intent on introducing anti-doping measures were playing catch-up. It was not until the beginning of the twenty-first century, with the formation of the World Anti-Doping Agency (WADA), that the anti-doping movement sought to gain the upper hand.

Not only have individual athletes been culpable of doping, but entire teams and even state-sponsored doping has been evident, posing significant challenges to anti-doping organisations.

Figure 2.1 shows a time-line for many of the significant events related to doping and anti-doping within sport, from the ancient Olympics to the current time.

This chapter describes these events in more detail, highlighting the key lessons that have been learned from such landmark events.

2.2 The ancient Olympic and Roman Games

The ancient Olympic Games began in 776 BC and were the most important of the Panhellenic Games. Initially, the Games comprised just running events. Over the centuries other sports, such as wrestling, boxing, chariot racing, long jump, javelin and discus throwing were introduced. Participants represented their city-states and the victors were rewarded with rich

Doping–related events	Time	Anti-doping events
Ancient Olympics	800 BC	
6-day cycle races	1850	
Thomas Hicks	1904	
Amphetamines introduced	1920s	
	1928	IAAF bans doping
Anabolic Steroids introduced	1954	
Knud Jensen	1960	
	1963	France introduces anti-doping legislation
	1966	FIFA and UCI introduce testing
Tommy Simpson	1967	IOC Medical Commission and first Prohibited List
	1968	IOC testing at Grenoble Winter Games
GDR doping programme	1970s	
	1972	Comprehensive testing at Munich Olympics
	1976	Anabolic steroids prohibited
	1980s	Therapeutic Use Exemption introduced
Athlete withdrawal from Pan-Am Games	1983	
	1984	CAS operational
	1985	Blood doping prohibited
Ben Johnson	1988	
Recombinant EPO introduced	1989	
	1992	TUE Committee at Barcelona Olympics
	1994	Blood testing introduced
Festina affair	1998	
	1999	Lausanne Declaration/WADA established
	2000	EPO test validated
Alain Baxter	2002	
BALCO	2003	First World Anti-Doping Code
	2003	Gene Doping prohibited
	2005	UNESCO Convention
Operación Puerto	2006	
	2008	Athlete Biological Passports introduced
Lance Armstrong	2012	
	2015	Third World Anti-Doping Code
Maria Sharapova	2016	
Russian doping programme	2016	McLaren Report
	2017	Sanctions for Athlete Support Personnel

Figure 2.1 Time-line for significant events related to sport, doping and anti-doping

prizes and high esteem. The use of supplements to enhance athletic performance dates back to this period, when herbal preparations and animal extracts were experimented with.

2.3 Nineteenth century

The increasing industrialisation of society altered peoples' lifestyles. Transport systems improved and leisure time increased along with peoples' disposable income. Sport became more organised, with the formation of sports clubs and societies. Some sports became more professional and stadia were built where spectators could pay to watch events.

Most medicinal products were extracted from plant and animal sources. Those used by athletes included stimulants such as caffeine (from tea and coffee), strychnine (from the seeds of Strychnos Nux Vomica) and cocaine (from the leaves of the coca plant). The analgesic morphine (from the opium poppy) and the depressant, alcohol (brewed and/or distilled from a variety of sources), were also used. It is widely accepted that the word "doping" derives from "dop", an alcoholic beverage made from grape skins that was used in South Africa and exported by the Dutch in the nineteenth century.

Few reports of drug use in sport were recorded, although cycle racing, a sport long associated with substance misuse, had its roots in the second half of the nineteenth century when gruelling six-day cycle races took place in Europe and North America and involved cyclists taking cocktails of substances, including Vin Mariani, a mixture of coca leaf extract in wine (Murray, 1983).

2.4 Early twentieth century

The first recorded instance of drug use in the Modern Olympics occurred in the 1904 Games in St. Louis, where the marathon runner, Thomas Hicks, received doses of strychnine and brandy during the closing stages of the race.

Amphetamine, in 1920, was one of the earliest drugs to be produced synthetically in the laboratory. By 1935 it was being used to treat narcolepsy, depression, anxiety and hyperactivity in children (George, 2005). There was little regulation of drug use in sport. The first International Sport Federation to ban the use of doping (stimulants) was the International Amateur Athletic Federation, in 1928, although restrictions remained ineffective because no tests were made (Fraser, 2004).

2.5 The 1940s and '50s

Amphetamine was used widely in society to enhance mental awareness, a property that was exploited during the Second World War to delay fatigue in combat troops and air crew. This non-therapeutic use of drugs was then mirrored in sport, where athletes experimented with amphetamines to enhance performance (Verroken, 1996).

The use of anabolic steroids in sport dates back to the 1950s. Dr. John Ziegler, a physician to the American Weightlifting Team, suspected the Soviet team of using testosterone at the 1954 World Weightlifting Championships in Vienna (Hoberman, 1992). In the 1950s, multi-national drug companies evolved and invested huge sums of money on research into new classes of drugs for the treatment of diseases. The anabolic steroid, Dianabol, was synthesised in 1958 and was used by the American weightlifters at the 1962 World Championships.

2.6 The 1960s

Several major new classes of drugs were developed by the pharmaceutical industry. These included oral contraceptives, corticosteroids, beta blockers, tranquilizers and antidepressants. The 1960s heralded the era of experimentation into the non-therapeutic use of drugs both socially and in sport.

Although it is difficult to attribute mortality and morbidity directly to drug use, as there may be other contributory factors, there were a number of deaths of athletes directly associated with drug taking during the 1960s. The cyclist Knud Jensen died in the 100 km Team Time Trial at the 1960 Rome Olympic Games and Tommy Simpson during the 1967 Tour de France. Both deaths were associated with amphetamine use but both occurred under exceptional conditions of heat and exhaustion (George, 2005).

The fear of bringing sport into disrepute meant that many sporting authorities denied the possibility that doping took place, therefore anti-doping testing was, at best, haphazard. The International Federations for football (FIFA) and cycling (UCI) introduced doping tests into their respective World Championships in 1966.

In 1967, the International Olympic Committee (IOC) instituted its Medical Commission with three guiding principles: protection of the health of athletes, respect for medical and sport ethics, and equality for competing athletes (IOC, 2016). The IOC also set up a list of prohibited substances (Table 2.1). The first mandatory tests at Olympic events were in 1968 at the Winter Olympics in Grenoble and at the Summer Games in Mexico (Fraser, 2004).

Table 2.1 Major changes to the IOC Prohibited List 1967–2003

Year	Classes of substances and methods prohibited	Major changes
1967	1 Central nervous system stimulants 2 Psychomotor stimulants 3 Sympathomimetic amines 4 Narcotic analgesics	
1976		• Anabolic steroids added
1985		• Beta blockers and diuretics added • Prohibited methods added, including; blood doping and pharmacological, chemical and physical manipulation
1987		• Probenecid and other masking agents added
1988	I Doping classes Stimulants Narcotic analgesics Anabolic steroids Beta blockers Diuretics II Doping methods Blood doping Pharmacological, chemical and physical manipulation III Classes of drugs subject to certain restrictions Alcohol Local anaesthetics Corticosteroids	• CNS and psychomotor stimulants and sympathomimetics grouped under stimulants • Classes of drugs subject to certain restrictions added

1989		• Peptide hormones and analogues added
1993		• Beta blockers moved to "Drugs subject to certain restrictions" • Anabolic steroid class re-named as anabolic agents to incorporate Clenbuterol • Codeine removed from the list
1998		• Insulin added
2000		• Oxygen carriers and plasma expanders added • Erythropoietin added to peptide hormones
2003	I Prohibited classes of substances Stimulants Narcotics Anabolic agents Diuretics Peptide hormones, mimetics and analogues Agents with anti-oestrogenic activity Masking agents II Prohibited methods Enhancement of oxygen transfer Pharmacological, chemical and physical manipulation Gene doping III Classes of prohibited substances in certain sports Alcohol Cannabinoids Local anaesthetics Glucocorticosteroids Beta blockers	• The IOC and WADA produce a joint Prohibited List • Agents with anti-oestrogenic activity added • A separate class of masking agents added • Gene doping added as a prohibited method • Enhancement of oxygen transfer added to include blood doping and the administration of products that enhance the uptake, transport or delivery of oxygen • The title of Section III changed • Marijuana changed to cannabinoids

2.7 The 1970s

The paper by Franke and Berendonk (1997), written after the reunification of Germany, provides a startling account of state controlled doping by the German Democratic Republic (GDR) during the late 1960s and 1970s.

Table 2.2 German Democratic Republic doping programme (1970s and 1980s)

German Democratic Republic doping programme (1970s and 1980s)	
Key factors	Lessons learnt
• Over 2000 athletes, preparing for international competition, were systematically dosed with performance-enhancing drugs, including androgenic hormones • Special emphasis was placed on administering androgens to women and adolescent girls	• State controlled doping can occur • Athletes are exposed to significant health risks arising from doping • Physicians and scientists may collaborate in doping

Scientists and physicians were implicated in the GDR doping programme.

Most international sports federations had introduced systems for drug testing by the 1970s. However, the IOC Prohibited List only comprised narcotic analgesics and three classes of stimulants (sympathomimetic amines, psychomotor stimulants and central nervous system stimulants). The first comprehensive testing at an Olympic games took place in Munich in 1972. Nine positive results, for stimulants, were detected from 2,079 tests.

The IOC added anabolic steroids to the Prohibited List in 1976, following ground-breaking research by Brooks and colleagues using radio-immunoassays to identify andro-genic anabolic steroids (Brooks et al., 1975). Steroid testing was conducted for the first time at the 1976 Montreal Olympic Games.

2.8 The 1980s

The 1980s was a turbulent time for sport, with political differences being manifested through boycotts at the Olympic Games of 1980 in Moscow and 1984 in Los Angeles. In addition, there were accusations of a cover up at the 1983 World Track and Field Championships and the withdrawal of athletes from the 1983 Pan American Games, in Caracas, Venezuela, when word got through that drug testing was to be included (Hunt, 2008).

Blood doping, in 1985, was the first doping method to be added to the IOC Prohibited List, following reports of its use by the US cycling team at the 1984 Los Angeles Olympics. In 1985, the IOC amended the Prohibited List to include beta blockers and diuretics as dop-ing agents and pharmacological, chemical and physical manipulation as prohibited meth-ods. Despite this, in the 1988 Tour de France the cyclist Pedro Delgado tested positive for probenecid, a masking agent that was banned according to the IOC Prohibited List but was not on the banned list for the International Cycling Union. This inconsistency between sporting authorities meant that Delgado was not disqualified and eventually won the race.

During the 1980s, Therapeutic Use Exemptions (TUEs) were introduced to allow ath-letes to take prohibited drugs for genuine medical conditions and still compete in sport (Fitch, 2012).

In the late 1980s, a number of countries, particularly in Scandinavia, developed national anti-doping organisations (NADOs) in an attempt to strengthen anti-doping activity across the boundaries of individual sports (Vance, 2007). Doping sanctions were often disputed by athletes and sometimes overruled in civil courts. The Court for Arbitration for Sports (CAS) became operational in June 1984.

The most significant event of the 1980s occurred at the Seoul Olympic Games in 1988, when Ben Johnson tested positive for the anabolic steroid, Stanazolol.

Table 2.3 Ben Johnson case (1988)

Ben Johnson case (1988)	
Key factors	Lessons learnt
• Johnson won the 100m Olympic Gold medal then tested positive for Stanazolol	• Doping occurs at the highest level of sport • Anabolic steroids may be used in any sport • Physicians and scientists may collaborate in doping • The Dubin inquiry was set up (Dubin, 1990)

This was significant for a number of reasons. It showed that athletes in disciplines other than pure strength events were using steroids and that athletes who thought that they could avoid detection were vulnerable to testing regimes. The Ben Johnson affair drew the attention of the world to the issue of doping in sport.

Subsequent events implicated six of the eight sprinters who competed in the Seoul 100m final in activities involving performance-enhancing substances (Cooper, 2012)

In the late 1980s a cluster of sudden deaths of European cyclists was associated with the appearance of recombinant erythropoietin on the market (Eichner, 2007).

2.9 The 1990s

Many doping cases illustrated the inconsistencies that existed between the IOC and individual sports federations regarding their respective prohibited lists and the application of regulations.

Evidence for the use of the hormone erythropoietin (EPO) to enhance oxygen transport, by increasing red blood cell production, led to its addition to the IOC Prohibited List, despite the absence of a validated test.

In 1992, the sprinter Diane Modahl received a four-year ban when she tested positive for testosterone during an event in Portugal. However, after a protracted appeal her suspension was lifted, the laboratory having failed to follow the accredited procedures for testing.

The IOC first operated a Therapeutic Use Exemption Committee, to approve or reject TUE applications by athletes, at the 1992 Olympic Games (Catlin et al., 2008).

The pre-testing of two British weightlifters, prior to the 1992 Olympic Games in Barcelona, led to their ban for using clenbuterol. This drug is a beta-2 agonist, classed under stimulants. However, clenbuterol was being used for anabolic effects, a secondary pharmacological property that a number of beta-2 agonists possess. The chemical nature of beta-2 agonists does not permit their classification as anabolic steroids. Consequently, in 1993, the IOC changed its prohibited list to include the class of anabolic agents, which include anabolic steroids and other agents with anabolic properties.

Blood testing of athletes was first implemented at the 1994 Winter Olympic Games in Lillehammer, Norway. Initially, blood testing was used to define acceptable upper limits for blood parameters in an attempt to control the use of drugs such as erythropoietin (EPO), for which a validated urine test was not available. An example where upper limits were used was the "no-start" rule in cycling where a percentage of red blood cells, the haematocrit, higher than 50 per cent precluded the cyclist from competing (Saugy et al., 2011). Blood testing eventually led to the development of the "Athlete Biological Passport".

Although unpublished evidence existed, particularly in East Germany, that anabolic steroids were effective as doping agents, it was not until 1996 that scientifically robust evidence showed that increased muscle bulk and strength resulted from supraphysiological doses of testosterone (Bashin et al., 1996).

The majority of athletes use supplements. However, the production and marketing of supplements is not always reliable. In the late 1990s, a spate of positive dope tests for the anabolic steroid nandrolone occurred which, it was claimed, had been taken inadvertently in supplements. This was substantiated by a study showing that many supplements did contain hormonal-based constituents (Schänzer, 2002).

In 1963, the French government had enacted national anti-doping legislation. This allowed the French police to undertake a raid during the 1998 Tour de France. This became known as the "Festina affair".

Table 2.4 The Festina affair (1998)

The Festina affair (1998)	
Key factors	Lessons learnt
• A French Police raid revealed significant quantities of prohibited substances in a Festina Team car • Several drugs were identified, particularly erythropoietin (EPO)	• Willy Voet published his revealing account of the affair (Voet, 2001) • Teams undertook systematic doping • This affair highlighted the need for a world-wide anti-doping agency

Table 2.5 Ross Ribagliati case (1998)

Ross Ribagliati case (1998)	
Key factors	Lessons learnt
• Ribagliati tested positive for marijuana and the IOC stripped him of his gold medal • His medal was reinstated as the FIS did not ban the drug • Ribagliati claimed the drug entered his body through passive inhalation	• Lack of harmonisation between anti-doping organisations can lead to confusion and miscarriage of rules • Inadvertent doping may take place

At the 1998 Winter Olympic Games in Nagano, the Canadian snowboarder, Ross Ribagliati, tested positive for marijuana and in so doing triggered a bizarre series of events.

By the end of the 1990s, questions were being asked as to whether the IOC Prohibited List needed updating (Mottram, 1999). More significantly, the whole question of the harmonisation of doping control was called into question. The IOC convened the World Conference on Doping in Sport, in Lausanne, in February 1999 resulting in the Lausanne Declaration on Doping in Sport (https://www.wada-ama.org/en/resources/general-anti-doping-information/lausanne-declaration-on-doping-in-sport; accessed October 2017). The World Anti-Doping Agency (WADA) was then established on 10 November 1999 as a direct result of the Lausanne Declaration.

Previously, different international sport federations and national anti-doping organisations were operating different rules, leading to doping cases being contested in courts; there was a lack of a coordinated research policy, particularly with respect to new analytical methods; little had been done to promote anti-doping activities internationally (Catlin et al., 2008). WADA's mission was to lead a collaborative, worldwide movement for doping-free sport. WADA provided harmonisation between anti-doping agencies and its creation triggered the foundation of National Anti-Doping Organisations (NADOs) and Regional Anti-Doping Organisations (RADOs), key agencies in the worldwide fight against doping in sport (Kamber, 2011).

2.10 2000 to 2010

The first decade of the new millennium heralded a number of significant events associated with doping and anti-doping.

A validated test for EPO was introduced at the 2000 Olympic Games in Sydney (Lasne and Ceaurriz, 2000). This may have prompted the withdrawal of six Chinese female track and field athletes from these Games. Athletes turned to darbepoetin, a second-generation EPO, in 2002, and at the 2008 Beijing Olympics five athletes were disqualified for using the third-generation EPO, Continuous Erythropoietin Receptor Activator (CERA) (Fitch, 2012).

Improvements continued to be made in testing procedures, not least being the development of Isotope Ratio Mass Spectrometry (IRMS) for the detection of testosterone misuse (Aguilera et al., 2001).

The use by athletes of over-the-counter (OTC) medicines, containing minor stimulants such as ephedrine, to treat minor conditions has created serious problems. Andreea Raducan, a gymnast lost her gold medal from the Sydney Olympics in 2000 for using pseudoephedrine, despite the fact that she had been given the drug by her team doctor and, in 2002, Alain Baxter, the Scottish skier tested positive for metamfetamine at the 2002 Winter Olympics in Salt Lake City (Armstrong and Chester, 2005).

These and other cases led to the removal of most of these OTC drugs from the first Prohibited List produced by WADA in 2004. These drugs were placed on a Monitoring List. Evidence suggested that some of these OTC drugs became a target for performance enhancement (Mottram et al., 2008). This led WADA to reconsider their prohibited status and in January 2010, WADA re-introduced pseudoephedrine on to the Prohibited List, subject to a urinary threshold limit.

From 2004, WADA has undertaken an annual review of the Prohibited List, major changes which are presented in Table 2.7 and Table 2.8.

A review of the processes involved in its annual revision is presented by Mazzoni et al. (2011).

Underground drug suppliers were attempting to produce "designer" drugs that were ostensibly "undetectable". A key example was Tetrahydrogestrinone (THG), produced by the Bay Area Laboratory Co-operative (BALCO) (Catlin et al., 2004). An extensive investigation, undertaken by US government agencies, resulted in several prosecutions for doping offences despite the absence of any adverse analytical chemical evidence, an unprecedented event in the history of doping at that time (Marclay et al., 2013)

Research into gene technology had been undertaken to develop non-drug based prevention and treatment of disease. In anticipation of this technology being applied to enhance sporting performance, the IOC and WADA added Gene Doping to the Prohibited List in 2003. Monitoring technological advances in this field remains imperative (Wells, 2008).

WADA has consolidated several agreements with representatives from the pharmaceutical and biotechnological industries to facilitate the identification and transfer of information on drugs and biotechnological methods in development (Rabin, 2011).

Table 2.6 Alain Baxter case (2002)

Alain Baxter case (2002)	
Key factors	Lessons learnt
• Baxter tested positive for Levmethamfetamine from a medicine purchased over-the-counter (OTC) in the USA • He was stripped of his Olympic Medal but an appeal hearing acknowledged that he had not attempted to cheat since the same medicine available in his home country did not contain Levmethamfetamine	• OTC medicines pose a significant problem to athletes • All medications taken by athletes should be checked by a healthcare professional • WADA introduced the "Specified Substances" clause for those prohibited substances that may be taken inadvertently

Table 2.7 Major changes to the WADA Prohibited List 2004–2012

Year	Classes of substances and methods prohibited	Major changes
2004	I Substances and methods prohibited in-competition S1 Stimulants S2 Narcotics S3 Cannabinoids S4 Anabolic agents S5 Peptide hormones S6 Beta-2 agonists S7 Agents with anti-oestrogenic activity S8 Masking agents S9 Glucocorticosteroids M1 Enhancement of oxygen transfer M2 Pharmacological, chemical and physical manipulation M3 Gene doping II Substances and methods prohibited in- and out-of-competition Sections S4 to S8 and M1 to M3 above III Substances prohibited in particular sports P1 Alcohol P2 Beta blockers P3 Diuretics IV Specified substances	• Beta-2 agonists now a separate class • Diuretics included in S8 as masking agents but also prohibited in sports (P3) when used to reduce weight • Most over-the-counter stimulants (e.g. caffeine, pseudoephedrine) removed but placed on a monitoring list • Therapeutic Use Exemption introduced for some classes such as beta-2 agonists and glucocorticosteroids • Specified substances added where some classes or specific substances within classes are subject to reduced sanctions if taken inadvertently • Glucocorticosteroids now prohibited in all sports
2005		• Re-arrangement of how substances and methods prohibited in-competition and out-of-competition were presented • Beta-2 agonists now prohibited in- and out-of-competition • Diuretics removed from section III and specifically mentioned with masking agents
2008		• Class S4 changed to Hormone antagonists and modulators to include other groups of drugs that affect endogenous hormones • Selective androgen receptor modulators added to S1 Anabolic agents
2009		• Section IV Specified substances removed as the definition was changed • Abbreviated TUEs removed
2010		• Class S2 changed to Peptide hormones, growth factors and related substances • Salbutamol and Salmeterol no longer require a TUE • Pseudoephedrine returned to the list
2011		• Class S0 added to cover drugs with no official approval • Methods that consist of sequentially withdrawing, manipulating and re-infusing whole blood added to M2 Chemical and physical manipulation

2012		• Formoterol excepted from prohibition, subject to restrictions on administration • S4 Hormone antagonists and modulators changed to S4 Hormone and metabolic modulators

Table 2.8 Major changes to the WADA Prohibited List 2013–2017

Year	Classes of substances and methods prohibited	Major changes
2013	I Substances and methods prohibited at all times (in- and out-of-competition) S0 Non-approved substances S1 Anabolic agents S2 Peptide hormones, growth factors and related substances S3 Beta-2 agonists S4 Hormone and metabolic modulators S5 Diuretics and other masking agents M1 Manipulation of blood and blood components M2 Chemical and physical manipulation M3 Gene doping II Substances and methods prohibited in-competition All categories in Section I plus S6 Stimulants S7 Narcotics S8 Cannabinoids S9 Glucocorticosteroids III Substances prohibited in particular sports P1 Alcohol P2 Beta blockers	• Insulins moved from S2 to S4 Hormone and metabolic modulators • M1 Enhancement of oxygen transfer changed to M1 Manipulation of blood and blood components
2014		• Re-classification of some stimulants to reflect their use in society and in sport • Changes made to the definition of "exogenous" and "endogenous" anabolic agents • Hypoxia-inducible factor (HIF) activators, xenon and argon added to Class 2.1
2015		• Class S2 changed to Peptide hormones, growth factors, related substances and mimetics to reflect the fact that synthetic analogs are also prohibited • Class S5 – removal of "other" to reflect that diuretics are abused other than as masking agents • Class S9 changed from Glucocorticosteroids to Glucocorticoids
2016		• Insulin mimetics added to Class S4 to include all insulin-receptor agonists • Meldonium (mildronate) added to Class S4
2017		• In Class S3, clarification was given to the selectivity and to dosage regimens for beta-2 agonists

Table 2.9 The BALCO affair (2003)

The BALCO affair (2003)	
Key factors	**Lessons learnt**
• The BALCO laboratory supplied drugs, including the "undetectable" steroid THG ("The Clear") • THG was discovered and several high profile athletes were sanctioned • Governmental law enforcement agencies were used to investigate doping	• Back-street laboratories produce "designer" drugs that have not undergone strict safety checks • Athletes can be prosecuted for doping offences in the absence of testing evidence

WADA produced the first World Anti-Doping Code (WADC) in 2003, a document endorsed by delegates at the Second World Conference on Doping in Sport in Copenhagen. The IOC transferred management of the Prohibited List to WADA in January 2004 (Table 2.7). WADA invited all stakeholders to comply with the Code. This included athletes and their supporters, sports federations, the Olympic movement and governments. The Code was implemented for the first time at the Olympic Games in Athens in 2004. By the end of the decade, most sports, apart from some professional sports in the United States of America, had declared their support for WADA and many governments had signed up in support of the UNESCO, 2005, International Convention against Doping in Sport (http://www.unesco.org/new/en/social-and-human-sciences/themes/anti-doping/international-convention-against-doping-in-sport/). Furthermore, since 2006, WADA had been working closely with international enforcement agencies to uncover doping activities such as trafficking. This was exemplified by the US Enforcement Administration's operation, Raw Deal, which involved ten countries and resulted in 124 arrests and the seizure of large quantities of steroids from 56 laboratories across the US, mainly supplied from companies in China (Vance, 2007).

Another significant law enforcement agency swoop, "Operación Puerto", involved an investigation of a laboratory in Spain (Soule and Lestrelin, 2011).

In 2007, the sprinter Marion Jones admitted to previous steroid use, leading up to the 2000 Sydney Olympic Games. She also admitted to using the BALCO steroid "The Clear". The IOC stripped Marion Jones of the three gold and two bronze medals she won in 2000.

A further strengthening of the testing procedures was implemented through athletes having to declare their whereabouts for a one-hour period each day in order to facilitate no-notice, out-of-competition testing with penalties for missed tests. Testing authorities increased their use of "intelligence" testing where, instead of randomly testing athletes, resources are more focussed on athletes who are either in higher risk sports and/or by their own behaviour or biological profile (Athlete Biological Passports) trigger an element of suspicion (Vance, 2007; Schumacher et al., 2012).

The Global Drug Reference Online (Global DRO), web-based reference resource (http://www.globaldro.com; accessed October 2017) was established through the partnership of United Kingdom Anti-Doping (UKAD), Canadian Centre for Ethics in Sport (CCES) and United States Anti-Doping Agency (USADA). It provided athletes and support personnel with details on the prohibited status of medicines commonly used in the three partner countries. Other countries have subsequently become partners for Global DRO.

Table 2.10 Operación Puerto (2006)

Operación Puerto (2006)

Key factors	Lessons learnt
• Spanish Police discovered frozen blood packs and prohibited substances, such as anabolic steroids and growth hormone • Several cyclists were implicated leading to withdrawal from the Tour de France	• This case showed the effectiveness of collaboration between anti-doping organisations and criminal investigation authorities • Evidence revealed medical practitioners' involvement in doping

2.11 2011 and onwards

A significant advance in anti-doping was achieved at the London 2012 Olympic and Paralympic Games when the biomarker test for human growth hormone (Erotokritou-Mulligan et al., 2007; Powrie et al., 2007) was introduced, resulting in the eviction from the Games of two paralympian athletes.

Perhaps the most significant doping case revealed to date came on 24 August 2012, when the United States Anti-Doping Agency (USADA) announced that it had imposed on Lance Armstrong a sanction of lifetime ineligibility and disqualification of competitive results achieved since 1 August 1998 (Mottram, 2013). On 10 October 2012, USADA published their "Reasoned Decision" on the Lance Armstrong case, stating that the evidence showed beyond any doubt that the US Postal Service Pro Cycling Team "ran the most sophisticated, professionalized and successful doping programme that sport has ever seen" (http://www.usada.org/cyclinginvestigationstatement.html; accessed October 2017). On 22 October 2012, the Union Cycliste International (UCI) accepted the USADA findings and formally stripped Lance Armstrong of his seven Tour de France titles.

Lance Armstrong claimed to have been one of the most frequently tested athletes in the world and that the results of his tests had never shown the presence of a prohibited drug. However, USADA's charge against Lance Armstrong was based on a wide variety of evidence, including:

- Sworn statements from professional cyclists
- Banking and accounting records
- Email communications
- Laboratory test results and expert analysis

Table 2.11 Lance Armstrong case (2012)

Lance Armstrong case (2012)

Key factors	Lessons learnt
• USADA announced a lifetime ban and disqualification of Armstrong's results since 1998 • Armstrong was stripped of his seven Tour de France titles • Evidence was based, primarily, on sworn testimonies	• Evidence of extensive team doping in sport • Sanction can be applied for anti-doping rules violations other than analytical tests • Commercial sponsorship can be rapidly withdrawn where doping is proven

One might ask the question "Why were Lance Armstrong and his team not sanctioned earlier?" There are two principal reasons:

- The nature of the substances and methods used
- The inadequacies of the testing procedures

The substances and methods used included testosterone, erythropoietin, blood transfusions, human growth hormone and corticosteroids. These are substances and methods for which there is a naturally occurring component in the body and for which analytical testing provides significant challenges to the testers. Regarding inadequacies of the testing procedures, it was reported in USADA's Reasoned Decision document that the team riders overcame what little out-of-competition testing there was at the time by simply using their wits to avoid the testers.

Further evidence for the reasons why Lance Armstrong avoided earlier detection and sanctioning was revealed in the report, in March 2015, of the UCI's Independent Commission for Reform in Cycling (UCI, 2015). In this report it was stated that

> Numerous examples have been identified showing that the UCI leadership 'defended' or 'protected' Lance Armstrong and took decisions because they were favourable to him. This was in circumstances where there was strong reason to suspect him of doping, which should have led UCI to be more circumspect in its dealings with him.

The 2013 Australian Crime Commission Report (http://www.acic.gov.au; accessed October 2012) revealed that scientists, coaches and support staff had been involved in providing drugs across multiple sporting codes within Australia. In addition, medical practitioners were implicated in unethical prescribing, including the use of drugs that, at the time, had not been approved for human use.

Anti-doping policies continue to be centred on a strategy of testing and punishment (Mazanov and Connor, 2010; Hunt et al., 2012). This fact has been acknowledged by WADA who, in 2012, established a working group to investigate and report on the "Lack of Effectiveness of Testing Programs" (WADA, 2013).

With respect to WADA's policy of global harmonisation of anti-doping work, a survey of members of Associations of National Anti-Doping Organisations revealed that, in many countries, the WADA Code was not implemented in accordance with prescribed policy with regards to registered testing pools, the requirements of availability for testing athletes and the requirements on sanctions (Hanstad et al., 2010).

Following an extensive consultation period between WADA and its stakeholders, the World Conference on Doping in Sport, held in December 2013 in Johannesburg, approved the 2015 World Anti-Doping Code (http://www.wada-ama.org/code; accessed October 2017). A number of significant changes to the rules and regulations were embodied within the 2015 Code (http://www.wada-ama.org/en/resources/the-code/significant-changes-between-the-2009-code-and-the-2015-code; accessed October 2017). Some of these changes are summarised in Table 2.12.

In 2013, the Steroidal Module for Athlete Biological Passports was introduced in order to monitor endogenous steroids, such as testosterone.

In 2014, a number of investigations by journalists alleged widespread infringements of doping rules and regulations by Russian athletes and their national anti-doping organisation. These allegations were investigated by WADA, resulting in the publication of the McLaren Independent Investigation Report (http://www.wada-ama.org/en/resources/doping-control-process/mclaren-independent-investigations-report-into-sochi-allegations; accessed October 2017). The key findings of part 1 this report are shown in Table 2.13.

Table 2.12 Significant changes introduced in the 2015 World Anti-Doping Code

- Target testing of athletes based on improved anti-doping intelligence
- Incorporation of Investigations as part of the International Standard on Testing and Investigations (www.wada-ama.org/en/resources/world-anti-doping-program/international-standard-for-testing-and-investigations-isti-0)
- Sanctions for deliberate cheating increased to four years
- Reduced sanction for athletes who can establish "No Significant Fault"
- Statute of limitations, through which doping investigations and retrospective testing may continue, increased from eight to 10 years
- Two new Anti-Doping Rule Violations introduced to address the problem of the involvement of Athlete Support Personnel in doping
- The window within which an athlete may accumulate three whereabouts filings (filing failures or missed tests) reduced from 18 months to 12 months

Table 2.13 Key findings of the McLaren Independent Person 1st Report

- The Moscow Laboratory operated, for the protection of doped Russian athletes, within a State-dictated failsafe system, described in the report as the Disappearing Positive Methodology.
- The Sochi Laboratory operated a unique sample swapping methodology to enable doped Russian athletes to compete at the Games.
- The Ministry of Sport directed, controlled and oversaw the manipulation of athletes' analytical results or sample swapping, with the active participation and assistance of the Russian Federal Security Service (FSB), Center of Sports Preparation of National Teams of Russia (CSP), and both Moscow and Sochi Laboratories.

Based on the McLaren Report, WADA recommended "The IOC and IPC consider to decline entries for Rio 2016 of all Russian athletes". The two organisations adopted very different approaches to this recommendation. The IOC abrogated responsibility to international federations to decide on the technical eligibility of athletes to compete in the Rio Olympic Games, whereas the IPC suspended the Russian Paralympic Committee, who were therefore unable to send any athletes to the Rio 2016 Paralympic Games.

Subsequent findings of the McLaren Independent Investigation were published in December 2016 (https://www.wada-ama.org/en/resources/doping-control-process/mclaren-independent-investigation-report-part-ii; accessed October 2017). Some of the key findings from part 2 of the report are shown in Table 2.14.

In January 2016, Maria Sharapova tested positive for the drug meldonium (Table 2.15).

The Sharapova case identified the need for athletes to discuss with appropriate Athlete Support Personnel any substances that they may be taking, for whatever reason.

In September 2016, following the Rio 2016 Olympic Games, WADA confirmed illegal hacking into their Anti-Doping Administration and Management System (ADAMS) by a group of cyber hackers calling themselves "Fancy Bears". This group published data relating to the TUEs for many high profile athletes. This led to a significant review of the security for sensitive online data within anti-doping organisations.

A further development, following the Rio 2016 Games was the Declaration of the 5th Olympic Summit on 8 October 2016 (http://www.olympic.org/news/declaration-of-the-5th-olympic-summit; accessed October 2017) in which the IOC recommended that the anti-doping system should be independent from sports organisations and proposed:

- A new anti-doping testing authority within the framework of WADA
- Sanctions related to doping cases be delegated to the Court of Arbitration for Sport (CAS)

Table 2.14 Some key findings of the McLaren Independent Person 2nd Report

Institutionalised doping conspiracy and cover up

- An institutional conspiracy existed across summer and winter sports athletes who participated with Russian officials within the Ministry of Sport and its infrastructure, such as the RUSADA, CSP and the Moscow Laboratory, along with the FSB for the purposes of manipulating doping controls.
- This systematic and centralised cover up and manipulation of the doping control process evolved and was refined over the course of its use at London 2012 Summer Games, Universiade Games 2013, Moscow IAAF World Championships 2013 and the Winter Games in Sochi in 2014.
- The swapping of Russian athletes' urine samples further confirmed in this 2nd Report as occurring at Sochi, did not stop at the close of the Winter Olympics.

The athlete part of conspiracy and cover up

- Over 1,000 Russian athletes competing in summer, winter and Paralympic sport, can be identified as being involved in or benefiting from manipulations to conceal positive doping tests.

Table 2.15 Maria Sharapova case (2016)

Maria Sharapova case (2016)

Key factors	Lessons learnt
• Meldonium was a drug under review on WADA's Monitoring Program in 2015 • Significant numbers of athletes were using meldonium at the Baku 2015 European Games (Stuart et al., 2016) • Meldonium was placed on the WADA Prohibited List in January 2016 • Sharapova tested positive for meldonium in January 2016. She claimed to have been using it for therapeutic reasons for 10 years • Sharapova's sanction was reduced from two years to 15 months by CAS	• Some athletes use permitted therapeutic agents for performance enhancement • WADA's Monitoring Program is a useful tool to identify potential prohibited substances • Athletes should discuss their substance use with appropriate Athlete Support Personnel

In line with new Anti-Doping Rule Violation articles, aimed at Athlete Support Personnel (ASP), WADA introduced sanctions for ASP, many of which were imposed for life (https://www.wada-ama.org/en/resources/the-code/prohibited-association-list; accessed October 2017).

2.12 Summary

- The use of substances and methods to attempt to improve sport performance dates back to the ancient Olympics.
- The first IOC list of prohibited substances was introduced in 1967 with mandatory testing at Olympic Games in 1968.
- Landmark doping cases, at the individual athlete, team and even national levels were prevalent through the late twentieth and early twenty-first centuries.
- By the end of the 1990s, it was clear that a more harmonised approach to combating doping was required. The First World Conference on Doping in 1999 led to the establishment of the World Anti-Doping Agency (WADA).

- Significant changes to the WADA Prohibited List and improvements in testing regimes were introduced during the early twenty-first century. However, remarkable revelations of doping cases persisted.
- The current strategy for anti-doping agencies is to continue with robust analytical testing regimes but supported by collaboration with governments and other organisations to implement a more targeted, intelligence-based anti-doping approach.

2.13 References

Aguilera, R., Chapman, T.E., Starcevic, B. et al. (2001) Performance characteristics of a carbon isotope ratio method for detecting doping with testosterone based on urine diols: Controls and athletes with elevated testosterone/Epitestosterone ratios. *Clinical Chemistry* 47: 292–300.

Armstrong, D.J. (2005) Blood boosting and sport. In D.R. Mottram (ed.) *Drugs in Sport*, 4th edn. London, Routledge.

Armstrong, D.J. and Chester, N. (2005) Drugs used in respiratory tract disorders. In D.R. Mottram (ed.) *Drugs in Sport*, 4th edn. London, Routledge.

Bashin, S., Storer, T.W., Berman, N. et al. (1996) The effects of supraphysiological doses of testosterone on muscle size and strength in normal men. *New England Journal of Medicine* 335: 1–7.

Brooks, R.V., Firth, R.G. and Sumner, N.A. (1975) Detection of anabolic steroids by radioimmunoassay. *British Journal of Sports Medicine* 9: 89–92.

Catlin, D.H., Fitch, K.D. and Ljungqvist, A. (2008) Medicine and science in the fight against doping in sport. *Journal of Internal Medicine* 264: 99–114.

Catlin, D.H., Sekera, M.H.. Ahrens, B.D. et al. (2004) Tetrahydrogestrinone: Discovery, synthesis and detection in urine. *Rapid Communications in Mass Spectrometry* 18: 1245–1249.

Cooper, C. (2012) Prologue: A tale of two races. In *Run, Swim, Throw, Cheat*. Oxford, Oxford University Press.

Dubin, C.L. (1990) *Commission of Inquiry into the Use of Drugs and Banned Practices Intended to Increase Athletic Performance*. Ottawa, Canadian Publishing Centre.

Eichner, E.R. (2007) Blood doping: infusions, erythropoietin and artificial blood. *Sports Medicine* 37: 389–391.

Erotokritou-Mulligan, I., Bassett, E.E., Kniess, A. et al. (2007) Validation of the growth hormone (GH)-dependent marker method of detecting GH abuse in sport through the use of independent data sets. *Growth Hormone and IGF Research* 17: 416–423.

Fitch, K. (2012) Proscribed drugs at the Olympic Games: Permitted use and misuse (doping) by athletes. *Clinical Medicine* 12(3): 257–260.

Franke, W.W. and Berendonk, B. (1997) Hormonal doping and androgenization of athletes: A secret program of the German Democratic Republic government. *Clinical Chemistry* 43(7): 1262–1279.

Fraser, A.D. (2004) Doping control from a global and national perspective. *Therapeutic Drug Monitor* 26: 171–174.

George, A.J. (2005) CNS Stimulants. In D.R. Mottram (ed.) *Drugs in Sport*, 4th edn. London, Routledge.

Hanstad, D.V., Skille, E.A. and Loland, S. (2010) Harmonization of anti-doping work: Myth or reality. *Sport in Society* 13(3): 418–431.

Hoberman, J.M. (1992) Faster, higher stronger: A history of doping in sport. In J.M. Hoberman (ed.) *Mortal Engines: The Science of Performance and Dehumanization of Sport*. Toronto, Maxwell Macmillan Canada.

Hunt, T.M. (2008) The lessons of crisis: Olympic doping regulations during the 1980s. *Iron Game History* 10(2): 12–25.

Hunt, T.M., Dimeo, P. and Jedlicka, S.R. (2012) The historical roots of today's problems: A critical appraisal of the international anti-doping movement. *Perfomance Enhancement and Health* 1: 55–60.

IOC (2016) IOC Medical and Scientific Commision: Olympics. Available at https://www.olympic.org/medical-and-scientific-commission (Accessed October 2016).

Kamber, M. (2011) Development of the role of National Anti-Doping Organisations in the fight against doping: From past to future. *Forensic Science International* 213: 3–9.

Lasne, F. and Ceaurriz, J.D. (2000) Recombinant erythropoietin in urine. *Nature* 405: 635.

Marclay, F., Mangin, P., Margot, P. et al. (2013) Perspectives for forensic intelligence in anti-doping: Thinking outside the box. *Forensic Science International* 229: 133–144.

Mazanov, J. and Connor, J. (2010) Rethinking the management of drugs in sport. *International Journal of Sport Policy and Politics* 2: 49–63.

Mazzoni, I., Barroso, O. and Rabin, O. (2011) The list of prohibited substances and methods in sport: Structure and review process by the World Anti-Doping Agency. *Journal of Analytical Toxicology* 35: 608–612.

Mottram, D.R. (1999) Banned drugs in sport: Does the International Olympic Committee (IOC) list need updating? *Sports Medicine* 27(1): 1–10.

Mottram, D. (2013) The Lance Armstrong case: The evidence behind the headlines. *Aspetar Sports Medicine Journal* 2(1): 60–65.

Mottram, D., Chester, N., Atkinson, G. et al. (2008) Athletes' knowledge and views on OTC medication. *International Journal of Sports Medicine* 29: 851–855.

Murray, T.H. (1983) The coercive power of drugs in sport. *The Hastings Center Report* 13(4): 24–30.

Powrie, J.K., Bassett, E.E., Rosen, T. et al. (2007) Detection of growth hormone abuse in sport. *Growth Hormone and IGF Research* 17: 220–226.

Rabin, O. (2011) Involvement of the health industry in the fight against doping in sport. *Forensic Science International* 213: 10–14.

Saugy, M., Robinson, N., Grimm, K. et al. (2011) Future of the fight against doping: Risk assessment, biological profiling and intelligence. *Forensic Science International* 213: 1–2.

Schänzer, W. (2002) Analysis of non-hormonal nutritional supplements for anabolic-androgenic steroids: An international study. www.olympic.org.

Schumacher, Y.O., Saugy, M., Pottgiesser, T. et al. (2012) Detection of EPO, doping and blood doping: the haematological module of the Athlete Biological Passport. *Drug Testing and Analysis* 4: 846–853.

Soule, B. and Lestrelin, L. (2011) The Puerto Affair: Revealing the difficulties of the fight against doping. *Journal of Sport and Social Issues* 35: 186–208.

Stuart, M., Schneider, C. and Steinbach, K. (2016) Meldonium use by athletes at the Baku 2016 European Games. *British Journal of Sports Medicine* 50: 694–698.

UCI (2015) Cycling Independent Reform Commission. Report to the President of the Union Cycliste Internationale. Available at: http://www.uci.ch/mm/Document/News/CleanSport/16/87/99/CIRCReport2015_Neutral.pdf (Accessed January 2017).

Vance, N. (2007) Developments in anti-doping in elite sports. *Journal of Exercise Science and Fitness* 5(2): 75–78.

Verroken, M. (1996) Drug use and abuse in sport. In D.R. Mottram (ed.) *Drugs in Sport*, 2nd edn. London, E. & F.N. Spon.

Voet, W. (2001) *Breaking the Chain*. Yellow Jersey Press, London.

WADA (2013) Lack of effectiveness of testing programs. Available at http://playtrue.wada-ama.org/news/wada-seeks-stakeholder-feedback-on-working-group-report-lack-of-effectiveness-of-testing-programs/?utm_source=rss&utm_medium=rss&utm_campaign=wada-seeks-stakeholder-feedback-on-working-group-report-lack-of-effectiveness-of-testing-programs (Accessed June 2013).

Wells, D.J. (2008) Gene doping: The hype and the reality. *British Journal of Pharmacology* 154: 623–631.

Chapter 3

Prevalence of doping in sport

Kelsey Erickson and Susan H. Backhouse

3.1 Introduction

As the number of individuals competing in sport has increased, the types of doping and its pervasiveness have intensified (De Rose, 2008). Doping is no longer confined to professional sport (Zenic, Stipic and Sekulic, 2013); it is evident across the lifespan and fitness and sport contexts (Lippi, Franchini and Guidi, 2008; Uvacsek et al., 2011). Moreover, doping persists in the face of increasing public scrutiny (both nationally and internationally) and severe consequences for the doper (Buckman, Yusko, White and Pandina, 2009).

Doping is defined by the World Anti-Doping Agency (WADA) as "the occurrence of one or more of the anti-doping rule violations set forth in Article 2.1 through Article 2.10 of the Code" (p.18) (WADA, 2015). The anti-doping rule violations include: (2.1) the presence of a prohibited substance (or its metabolites or markers) in an athlete's sample following a drugs test, (2.2) use or attempted use of a prohibited substance or method, (2.3) evading, refusing or failing to submit to a sample when asked to undertake a drugs test, (2.4) as part of the whereabouts system, missing three tests and/or filing failures within a 12-month period by athletes who are part of a registered testing pool, (2.5) tampering or attempted tampering with doping control, (2.6) possession of a prohibited substance or method, (2.7) trafficking or attempted trafficking of a prohibited substance or method, (2.8) administration or attempted administration of any prohibited substance or method to any athlete in-competition or any substance that is also prohibited out-of-competition, (2.9) complicity – aiding, encouraging, assisting, abetting, conspiring or covering up any intentional complicity involving an anti-doping rule violations (ADRV) by another person, and (2.10) prohibited association – associating with any athlete support personnel (e.g., coach, doctor, physiotherapist) who are serving an ADRV or have been found guilty of a criminal or disciplinary offence that is equivalent to an ADRV. For the purpose of this chapter, we will focus on doping via the presence of a prohibited substance in an athlete's sample following a drugs test.

Despite growing recognition of the ubiquity of doping within (and beyond) sport and an exponential increase in the quantity of anti-doping research being conducted over the past decade (Backhouse et al., 2015), the prevalence of doping in sport is unknown. Establishing actual prevalence is confounded by issues of definition and measurement, along with the prevailing social norms around doping in sport and the stigma attached to doping use. Of relevance to all those involved in sport, the inability to establish accurate prevalence statistics renders it impossible to evaluate the effectiveness of current anti-doping policy and practice.

Reported positive drug tests from WADA-accredited laboratories remain relatively stable, at around 2 per cent year-on-year. Conversely, studies administering questionnaires reveal that self-declared doping and non-doping athletes provide doping estimations and doping use data that far exceeds official statistics (Moston, Engelberg and Skinner, 2015a; Uvacsek et al., 2011). Taking all available data into account, the prevalence of doping in elite sports is argued to be between 14 and 39 per cent, although this figure can differ widely in various sub-groups (e.g., sport, national, training group) of athletes (de Hon, Kuipers and van Bottenburg, 2015).

This chapter sets out to provide an updated (since 2013) review and discussion of current estimates of doping prevalence in elite sport. Specifically, we cover analytical data from WADA-accredited laboratories, along with direct and indirect estimates of doping use reported in the literature. These findings are then brought together to conclude the chapter and consider the future of doping prevalence estimation.

3.2 WADA-accredited laboratory anti-doping testing figures

WADA is the global governing body for anti-doping in sport and aims to "bring consistency to anti-doping policies and regulations within sport organizations and governments" worldwide (WADA, 2017). In line with their mandate, WADA has annually published testing statistics from their official WADA-accredited laboratories since 2003 (based on either urine or blood analysis). These reports encompass more than 50 different sports, including all Olympic and Paralympic sports (de Hon et al., 2015). The most recent testing figures from 2015 are publicly available on the WADA website (https://www.wada-ama. org/en/resources/search?f[0]=field_resource_collections%3A202) and include data from 35 WADA-accredited laboratories. For the 2015 report, the Cologne (Germany) laboratory analysed the most samples (N = 25,922), followed by Beijing (China; N = 17,619) and Moscow (Russia; N = 16,961).

Annual adverse analytical and atypical findings

Table 3.1 illustrates that the percentage of adverse analytical findings (AAFs) and atypical findings across WADA-accredited laboratories between 2003 and 2015 has remained relatively stable and low at ~1.9 per cent (SD = 0.2, range 1.36–2.21%). This is despite the doubling of testing efforts (number of samples analysed) across this same time period (151, 210 samples analysed in 2003 compared to 303, 369 in 2015; 101% increase). At the same time, there has been an increase in the number of substances/methods included in the list of prohibited substances in sport (Aguilar, Muñoz-GuerraPlata and Del Coso, 2017). Further, when interpreting the data, it is important to note that an adverse analytical and atypical finding does not necessarily imply that an ADRV has been committed; for example, the athlete may have a Therapeutic Use Exemption allowing them to legitimately use the substance detected in their sample. Therefore, comparing the data longitudinally in a bid to comment on the prevalence of doping in sport is futile because rule changes have occurred over this period and it is impossible to derive the level of intentionality of doping use on the basis of AAFs (de Hon et al., 2015).

These limitations notwithstanding, Table 3.2 breaks down the reported AAFs according to each drug class for all sport. Anabolic agents represent the largest percentage of positive tests (~ 58%) between the years 2003 and 2015 but this percentage is decreasing following

Table 3.1 Adverse and atypical findings, for all sports, by WADA-accredited laboratories from 2003–2015

Year	A-samples analysed (n)[a]	Adverse analytical findings (AAFs) (n)[b]	Atypical findings (ATFs) (n)[b]	Total findings (AAFs + ATFs)	% Adverse findings
2015	303,369	3,809	2,103	5,912	1.95
2014	283,304	3,153	713	3,866	1.36
2013	269,878	3,529	2,433	5,962	2.21
2012	267,645	3,190	1,533	4,723	1.76
2011	243,193	2,885	1,971	4,856	2.0
2010	258,267	2,790	2,027	4,817	1.87
2009	277,928	3,091	2,519	5,610	2.02
2008	274,615	2,956	2,105	5,061	1.84
2007	223,898			4,402	1.97
2006	198,143			3,887	1.96
2005	183,337			3,909	2.13
2004	169,187			2,909	1.72
2003	151,210			2,447	1.62

a Includes non-ADAMS samples, which refers to anti-doping results that were not reported in ADAMS (e.g. North American professional leagues).

b Available since 2008.

the 2014 introduction of the steroidal module within the Athlete Biological Passport (ABP) (Aguilar et al., 2017). The ABP is used to monitor selected biological variables over time that can indirectly reveal the effects of doping rather than attempting to detect the doping substance or method itself. Stimulants, a large category of substances that speed up activity in the central nervous system, have generally represented the second most identified category of substances (on average ~12% from 2003 to 2015). In comparison to anabolic androgenic steroids, stimulants are banned *only* in-competition while anabolic steroids are banned in- *and* out-of-competition. Finally, cannabinoids commonly represent the third most identified substance across the time period, but there has been a noticeable decrease in prevalence across the years, particularly since 2012. However, this shift can likely be explained by changes in WADA's testing procedures and policies rather than actual changes in athletes' behaviours (Aguilar et al., 2017). Similarly, the increase in detection of peptide hormones/growth factor AAFs during the year 2015 could be accounted for by changes in detection methods (Aguilar et al., 2017).

To conclude, the annual percentage of AAFs and atypical findings from WADA-accredited laboratories do not establish the actual prevalence of doping for a number of reasons clearly articulated by de Hon and colleagues (2015). These include issues relating to legitimate use of controlled substances, inability to identify intentional doping use through analytics alone, and failure of the doping control system to detect low thresholds of doping substances and keep up with pharmacological advancement in human performing enhancement substances. Nevertheless, in 2013 WADA added another layer to its global annual analytical reporting through the publication of its ADRV report. Specifically, the report includes the decisions of all AAFs for which the samples were received by the laboratories in the reporting year along with a breakdown of non-analytical ADRVs.

Table 3.2 Substances identified as AAFs in each drug class (all sports) by WADA-accredited laboratories from 2003–2015

	2003	2004	2005	2006	2007	2008	2009	2010	2011	2012	2013	2014	2015
Anabolic agents	872	1,191	1,864	1,966	2,322	3,259	3,297	3,374	3,325	2,279	3,320	1,479	1,728
Stimulants	516	382	509	490	793	472	325	574	718	697	530	474	528
Diuretics and masking agents	142	157	246	290	359	436	273	396	368	322	393	389	428
Glucocorticoids	286	548	325	282	288	316	265	234	274	365	330	252	215
Cannabinoids	378	518	503	553	576	496	399	533	445	406	188	73	127
Beta-2 agonists	297	381	609	631	399	350	303	209	225	131	138	122	115
Peptide hormones, growth factors and related substances [+]	79	78	162	42	41	106	100	86	125	181	202	91	98
Hormone antagonists and metabolic modulators [++]	6	8	21	30	18	29	50	75	70	74	93	145	152
Narcotics	26	15	17	16	21	28	24	20	20	26	43	26	21
Beta blockers	30	25	42	28	27	31	38	30	21	13	25	25	19
Manipulation of blood and blood components [+++]	–	2	–	–	3	–	–	–	1	–	–	–	–
Chemical and physical manipulation	2	–	–	4	3	–	5	6	3	1	1	3	1
Alcohol	–	–	–	–	–	–	5	9	5	5	8	–	–
Total	2,716	3,305	4,298	4,332	4,850	5,523	5,084	5,546	5,600	4,500	5,271	3,079	3,432

* The adverse analytical findings (AAFs) should not be confused with sanctioned Anti-Doping Rule Violations (ADRVs), as the figures given in the WADA reports may contain findings that underwent the Therapeutic Use Exemption (TUE) approval process or multiple findings on the same athlete.

+ Agents with Anti-Oestrogenic Activity prior to 2008; ++ Hormones and related substances prior to 2011; +++ Enhancement of oxygen transfer prior to 2013

Annual analytical anti-doping rule violations

In 2013, WADA published their first ADRV Report to further increase the transparency of global reporting of anti-doping activity through the Anti-Doping Administration and Management System (ADAMS) system. The reports include the decisions of all AAFs for which the samples were received by the WADA-accredited laboratories in each reporting year, as well as non-analytical ADRVs for decisions rendered in each year.

An analytical ADRV refers to a violation of Code Article 2.1 (Presence of a prohibited substance or its metabolites or markers in an athlete's sample) and is based on an AAF, which indicates the presence of a prohibited substance in a urine and/or blood sample collected from athletes and analysed by a WADA-accredited laboratory. In contrast, a non-analytical ADRV is where an athlete or athlete support person (coach, trainer, manager, agent, medical staff, parent, etc.) commits another type of ADRV that does not involve the detection of a prohibited substance in a urine or blood sample from athletes, as outlined in Code Articles 2.2 to 2.10 (e.g., trafficking prohibited substances, tampering with the sample collection process, complicity). Although beyond the scope of this chapter, the annual ADRV reports also include non-analytical ADRVs, which have increased from 266 in 2013 to 280 in 2015.

Table 3.3 shows the number of samples reported as AAFs through ADAMS (2013: 2,540; 2014: 2,287; 2015: 2,522) alongside the number of cases that actually resulted in an ADRV (2013: 1,687, 66%; 2014: 1,462, 64%; 2015: 1,649, 65%) between 2013 and 2015. The percentage of reported AAFs confirmed as ADRVs is consistent across this time period, ranging from 64 to 66 per cent.

Considering actual sanctions (i.e., ADRVs), Table 3.4 presents population demographics associated with recorded ADRVs during the period of 2013–2015. Across the three years, the number of ADRVs resulting from an AAF is relatively stable, ranging from 1,462 to 1,678. Considering gender differences, ADRVs were largely attributed to males (79–80%) and detected from samples collected in-competition (~77%). Since 2013, ADRVs have been committed by athletes representing over 110 nationalities and over 80 sports.

In terms of the sports represented in the ADRV report, in 2015, bodybuilding was the sport with the highest number of ADRVs (n = 270), followed by athletics (n = 242), weightlifting

Table 3.3 Summary of WADA Anti-Doping Rule Violation (ADRV) Reports for 2013–2015

	2013	2014	2015
Samples received and analysed	207,513	217,762	229,412
Samples reported as adverse analytical findings (AAFs)	2,540	2,287	2,522
Samples confirmed as ADRVs (sanctions applied)	1,687 (66%)	1,462 (64%)	1,649 (65%)
Samples dismissed because of a valid medical reason	223 (9%)	224 (10%)	300 (12%)
Categorised as "no case to answer" (valid non-medical reason)	347 (14%)	317 (14%)	178 (7%)
Samples returned as "no sanction" (athlete exonerated)	106 (4%)	132 (6%)	194 (8%)
Samples still pending	177 (7%)	152 (7%)	201 (8%)

Table 3.4 Profile of Anti-Doping Rule Violations (ADRVs) as a result of an adverse analytical finding (AAF)

	2013	2014	2015
Total number of ADRVs as a result of an AAF	1,678	1,462	1,649
Gender of athlete:			
Female	330 (20%)	303 (21%)	345 (21%)
Male	1,357 (80%)	1,159 (79%)	1,304 (79%)
When sample collected:			
Out-of-competition	366 (22%)	328 (22%)	390 (24%)
In-competition	1,321 (78%)	1,134 (78%)	1,259 (76%)
Sample type:			
Urine	1,684	1,458	1,644
Blood	3	4	5
Nationalities involved	112	109	121
Sports involved	84	82	80

(n = 239), and cycling (n = 200) (Figure 3.1). However, it is important to note that these sports were amongst those reporting the highest number of samples analysed. Importantly, for doping prevention, the 2015 ADRV report highlights that no sport is immune from the issue of doping. Finally, the nationalities recording the highest number of ADRVs – with over 100 ADRVs in 2015 – were the Russian Federation (n = 176), Italy (n = 129) and India (n = 117).

In sum, the anti-doping analytical procedures of blood and urine testing are not a reliable method for detecting all athletes who use prohibited substances and methods (de Hon et al., 2015). Furthermore, longitudinal comparisons of data collected since WADA began

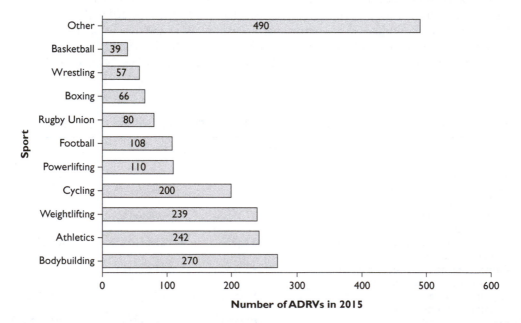

Figure 3.1 Sports with the highest number of ADRVs

reporting on AAFs and ADRVs are impractical as the rules governing anti-doping policy and practice continue to change with every published update to the Prohibited List and revision to the WADA Code. However, they do allow for comparison in relation to the number of tests currently being conducted globally on an annual basis. They also serve as a reminder that the considerable investment and burden of responsibility inherent in current doping control policies and practice may not be proportionate to the positive doping detection rate that ensues.

3.3 Indirect estimates of doping prevalence

Given the lack of reliable direct evidence of the use of prohibited substances in sport it is necessary to make indirect prevalence estimates. However, it is difficult to determine doping prevalence in elite sport because one of its defining features – its prohibition – means that doping users are "hidden" and are thus hard to identify. Even if all doping users can be located and interviewed, they may attempt to conceal their doping behaviour in order to protect themselves, and the reputation of their sport.

Currently, there are no widely accepted "gold standard" methods for producing credible estimates of the number of elite athletes who make up the "hidden population" of doping users in sport. In other fields, the preferred method for determining drug use prevalence is to look for convergence in estimates produced by a variety of different methods of estimation (EMCDDA, 1999). These methods are of two broad types, direct and indirect. Direct estimation methods attempt to estimate the number of doping users in representative samples of the population. Indirect estimation methods attempt to use information from known populations to estimate the size of the hidden population of doping users. However, prevalence data reported in peer-reviewed literature are scarce and often unrepresentative when it comes to doping in elite sport. In addition, the range of methodologies used makes comparisons between studies difficult (Backhouse et al., 2015).

Self-report surveys

Although we acknowledge that the methodological heterogeneity inherent in the cross-sectional studies of self-reported doping prevalence make it impossible to compare findings across studies, it is worth noting that studies generally converge in reporting higher percentages of self-reported banned substance use compared to official laboratory statistics. Within such studies, prevalence rates are reported to range from 1 to 70 per cent of all athletes having used banned substances at some point in their career, dependent on specific sport and competitive level (de Hon et al., 2015).

Studies presenting empirical data on the self-reported prevalence of doping in elite sport are scarce. Where data is available, wide ranging estimations are offered. For example, a study involving elite athletes from Greece presented a doping prevalence estimate of 10 per cent (Barkoukis, Lazuras, Tsorbatzoudis and Rodafinos, 2013). Of those athletes reporting the use of prohibited substances (N = 74), 32 athletes said they doped once but never since, 27 reported occasional use of prohibited substances and 15 reported systematic use of prohibited substances. In Australia, out of a sample of 1,237 elite athletes, 6.9 per cent declared lifetime use of prohibited substances and 3.4 per cent reported use within the last 12 months (Jalleh, Donovan and Jobling, 2013). These estimates are considerably lower than the 21 per cent estimate of lifetime use of anabolic steroids amongst former elite power sport athletes from Sweden competing in the era 1960–1979 (Lindqvist et al., 2013). A fundamental threat to establishing prevalence estimations from standard questionnaires is the risk of drawing socially accepted answers in a possibly biased response group (Petróczi et al., 2011; de Hon et al., 2015).

Projected questioning

In a bid to overcome socially desirable responding, studies utilising indirect methods – such as social projection of doping – are increasingly available in the literature (Backhouse et al., 2015). In this instance, participants are not asked to report on their own use of prohibited substances and methods, but others doping use instead. This is an indirect method of assessment because of the shift from the self to asking about others doping use (Petróczi, 2015). As with self-reported data, social projections of doping use also evidence-biased perception, where the bias is a function of involvement, sensitivity of the behaviour and the reference frame (i.e., in- and out-group) in which the estimation is solicited (Uvacsek et al., 2011; Petróczi, Mazanov and Naughton, 2011).

Typically, projected questioning leads to higher doping prevalence estimates compared to official laboratory estimates and self-reported doping behaviour. For example, among 488 elite multi-sport athletes (Mean age = 24.2 years; 76% male), the perceived prevalence rate of performance-enhancing drug use in all sports was found to be 18 per cent (SD = 19.1). Yet, within one's own sport, the perceived percentage of use decreased to 9.8 per cent (SD = 16.4) (Moston et al., 2015b). Studies consistently note athletes' beliefs that a significant proportion of professional and elite athletes are using prohibited substances, while self-declared doping users discuss doping as normalised in sport (Pappa and Kennedy, 2012).

This divergence in self-reported and socially projected doping use does not just apply to studies of athletes. In Spain, football coaches (N = 101), physical trainers (N = 68), and technical staff (N = 237) completed a survey exploring attitudes and behaviours towards doping. Within this sample, coaches (8.1%), physical trainers (6%) and technical staff (1.5%) admitted to using banned substances. Additionally, approximately 30–35 per cent of all support personnel indicated that they knew someone who had used banned substances and 14–16 per cent stated that they had observed people inciting others or being incited by others to use them (Morente-Sánchez and Zabala, 2015). In Australia, 92 coaches (76% male) were surveyed (Mean age = 37.8 years, SD = 13.7). Among the coaches, they perceived that the incidence of performance-enhancing drug use across all sports was 20.9 per cent (SD = 20.02), yet within their own sports this dropped to 9.97 per cent (SD = 15.86) (Moston Engelberg and Skinner, 2015b).

Random response techniques

Prevalence estimation models, using randomised or fuzzy responses, represent a useful research tool for studying behaviours that are prohibited and/or socially sensitive as they theoretically provide protection against exposure to respondents beyond anonymity (Nepusz et al., 2014). Unsurprisingly, these estimation models are beginning to receive increased attention in the doping field, owing to the absence of evidence pertaining to the prevalence of doping in sport and the inherent limitations of surveys directly questioning self-use of doping substances. All the studies conducted to date have yielded higher prevalence of doping use than previously found in standard self-report questionnaire research (de Hon et al., 2015).

The common feature of these models is that they instruct respondents how they should respond, based on the outcome of some randomisation (e.g., using a device involving cards, dice or spinner) or according to an unrelated question with known probability (e.g., someone's birthday or last digit of a phone number) (Nepusz et al., 2014). These item count techniques (ICT) protect the privacy of the respondents, because only the overall sum of outcomes of a sensitive characteristic and several innocuous characteristics are revealed. According to this privacy protection, we can expect the ICT to deliver more trustworthy estimates than direct questioning. To gather data on sensitive attributes, different alternatives are available in the literature (e.g., the randomised response technique (RRT); single sample count (SSC)).

In one of the first doping-related studies to utilise an ICT known as the RRT, Pitsch, Emrich and Klein (2007) examined intentional doping amongst elite adult athletes. They noted that between 26 and 48 per cent of a group of 448 German Olympic-level athletes admitted to having used doping at some point in their career. The last year prevalence was estimated at 20–39 per cent. Similarly, amongst a sample of 480 junior athletes in Germany, the RRT estimated the lifetime prevalence of doping to be between 3 and 11 per cent (Striegel et al., 2010). More recently, a study commissioned by WADA utilised random response methods to investigate the prevalence of doping in a sample of more than 2,000 track and field athletes participating in the 2011 World Championships and the 2011 Pan-Arab Games. The authors of the report estimate that 29 per cent of the athletes at the 2011 World Championships and 45 per cent of the athletes at the 2011 Pan-Arab Games had doped in the past year (Ulrich et al., 2017).

Although prevalence estimation models offer a promising avenue for the development of a harmonised approach to collecting prevalence data, unless the true value of a sensitive item in a certain population is known, the capacity of ICTs (e.g., SSC) in producing valid results is, at least partially, unclear, because even if ICT estimates are "better" than direct questioning methods, they can still be far off the mark from the actual value. To address this issue, validation studies with known individual values of sensitive behaviours need to be conducted in order to gain further insight into the power of ICT designs. However, given the prohibited and socially stigmatised nature of doping in sport, this presents a considerable challenge to researchers. Furthermore, owing to the complexity of the instructions of the estimation models, the likelihood of innocent noncompliance could be larger than it is with direct questioning, potentially having a distortion effect on the model outcomes and the prevalence estimates (Nepusz et al., 2014). Further research is required in order to fully understand the implications of the methodological nuances of this approach. Recognising the urgency of establishing robust prevalence estimates of doping in sport, WADA have established an expert group to explore such issues in a bid to develop a harmonised approach to data collection and analysis.

3.4 Summary

"How many athletes use prohibited substances in sport?" This is a deceptively easy question to ask, but a notoriously difficult one to answer. Despite increased testing efforts and changes in global anti-doping policy and practice, the prevalence of prohibited substance use in sport is still unknown. Routinely compiled testing statistics from WADA's global network of accredited laboratories, as well as population estimates based on biological parameters and cross-sectional surveys reporting self-declared doping use, provide a wealth of information, but do not afford clarity on the actual incidence and prevalence of prohibited substance use.

The importance of obtaining accurate information on the prevalence of doping in sport should not be underestimated. Such information is valuable both in terms of monitoring the impact of prohibited substance use at sub-group level (e.g., local and national levels) as well as in assessing the effectiveness of doping prevention efforts. The use of drugs in sport, and the policy and practice response to it, transcends national boundaries and therefore WADA needs to inform policy makers globally on the nature and extent of doping in different settings. To address this absence of evidence, comparable methods and definitions must be established and a clear agenda set.

Intelligence on the prevalence of doping in elite sport is critical to the development of anti-doping policy and practice, and the implementation and evaluation of interventions. Determining accurate prevalence rates for doping behaviour in sport is hindered by three key challenges: (1) chemical analyses cannot detect all banned substances (or methods), (2) study designs rely on (honest and willing) personal input from athletes regarding a prohibited behaviour, and (3) issues with the definition of 'doping'.

Whilst we might conceive that it is virtually impossible to uncover the exact prevalence of a largely hidden and socially undesirable behaviour, calls for research to systematically investigate convergence in prevalence estimates produced by a variety of methods of estimation (e.g., population estimates based on physiological data and RRTs) have been made (de Hon et al., 2015).

In summary, the field has not advanced since the sixth edition of *Drugs in Sport*, in which the following concluding statements were offered:

- Meaningful data on the prevalence of doping in sport is difficult to obtain.
- WADA laboratory statistics suggest that, annually, fewer than 2 per cent of samples analysed produce an adverse analytical finding.
- Results derived from statistical data from testing laboratories is very different from those obtained through surveys.
- Independent studies on prevalence of doping reveal higher levels of prohibited substance use in sport.

No matter what approach to doping prevalence estimation is taken, the portrait produced by any data triangulation process will only ever be an imperfect approximation of the real state of affairs.

3.5 References

Aguilar, M., Muñoz-Guerra, J., Plata, M.D.M. and Del Coso, J. (2017) Thirteen years of the fight against doping in figures. *Drug Testing and Analysis* 9(6): 866–869.

Backhouse, S.H., Whitaker, L., Patterson, L., Erickson, K. and McKenna, J. (2015) *Social Psychology of Doping in Sport: A Mixed Narrative Synthesis*. Available at: https://www.wada-ama.org/sites/default/files/resources/files/literature_review_update_-_final_2016.pdf (Accessed on 29 August 2017).

Barkoukis, V., Lazuras, L., Tsorbatzoudis, H. and Rodafinos, A. (2013) Motivational and social cognitive predictors of doping intentions in elite sports: An integrated approach. *Scandinavian Journal of Medicine and Science in Sports* 23(5): e330–340.

Buckman, J.F., Yusko, D.A., White, H.R. and Pandina, R.J. (2009) Risk profile of male college athletes who use performance-enhancing substances. *Journal of Studies on Alcohol and Drugs* 70(6): 919–923.

de Hon, O., Kuipers, H. and van Bottenburg, M. (2015) Prevalence of doping use in elite sports: A review of numbers and methods. *Sports Medicine* 45(1): 57–69.

De Rose, E.H. (2008) Doping in athletes: An update. *Clinics in Sports Medicine* 27(1): 107–130.

EMCDDA (1999) Annual report on the state of the drugs problem in the European Union. Available at: http://www.emcdda.europa.eu/html.cfm/index37340EN.html (Accessed on 29 August 2017).

Jalleh, G., Donovan, R. and Jobling, I. (2013) Predicting attitude towards performance enhancing substance use: A comprehensive test of the Sport Drug Control Model with elite Australian athletes. *Journal of Science and Medicine in Sport* 17(6): 574–579.

Lindqvist, A.S., Moberg, T, Eriksson B.O., Ehrnborg, C., Rosen, T. and Fahlke, C. (2013) A retrospective 30-year follow-up study of former Swedish-elite male athletes in power sports with a past anabolic steroids use: A focus on mental health. *British Journal of Sports Medicine* 47: 965–969.

Lippi, G., Franchini, M. and Guidi, G. C. (2008) Doping in competition or doping in sport? *British Medical Bulletin* 86: 95–107.

Morente-Sánchez, J. and Zabala, M. (2015) Knowledge, attitudes and beliefs of technical staff towards doping in Spanish football. *Journal of Sports Sciences* 33(12): 1,267–1,275.

Moston, S., Engelberg, T. and Skinner, J. (2015a) Self-fulfilling prophecy and the future of doping. *Psychology of Sport and Exercise* 16, Part 2 (0): 201–207.

Moston, S., Engelberg, T. and Skinner, J. (2015b) Perceived incidence of drug use in Australian sport: A survey of athletes and coaches. *Sport in Society* 18(1): 91–105.

Nepusz, T., Petróczi, A., Naughton, D., Epton, T. and Norman, P. (2014) Estimating the prevalence of socially sensitive behaviours: Attributing guilty and innocent noncompliance with the single sample count method. *Psychological Methods* 19: 334–355.

Pappa, E. and Kennedy, E. (2012) "It was my thought . . . he made it a reality": Normalization and responsibility in athletes' accounts of performance-enhancing drug use. *International Review for the Sociology of Sport* 48(3): 277–294.

Petróczi, A. (2015) Indirect measures in doping behaviour research. In V. Barkoukis, L. Lazuras and H. Tsorbatzoudis (eds) *The Psychology of Doping in Sport*. London, Routledge.

Petróczi, A., Mazanov, J., and Naughton, D.P. (2011) Inside athletes' minds: Preliminary results from a pilot study on mental representation of doping and implications for anti-doping. *Substance Abuse, Treatment Prevention and Policy* 6: 10.

Petróczi, A., Uvacsek, M., Nepusz, T., Deshmukh, N., Shah, I. et al. (2011) Incongruence in doping related attitudes, beliefs and opinions in the context of discordant behavioural data: In which measure do we trust? *PLOS ONE* 6(4): e18804.

Pitsch, W., Emrich, E. and Klein, M. (2007) Doping in elite sports in Germany: Results of a www survey. *European Journal for Sport and Society* 4(2): 89–102.

Striegel, H., Ulrich, R. and Simon, P. (2010) Randomised response estimates for doping and illicit drug use in elite athletes. *Drug and Alcohol Dependence* 106: 230–232.

Ulrich, R., Pope, H.G., Cleret, L., Petroczi, A., Nepusz, T., Schaffer, J. et al. (2017) Doping in elite sport assessed by randomised-response surveys. Unpublished manuscript available at: https://www.parliament.uk/documents/commons-committees/culture-media-and-sport/WADA%27s-athlete-doping-prevalence-survey.pdf (Accessed on 2 June 2017).

Uvacsek, M., Nepusz, T., Naughton, D. P., Mazanov, J., Ránky, M. Z. and Petróczi, A. (2011) Self-admitted behavior and perceived use of performance-enhancing vs psychoactive drugs among competitive athletes. *Scandinavian Journal of Medicine and Science in Sports* 21(2): 224–234.

WADA (2016) 2015 Anti-Doping Testing Figures. Available at: https://www.wada-ama.org/sites/default/files/resources/files/2015_wada_anti-doping_testing_figures_report_0.pdf (Accessed on 29 August 2017).

WADA (2017) 2015 Anti-Doping Rules Violations (ADRVs) Report. Available at: https://www.wada-ama.org/sites/default/files/resources/files/2015_adrvs_report_web_release_0.pdf (Accessed on 29 August 2017).

Zenic, N., Stipic, M. and Sekulic, D. (2013) Religiousness as a factor of hesitation against doping behavior in college-age athletes. *Journal of Religion and Health* 52(2): 386–396.

Chapter 4

Regulation of anti-doping in sport
International and national operational frameworks

Neil Chester and Nick Wojek

4.1 Introduction

Ever since drug use has been recognised as a significant issue in sport the need to regulate it has been seen as an important step in safeguarding both the welfare of athletes and the integrity of sport. As the prevalence of doping grew it was evident that sports governing bodies needed to impose rules and regulations to provide clear direction regarding the use of drugs by athletes. Following on from this was a clear need to impose a framework by which governance and sanctions may be applied. Whilst the need for regulation was apparent, the difficulty in establishing such an operational framework was evident in light of the numerous sports governing bodies and cultural differences that exist. In recent years the creation of the World Anti-Doping Agency (WADA) has helped in providing much uniformity to the anti-doping movement. Nevertheless, challenges remain in ensuring parity from an anti-doping governance perspective both nationally and internationally across different sports.

4.2 Why regulate drug use in sport?

From Chapter 1 it is clear that there are a number of reasons why athletes might use drugs. It is also evident that there exists a distinction between those used to enhance performance and those used for what they have been designed to do, that is, treat illness or injury. It is for this distinction that anti-doping regulation exists, to deter athletes from using drugs to enhance performance. Whether regulation should exist at all is typically viewed as an ethical issue and has been the topic of much philosophical debate.

Maintenance of the proverbial 'level playing field' is often quoted as a major reason to prohibit the use of drugs in sport, as those who use performance-enhancing drugs are deemed to have an advantage over those who don't. However, it is argued that even without drugs the 'level playing field' does not exist due to both biological and environmental inequalities (Kayser et al., 2007). Debate often surrounds the fact that the use of many performance-enhancing drugs is not illegal under state law yet is prohibited under the rules laid down by WADA. This generally means that those not competing in organised sport may freely use such drugs to enhance image and performance, and not fear any sanctions. There is clearly an ethical issue surrounding the use of drugs for non-therapeutic purposes, but this is often left to an individual decision and one that is often not legislated for, outside of organised sport. This is unless such drugs are deemed to have a significant impact on public health, for example some recreational psychoactive drugs such as amphetamine or cocaine.

A major argument in support of the regulation of drug use in sport is related to the welfare of athletes in terms of protecting their health. Despite the lack of empirical evidence, it is widely accepted that athletes who use drugs (and methods) to enhance sports performance are putting their health at significant risk. However, the opposing argument might be that participation in sport, particularly at an elite level, increases the chances of developing serious health problems such as injury (Kayser et al., 2007). One might argue that the risks of participating in sport might be made more apparent, allowing an individual to make a more informed decision as to whether they partake or not.

Whether one agrees with the ethical arguments put forward to justify the legislation of drug use in organised sport, the bottom line remains that the use of performance-enhancing drugs, and in most cases recreational drugs, is against the rules of sport. Therefore, much like the handball rule in soccer, the use of such drugs is prohibited. The whole basis of competitive sport relies on rules and without such rules sport would cease to function. The ethical arguments around drug use in sport therefore become secondary but nonetheless no less important.

4.3 The history of the anti-doping movement

Anti-doping has been a reactive movement in response to key incidents in sport that have highlighted not only the use of drugs as performance enhancers but also the dangers surrounding their use from a health perspective.

The International Association of Athletics Federations (IAAF), formerly known as the International Amateur Athletics Federation, was the first sports federation to implement anti-doping regulations when it banned stimulants in 1928. However, it wasn't until the 1960s following the untimely death of the Danish cyclist, Knud Jenson in the Rome Olympics, allegedly as a consequence of amphetamine use, that other sports federations took significant steps to legislate against the use of drugs in sport. In 1966 the Fédération Internationale de Football Association (FIFA) introduced a list of prohibited substances and the following year the Union Cycliste Internationale (UCI) and the International Union of Modern Pentathlon (UIPM) followed suit (Mazzoni et al., 2011). In the same year the IOC formalised its battle against drug misuse in sport by establishing a Medical Commission to oversee doping matters and introduce anti-doping regulations.

In 1967 saw the death of Tom Simpson, the British cyclist who died shortly after his collapse close to the summit of Mont Ventoux during the thirteenth stage of the Tour de France, which was attributed to the use of amphetamine and alcohol. At this time the UCI and FIFA were the first to introduce drug tests as a deterrent to their athletes in their respective World Championships in 1966. The IOC followed suit in 1968 by introducing a list of prohibited substances and drug testing in time for the Winter Olympic Games in Grenoble and the Summer Games in Mexico City. Initial urine tests could only detect the use of stimulants such as amphetamine and it was not until the mid-1970s that a test was established for the detection of anabolic androgenic steroids (AAS). Further advances in analytical chemistry enabled a growing list of prohibited substances to be detected in urine, however problems still remained in terms of the effectiveness of doping control methods.

In 1988, one of the most famous episodes of drug misuse in sport led the anti-doping movement to consider its efficacy once more. The positive test, for the AAS stanozolol by the Canadian track and field athlete, Ben Johnson, immediately after the

100m Olympic final, led to a large review of the use of performance-enhancing drugs by athletes. This review was led by the Canadian lawyer Charles Dubin and was known as the Dubin Inquiry. The inquiry was to last one year and unearthed widespread doping amongst athletes as well as marked inadequacies from a doping control perspective. It also put forward numerous recommendations in an attempt to control performance-enhancing drug use in sport (Moriarty et al., 1992).

In addition to improved testing and stricter penalties to act as a deterrent to those partaking in doping or considering it in the future, the Dubin Inquiry also put forward several ambitious recommendations that would attempt to stem the tide of widespread doping. Such recommendations focused on maintaining ethical standards including changing the emphasis away from extrinsic rewards, such as gold medals, towards intrinsic rewards and incorporating ethics and morality into coach education (Moriarty et al., 1992). By and large many of the recommendations made in the report form the basis of the anti-doping education that we see today. However, as elite sport attracts a wider audience the rewards that come with success continue to grow and therefore it would appear that a huge cultural change would be needed for motivation to shift towards those that are more intrinsically based.

Although the failed drug test of Ben Johnson put doping in sport in the media spotlight this was to be no isolated case. Indeed, less than two years later reports of systematic doping in the former German Democratic Republic (GDR) were to be uncovered as reunification of Germany was reached. Shocking reports were uncovered that provided evidence of a state-run doping programme that would be central to the GDR success from the mid-1960s until reunification of Germany in 1990.

Despite the horrific reports of systematic doping in the GDR it is interesting to note that the sporting community did relatively little in the aftermath to address such atrocities. The international federations and the IOC did not address the humanistic issues that the investigation into the GDR-system unearthed nor did they look to rescind any of the medals or records that were achieved by known doped athletes. Franke and Berondonk (1997) provide a comprehensive review of the doping practices in the former GDR and in doing so offer a sobering reflection that doping was unlikely to have been isolated to such a small state or that other individuals with similar support would not have done the same.

It was not until after the events of the Tour de France in 1998, where large-scale team doping was uncovered, that the anti-doping movement would be pushed to make a monumental shift and establish the World Anti-Doping Agency (WADA). This allowed anti-doping as a movement to function both independently of sports federations and, most importantly, globally to harmonise the fight against doping in sport. On 10 November 1999, the IOC convened the first World Conference on Doping in Sport, held in Lausanne, Switzerland, which led to the formation of WADA.

Throughout the proceeding years WADA, following extensive consultation, produced the first draft of the World Anti-Doping Code (WADC) which would provide the framework for the anti-doping movement throughout the twenty-first century. The second World Conference on Doping in Sport was held in November 2003 in Copenhagen. In addition to major international sports federations, stakeholders from 80 governments were represented, who formally agreed the Copenhagen Declaration on Anti-Doping in Sport. This declaration was a formal acceptance of the WADC (and of WADA) by governments which was to come into effect on 1 January 2004. As part of the Code, international standards including a new List of Prohibited Substances and Methods (formally produced by the IOC Medical Commission) were introduced.

Since the WADC is a non-government document and therefore not legally binding for governments, the Copenhagen Declaration was further developed by the United Nations Educational, Scientific and Cultural Organisation (UNESCO). Indeed, the UNESCO International Convention against Doping in Sport was developed to provide an internationally recognised legal framework for governments to attend to doping in sport and to recognise the WADC. On 19 October 2005, the UNESCO Convention was adopted and took effect from 1 February 2007.

Further World Conferences on Doping in Sport in 2007 and 2013 have seen two revisions of the WADC and International Standards to adapt to the ever-changing doping landscape and further harmonise anti-doping regulations.

4.4 Anti-doping structure

Anti-doping from an organisational perspective is led by WADA, which links both international sporting organisations and state governments. There are few institutions that successfully combine such varied organisations with a unified goal to protect athletes against doping and provide a level playing field globally, across all sports. Clearly by combining both sports organisations and governments the fight against doping in sport benefits from not only a unified and consistent approach, but also from the resources that each organisation individually brings to the table.

Whilst WADA brings together both sports organisations, such as the IOC, and state governments in a unique partnership, its role is largely to manage the World Anti-Doping Program which has been developed to ensure that the WADC is adhered to by all those who sign up to it (Figure 4.1). As an independent body, WADA facilitates and monitors the efforts of all signatories (i.e. governments and sports federations) in terms of their compliance with the WADC and, where necessary, sanctions maybe imposed where non-compliance is evident. A set of international standards have also been developed to help to operationalise the Code together with models of best practice which provide guidelines and solutions for many anti-doping issues.

Regional and national anti-doping organisations (RADOs and NADOs) are in place to ensure that countries comply with the WADC. States that do not have the funds to commit to a fully operational NADO may be served by a RADO which ensures Code compliance across several states within a particular region. In the UK, UK Anti-Doping is the NADO responsible for all anti-doping matters and ensures effective governance of a national anti-doping programme set up to enable compliance with the Code.

The power afforded to WADA lies in the fact that the participation of specific sports and nations at major international competitions including the Olympics, Paralympics and World Championships (of various sports) is dependent on both the acceptance and implementation of the WADC.

From a legislative perspective, some countries have specific laws to help govern drug use in sport (e.g. France, Germany and Italy) whilst others have laws to help govern societal drug use as a whole and may be applied to doping (e.g. UK and USA). Nevertheless, the UNESCO convention is in place to provide a legal framework for those governments that have ratified it.

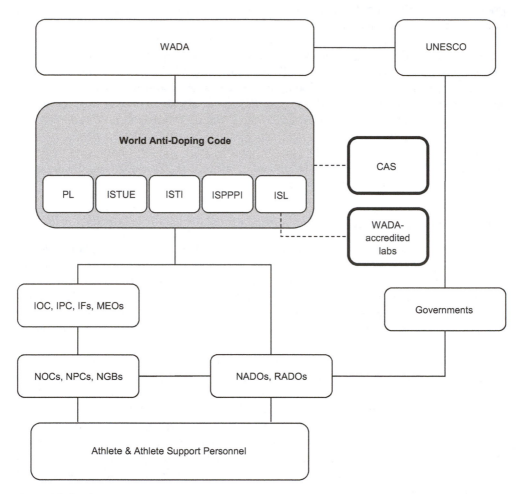

Figure 4.1 A schematic representation of the structure of anti-doping within the context of the World Anti-Doping Code

CAS, Court of Arbitration in Sport; IOC, International Olympic Committee; IPC, International Paralympic Committee; ISL, International Standard for Laboratories; ISPPPI, International Standard for Protection of Privacy and Personal Information; ISTUE, International Standard for Therapeutic Use Exemptions; ISTI, International Standard for Testing and Investigations; MEOs, Major Event Organisers; NADO, National Anti-Doping Organisation; NGBs, National Governing Bodies; RADO, Regional Anti-Doping Organisation; NOCs, National Olympic Committees; NPCs, National Paralympic Committees; PL, Prohibited List; UNESCO, United Nations Educational, Scientific and Cultural Organisation.

4.5 The World Anti-Doping Agency

In 1999 at the first World Conference on Doping in Sport, convened by the IOC in Lausanne, the World Anti-Doping Agency was founded and according to its constitution (WADA, 2016a), its purpose at an international level is to:

1 Promote and coordinate anti-doping in sport both in- and out-of-competition;
2 Reinforce ethical principles to underpin doping-free sport and protect the health of athletes;
3 Establish and update annually a list of prohibited substances and methods in sport;
4 Support and coordinate an out-of-competition drug testing programme;

5   Develop and harmonise a scientific approach to drug testing through technical standards and procedures in sampling and analysis;

6   Promote harmonised rules, disciplinary procedures and sanctions to combat doping in sport;

7   Develop an education programme to promote doping-free sport based on ethical principles; and

8   Promote and coordinate research into anti-doping.

Members of the WADA Foundation Board are made up, essentially, of representatives from the IOC and public authorities (i.e. government) to form an equal partnership. The president of WADA is an honorary position that lasts for a maximum of two 3-year terms. The position, appointed by the Foundation Board, alternates between representation from the IOC and public authorities. In addition to the Foundation Board an Executive Committee takes charge of the actual management and running of the organisation. There are also several additional committees with specialist roles, including: the Athlete Committee; the Education Committee; the Finance and Administration Committee; and the Health, Medical and Research Committee. Further groups have been formed to provide expert opinion in specialist areas and serve important roles with respect to the Code, including: The Prohibited List; Therapeutic Use Exemptions; Laboratories; Technical Document for Sport Specific Analysis; Gene Doping; and Ethical Issues.

As a partnership between governments and the IOC, WADAs budget is funded equally by both parties. In 2015 the WADA budget amounted to a total of over 26 million US dollars (WADA, 2016b).

4.6 The UNESCO International Convention against Doping in Sport

UNESCO introduced the International Convention against Doping in Sport on 1 February 2007. The convention provides the legal framework to enable governments to address anti-doping in sport. Whilst sports organisations may be able to progress so far with regards to anti-doping and sanctioning athletes there is a necessity for government to be able to support this work. Indeed, many doping programmes are so extensive that only governments have the authority to deal with them. Clearly to tackle a doping culture there is a need to focus on issues surrounding drug availability and distribution and to address the part in which athlete support personnel play in a doping case. Essentially the Convention highlights the importance of anti-doping and ensures that governments play a concerted effort in tackling the problem. According to the 2015 WADA Annual Report, 182 of 195 UNESCO member states, including all of the Americas and Europe, have ratified the UNESCO convention (WADA, 2016b).

4.7 The World Anti-Doping Code

Since its inception in 2004 over 660 organisations have signed up to the World Anti-Doping Code (WADA, 2017a) including, amongst others, the IOC, the International Paralympic Committee (IPC), International Sports Federations (IFs), National Olympic and Paralympic Committees (NOCs and NPCs), Regional and National Anti-Doping Organisations (RADOs and NADOs) and event organisations (e.g. Commonwealth Games Federation). The Code provides a universal standard for anti-doping practice which includes a wide range of activities ranging from drug testing to education and research. In addition to the WADC there are a number of mandatory documents which outline the international standards of operation for the key activities of anti-doping organisations and personnel, including:

1   The List of Prohibited Substances and Methods;
2   Therapeutic Use Exemptions;
3   Testing and investigations;
4   Laboratories;
5   Protection of privacy and personal information.

Models of best practice and guidelines relating to the Code and its implementation are also available to use by signatories, but are not mandatory (WADA, 2017b).

As the anti-doping landscape changes WADA must adapt accordingly and it does this most notably through regular revisions to the Code. Whilst the first WADC was introduced in 2004, the most recent revision of the Code was approved in 2013 at the fourth World Conference on Doping in Sport, in Johannesburg, following a widespread consultation process involving stakeholders.

The revised Code came into effect on 1 January 2015 and includes several changes to the 2009 version. The most significant changes include increased sanctions for those who commit a first doping offence, a recognition of the role of non-analytical evidence in investigations into potential ADRVs, and the role of athlete support personnel in doping offences. Further detail summarising the significant changes between the 2009 and 2015 Codes can be found in an overview document on the WADA website (WADA, 2013a).

Compliance with the Code is essential and thus a major element of the Code itself. Clearly in order for the anti-doping movement to function all signatories of the Code must adhere to the rules and regulations set out in the document. In doing so signatories must put in place policy that ensures that the rules, regulations and procedures set out in the Code are followed by all stakeholders. Governance relating to Code compliance is therefore an important aspect of WADA's role.

The following sections will include a brief description of the key elements of the WADC, including: doping control, education and research, and roles, responsibilities and compliance.

Doping control

A major portion of the Code is focused on anti-doping rules and regulations and the procedures required in order to enforce such rules. The Code outlines a wide range of rules and regulations that athletes must follow and sports organisations must implement. Further detail in relation to doping control procedure is provided in Chapter 5.

What is doping?

According to the Code (WADA, 2015a), doping is the occurrence of one or more of the following anti-doping rule violations (ADRVs):

1   The presence of a prohibited substance or its metabolites or markers in an athlete's sample;

2   The use of or attempted use by an athlete of a prohibited substance or method;

3   Refusing or failing to provide a sample, after notification without compelling justification;

4   Violation of applicable requirements regarding athlete availability for out of competition testing, including failure to file sufficient whereabouts information and missed tests;

5   Tampering or attempted tampering with any part of the doping control procedures;

6   Possession of prohibited substances or methods;

7   Trafficking or attempted trafficking in any prohibited substance or method;

8   Administration, attempted administration or assisting in the administration of any prohibited substance or method;

9   Intentional complicity (e.g. aiding, abetting, conspiring, covering up) to commit an ADR; and

10 Association in a professional or sport-related capacity of an athlete with support personnel who are serving a period of ineligibility or who have been convicted in a criminal proceeding for conduct that would constitute doping.

Proof of doping can be rather difficult to establish since many ADRVs do not involve the determination of a prohibited substance or use of a prohibited method via a positive drugs test. In attempts to establish non-analytical ADRV, evidence may be gathered from a variety of sources, including the admission by an athlete, the testimony by a third person as well as other documentary evidence. Where an ADRV is alleged to have occurred, an anti-doping organisation must establish that the proof is greater than the balance of probability for a case to proceed. The individual accused of an ADRV may then refute the claims at a hearing.

The Prohibited List

Whilst not all ADRVs involve the use of a prohibited substance or method the Prohibited List is fundamental to doping control since it clearly outlines what is deemed to be unacceptable both in- and out-of-competition (refer to Table 1.1 of this book). As with the Code, the Prohibited List is an evolving document. New pharmacological agents and potential performance-enhancing methods are continually being developed and becoming available and therefore the List must be updated regularly to keep pace with the rapidly changing landscape.

A specific expert committee has been established by WADA to oversee the development of the List and consider the inclusion or exclusion of specific substances or methods on an annual basis. Each year the List Expert Group initiates a consultation process to all WADA stakeholders asking them to consider potential modifications to the List. Modifications may take the form of changes to the terminology of the document (including the use of particular drug names) to help in the understanding and thus compliance of the List or changes to the actual content in terms of introducing or removing substances or methods to the List. In addition, the List Expert Group will also consider the inclusion of particular thresholds for specific substances or the reclassification of particular substances.

The criteria by which the List Expert Group make decisions as to whether a substance or method is to be considered for inclusion on the List are as follows:

1   The use of a substance or method has the potential to enhance performance in sport;
2   The use of a substance or method has the potential to adversely affect health; and
3   The use of a substance or method contravenes the 'spirit of sport'.

A substance or method is considered for inclusion by the List Expert Group if it meets any two of the above criteria. In addition, substances or methods that have the potential to mask the presence or use of a prohibited substance or method would also be considered for inclusion on the Prohibited List.

The List Expert Group will consider the comments made during the consultation process and also consider data made available to them from WADA-accredited laboratories, the WADA Monitoring Program and from research publications, particularly from those funded by WADA research grants.

The Monitoring Program

In addition to the List of Prohibited Substances and Methods, WADA also conducts a Monitoring Program which allows for monitoring of substances beyond that of the Prohibited List to determine patterns of use that may reflect possible misuse (WADA, 2016c). The programme typically includes substances that are not prohibited but have the potential to be misused in sport for possible performance-enhancing purposes. There are however a number of substances that are part of the Monitoring Program which are also present on the Prohibited List, although subject to only partial prohibition (i.e. only in-competition and/ or above a particular threshold).

Therapeutic Use Exemptions

Clearly doping by athletes is not to be confused with the use of drugs for therapeutic purposes. Whilst drug use in sport is synonymous with doping there are numerous instances when drug use by athletes is entirely legitimate. Indeed, WADA have outlined a process whereby athletes may apply for, and be granted an exemption for the use of a particular prohibited substance or method specifically for therapeutic purposes. This process is known as Therapeutic Use Exemption (TUE) and is outlined in detail in the International Standard for Therapeutic Use Exemptions (WADA, 2015b). The procedure involved in obtaining a TUE requires an athlete to make a request with supporting medical evidence. Each application is then considered according to the guidelines set out by the International Standards document, by an independent TUE Committee that is formed by the respective NADO, IF or major event organiser. TUE Committees are made up of physicians with experience in the field of sports medicine and specialists with expertise in treating specific medical conditions. TUE Committees make decisions as to whether to grant a TUE based on the following four criteria (WADA, 2015b):

•   The athlete would experience significant health problems without taking the prohibited substance or method;
•   The therapeutic use of the substance would not produce significant enhancement of performance;
•   There is no reasonable therapeutic alternative to the use of the otherwise prohibited substance or method; and
•   The necessity for the use of the prohibited substance or method is not a consequence of the prior use of a substance or method which was prohibited at the time of such use.

Decisions made by each committee are then reported to WADA who may then decide to confirm or rescind the initial decision according to whether or not the TUE Committee complied with procedures set out in the International Standards document. There is also an appeals process which can be used by athletes to contest a Committee decision.

Testing

In order to enforce the rules set out in the Code and International Standards a robust testing procedure is necessary. Indeed, so that the Prohibited List may serve as an effective deterrent testing is required to be a covert operation that follows strict guidelines in terms of sampling and analysis as outlined in the International Standard for Testing and Investigations (WADA, 2016d) and for Laboratories (WADA, 2016e).

Sample analysis is carried out in specific laboratories that follow approved procedures and are formally accredited by WADA. Strict accreditation and regular assessment procedures ensure both validity and harmonisation of test results across all laboratories and that the highest standards are maintained. In recent times, a few laboratories have had their accreditations suspended and even revoked following non-conformities with the International Standard for Laboratories.

There are currently 34 WADA-accredited laboratories that are distributed in cities across the globe (WADA, 2017c). More than half (19 out of 34) of the accredited laboratories are based in Europe whereas the African and South American regions are considered underserved. As a result, WADA are discouraging the set-up of further laboratories in Europe and are exploring opportunities to establish additional laboratories in South America and Africa (WADA, 2013b).

Results management

Allied to the high standards maintained by a laboratory is a results management system which ensures a clear chain of events whereby an athlete is notified as soon as their sample returns an adverse analytical finding that is not supported by a valid TUE nor is there any reported deviation from the procedures as outlined in the International Standards for Testing or Laboratories. The athlete may then request the analysis of their B-sample which, if confirms the analytical results of the A sample an adverse analytical finding is established.

In the event of an adverse analytical finding there is a requirement for an anti-doping organisation to provide a fair hearing process to establish if an ADRV has occurred and what sanctions are to be imposed. Where the hearing confirms the evidence put forward by the anti-doping organisation and a sanction is applied an appeals process must be made available. A disciplinary case for doping might be dealt with, initially between the NADO, IF and athlete and a subsequent appeal might be lodged with the Court of Arbitration for Sport (CAS).

Sanctions

The Code clearly outlines the sanctions to be imposed on individuals, teams and sporting organisations implicated in an ADRV. The provision of clear sanctions is imperative to ensure harmonisation and act as a real deterrent to all those tempted by doping. Current sanctions include disqualification and forfeiture of points, medals and prizes where an ADRV has occurred in-competition. In addition, a period of ineligibility is typically imposed which varies according to the nature of the ADRV and whether the athlete has committed a previous ADRV. The criteria for increasing or reducing the standard four-year period of ineligibility can be rather complex and are outlined in Chapter 5. A public disclosure of those individuals committing an ADRV is arguably the most impactful from both a professional and personal perspective. An athlete who is deemed to have committed an ADRV should be publicly identified after such a time that a hearing and subsequent appeal may have been concluded.

In addition to sanctions imposed on individuals there are circumstances whereby a team may be sanctioned particularly in circumstances where two or more members of a team commit an ADRV. In such instances likely sanctions would include loss of points or disqualification from a competition.

Whereabouts

As a means of conducting an effective and efficient out-of-competition testing programme a system whereby athletes must report their prospective location for one hour a day, each day throughout their competitive career has been established. This system, where athletes notify either their IF or NADO of their location is known as 'whereabouts'. Only elite athletes competing at the highest level who are identified by their respective IF or NADO are required to undertake such reporting and as such are part of a 'registered testing pool'. The accuracy of the information provided is critical and those athletes who fail to file information or file inaccurate information (i.e. they are found not to be at the location, at the time that they have stated in their whereabouts information) on three separate occasions over a 12-month period will be deemed to have committed an ADRV.

Doping control for animals competing in sport

Sports that involve animals such as horse racing implement anti-doping rules and procedures specific to the animals via their IF. However, testing of humans is under the jurisdiction of WADA where the specific federation has signed up to the Code.

Statute of limitations

There is a period of ten years during which an alleged anti-doping violation may have taken place and throughout which action against an athlete may proceed. This duration of time acknowledges that sophisticated doping can sometimes take a long time to uncover. In addition, where multiple ADRVs are to be considered in determining the sanction (i.e. length of period of ineligibility) these must occur within the same ten-year period.

Education and research

A key element of the WADC is seen to be the promotion of proactive or preventative measures in an attempt to limit both intentional and unintentional ADRVs. In the Code both research and education are highlighted as key preventative measures in which all signatories are expected to engage.

WADA have established two funding streams in an attempt to promote research in the physiological and analytical sciences and the social sciences. Funding is assigned to the two programmes on an annual basis and researchers are encouraged to apply for funds through an application process involving the submission of a detailed project proposal. Following review by the appropriate WADA committee, approval is given to those projects that are deemed to answer important questions or add key information to new and emerging areas within the field of anti-doping. Funds committed to research since 2001 has been over 69 million US dollars with 8.8 million US dollars paid out in 2014 and 2015 (WADA, 2016b).

The criticism levelled at many research studies that attempt to examine the reputed effects of prohibited substances and methods is that findings are those from recreational or non-elite athletic subjects and thus not representative of elite athletes. Whilst there might be a drive to redress this issue there is a need to be cognisant of the issues that this might raise. Indeed recruiting athletes to studies that include the supplementation of a prohibited substance or use of a prohibited method should be avoided due to the potential performance-enhancing effects and adverse side-effects and also the potential of a failed drugs test as a consequence of participation in a research study (Howman, 2013).

Roles, responsibilities and compliance

Clearly one of WADA's key roles is to monitor and ensure that its signatories adhere to the rules and procedures set out in the WADC. Nevertheless, ultimately each organisation that is governed by the Code must not only ensure its own compliance with the Code but also that of those organisations that it governs. The consequences of non-compliance should also be visible, with a clear penalty for perpetrators such as ineligibility to participate in major competitions or indeed to bid to host such events (WADA, 2015a). There is a clear chain of command in terms of roles and responsibilities from a Code compliance perspective which filters down from WADA, the IOC and the IPC to IFs, NADOs, NOAs and NPAs and ultimately to NGBs and athletes. The chain of command which also includes Government and major event organisers, is complex (see Figure 4.1), yet essential if anti-doping is to be effective. Devolution of governance ensures that there is engagement with anti-doping at all levels.

Whilst acceptance of the Code by signatories has been particularly encouraging, Houlihan (2013) argues that the degree of compliance is less so. Clearly such an issue places the core WADA principle of harmonisation in doubt. Further efforts are required to address issues concerning the capacity and commitment of stakeholders in terms of Code compliance. Indeed, a Code compliance framework culminating in the drafting of a new International Standard on the Code Compliance of Signatories is currently being developed by WADA for 2018. This new International Standard will outline (WADA, 2017d):

- Code signatories' rights and responsibilities;
- The ways WADA supports signatories in achieving and maintaining Code compliance;
- A range of consequences that could be imposed in situations of non-compliance; and
- A process whereby the consequences can be imposed by an independent tribunal.

WADA has also recently introduced a Compliance Monitoring Program to strengthen its ability to monitor and scrutinise signatories' enforcement of the Code. Monitoring will be achieved through questionnaires sent to signatories, the independent collection of information that is available to WADA (e.g. through investigations, tip-offs, and the mandatory input of drug test results into WADA's Anti-Doping Administration and Management System by Anti-Doping Organisations), and through audits of NADOs' and IFs' anti-doping programmes.

4.8 Court of Arbitration for Sport

CAS has an important role within the structure of anti-doping since it provides an independent means, where necessary, for the resolution of disputes associated with ADRVs and related sanctions. It is available to both athletes and federations for all sports-related disputes including those linked to disciplinary charges such as doping and those that are commercial in nature such as sponsorship and relationship disputes between athletes, coaches, clubs and agents.

The concept of CAS was introduced by the IOC and established in 1984. Based in Lausanne it was comprised of 60 members that were appointed by the IOC, IFs and national Olympic Associations. However, the independence of CAS was later questioned and in 1994, following major reform, it became both structurally and financially autonomous.

4.9 Summary

The anti-doping movement has made huge strides over recent decades in an attempt to address the increasingly complex nature of doping practice. The establishment of policies and practices to address doping in sport is now led by the World Anti-Doping Agency through the World Anti-Doping Code. International Federations, international and national Olympic and Paralympic committees, major event organisations and national anti-doping organisations are all signatories to the Code. Governments accept the Code through signing up to the UNESCO Convention which provides the legal framework to enable governments to address anti-doping in sport. Whilst sports organisations may be able to progress so far with regards to anti-doping and sanctioning athletes there is a necessity for governments to be able to support this work aligning their domestic policies with the Code. However, challenges exist to guarantee that such a model can be implemented across all states thus ensuring harmonisation, a fundamental objective of the Code.

4.10 References

Franke, W.W. and Berendonk, B. (1997) Hormonal doping and androgenization of athletes: A secret program of the German Democratic Republic government. *Clinical Chemistry* 43: 1,262–1,279.

Houlihan, B. (2013) Achieving compliance in international anti-doping policy: An analysis of the 2009 World Anti-Doping Code. *Sport Management Review* 17(3): 265–276.

Howman, D. (2013) Scientific research using elite athletes: WADA point of view. *Journal of Applied Physiology* 114(10): 1,365.

Kayser, B., Mauren, A. and Miah, A. (2007) Current anti-doping policy: a critical appraisal. *BMC Medical Ethics* 8(2): 1–10.

Moriarty, D., Fairall, D. and Galasso, P.J. (1992) The Canadian Commission of Inquiry into the use of drugs and banned practices intended to increase athletic performance. *Journal of Legal Aspects of Sport* 2(1): 23–31.

WADA (2013a) Significant changes between the 2009 Code and 2015 Code. Available at: https://www.wada-ama.org/en/resources/the-code/significant-changes-between-the-2009-code-and-the-2015-code (Accessed on 28 July 2017).

WADA (2013b) Laboratory Network Strategy. Available at: https://www.wada-ama.org/en/resources/science-medicine/laboratory-network-strategy (Accessed on 28 July 2017).

WADA (2015a) World Anti-Doping Code 2015. Available at: https://www.wada-ama.org/en/resources/the-code/world-anti-doping-code (Accessed on 28 July 2017).

WADA (2015b) International Standard for Therapeutic Use Exemptions. Available at: https://www.wada-ama.org/en/resources/therapeutic-use-exemption-tue/international-standard-for-therapeutic-use-exemptions-istue (Accessed on 28 July 2017).

WADA (2016a) Constitutive Instrument of Foundation of the World Anti-Doping Code. Available at: https://www.wada-ama.org/en/resources/legal/revised-statutes (Accessed on 28 July 2017).

WADA (2016b) 2015 Annual Report. Available at: https://www.wada-ama.org/en/resources/finance/annual-report (Accessed on 28 July 2017).

WADA (2016c) The 2017 Monitoring Program. Available at: https://www.wada-ama.org/en/resources/science-medicine/monitoring-program (Accessed on 28 July 2017).

WADA (2016d) International Standard for Testing. Available at: https://www.wada-ama.org/en/resources/world-anti-doping-program/international-standard-for-testing-and-investigations-isti-0 (Accessed on 28 July 2017).

WADA (2016e) International Standard for Laboratories. Available at: https://www.wada-ama.org/en/resources/laboratories/international-standard-for-laboratories-isl (Accessed on 28 July 2017).

WADA (2017a) Code Compliance. Available at: https://www.wada-ama.org/en/what-we-do/the-code (Accessed on 28 July 2017).

WADA (2017b) Model Rules, Guidelines and Protocols. Available at: https://www.wada-ama.org/en/model-rules-guidelines-and-protocols (Accessed on 28 July 2017).

WADA (2017c) List of WADA Accredited Laboratories. Available at: https://www.wada-ama.org/en/resources/laboratories/list-of-wada-accredited-laboratories (Accessed on 28 July 2017).

WADA (2017d) Code compliance and development of an International Standard for Code Compliance by Signatories. Available at: https://www.wada-ama.org/en/resources/the-code/backgrounder-code-and-is-review (Accessed on 28 July 2017).

Chapter 5

Doping control in sport

Neil Chester, Nick Wojek and Yorck Olaf Schumacher

5.1 Introduction

The anti-doping rules outlined in Chapter 4 are central to the World Anti-Doping Code in providing a clear definition of doping. Procedures that enable the determination of anti-doping rule violations (ADRV) are critical in ensuring a reliable and effective anti-doping programme. Doping control is an intrinsic element of any anti-doping programme. In addition, the consistency of approach across different nations and sports ensures that doping control acts as a credible and effective deterrent. Nevertheless, a programme that is proactive and centred around prevention rather than detection may be considered desirable.

Tackling doping in sport is continually developing and involves a wide range of strategies. Those aimed at identifying anti-doping rule violations through both analytical and non-analytical means are important not only in catching the perpetrators but also in acting as a deterrent to others. In addition, education is central to an effective pro-active approach to doping control. Acknowledgment of the importance placed upon education is clear by its presence in the Code. All signatories and stakeholders are bound to develop and implement appropriate information and education programmes for the purpose of doping prevention. Athletes and their support staff also have responsibilities around compliance with anti-doping rules and procedures and therefore must be pro-active in terms of their own education and knowledge.

This chapter seeks to provide an overview of the strategies in place designed to control doping through the detection or determination of anti-doping rule violations and via a more preventative approach (e.g. education). A comprehensive review of the analytical approaches including the processes involved in the detection of prohibited substances and in the detection of biomarkers (i.e. the Athlete Biological Passport) will be included as well as the recent focus towards non-analytical, intelligence-led approaches to doping control.

5.2 Analytical investigations

Historically the analysis of athlete samples, namely urine, enabled the determination of doping. Around the time of the publication of the list of prohibited substances by several International Federations and the IOC Medical Commission in the late 1960s came the advent of drug detection. Scientists first developed tests for the detection of stimulants in urine, closely followed by anabolic androgenic steroids in the mid-1970s. Since this time research has enabled the detection of an ever-increasing list of prohibited substances using both urine and blood as the preferred matrices. In more recent times the detection of biomarkers that are indicative of doping has also been added to the armoury of those involved in doping control in the form of the Athlete Biological Passport and biomarker test to detect growth hormone.

Drug detection

As outlined in Chapter 4, doping is defined as the infringement of at least one of ten anti-doping rules. Whilst the most notable rules relate to the prohibition of substances and methods as specified by the Prohibited List other rules include those that relate to the requirement of all athletes to engage appropriately in doping control procedures including routine urine and blood sample collection. In cases where there is evidence of an ADRV as a consequence of a positive drug test, the principle of 'strict liability' is upheld. In such cases the athlete receives a reprimand and where the test is 'in-competition', automatic disqualification of individual results, as well as forfeiture of any medals, points or prizes that may have been accrued is likely. In addition, further sanctions include a period of ineligibility which may last four years for a first offence. Only in exceptional circumstances is the potential sanction eliminated where an athlete can provide evidence to demonstrate that they bear no significant fault or negligence and can prove how the prohibited substance has entered their body (WADA, 2015a).

Test distribution plan

An important aspect of an effective doping control programme is the development of a test distribution plan, which not only has the best chance of success (i.e. detection of those athletes that practice doping) but is also the most cost-effective. Traditional methods of doping control are inherently ineffective, particularly when it is considered that the proportion of positive drug tests is between 1 and 2 per cent yet the prevalence of doping is considered to be much higher (de Hon et al., 2015).

It was assumed that increased tests would lead to greater success in terms of exposing those involved in doping; however the cost of increasing the number of tests is not economically viable. Moreover, the distribution of tests as opposed to the volume of tests is thought to have a much greater impact on the effectiveness of a testing programme. This change in philosophy has led to the focus of current testing programmes on increasing the proportion of target tests. Target tests are essentially tests that target specific individuals and sports at particular times according to the reputed risk of likely doping practice. Whilst random testing still has a place in drug testing, the development of a target testing scheme enables a much more proactive approach towards doping control. According to the International Standard for Testing and Investigations (WADA, 2016a) the following factors are considered when determining whom tests should be targeted towards:

1 Athletes competing at the highest level i.e. Olympics or World Championships;
2 Athletes receiving public funding;
3 Athletes presenting abnormal biological parameters arising from the Athlete Biological Passport;
4 Athletes displaying significant, acute and sustained improvements in performance;
5 Athletes repeatedly failing to file whereabouts information or demonstrating suspicious patterns of filing information e.g. last-minute updates or isolated locations;

6   Injured athletes;
7   Athletes that withdraw or are absent from expected competition;
8   Athletes moving into a different age category (e.g. junior athletes moving into the senior ranks) and those approaching retirement or wishing to return to competition following retirement;
9   Athletes currently serving a period of ineligibility as a consequence of an ADRV or those who have served a period of ineligibility for a prior ADRV;
10 Athletes subject to significant financial incentives for improvements in performance;
11 Athletes associated with team mates or support personnel who have a history of involvement in doping; and
12 Athletes identified by information obtained from a third party or intelligence as part of a non-analytical doping investigation.

As part of an effective doping control strategy, a risk assessment is performed to assess which sports or specific athletes might be liable to doping practice and whether this is likely at particular times of the year. A risk assessment to evaluate the potential doping practice of a particular sport should be based upon the following factors, as outlined in the International Standard for Testing and Investigations (WADA, 2016a):

1   The demands of the sport and the potential performance-enhancing effects of doping;
2   The rewards available within a particular sport and other incentives for doping;
3   The history of doping and any research available on doping trends in a specified sport;
4   The prohibited substances and methods considered useful in eliciting an appropriate benefit within a particular sport;
5   The training and competition calendar of the sport to identify particular times of the year when doping might be most advantageous;
6   The particular time points within an athletes career when doping might be perceived to be most profitable;
7   Any available information/intelligence on doping practice attributed to the sport (e.g. athlete testimonies and intelligence from a non-analytical doping investigation or criminal investigation); and
8   Outcomes from previous test distribution planning cycles.

This information is imperative in informing a robust target testing strategy. In addition to prioritising target testing and a test distribution plan, the National Anti-Doping Organisation (NADO) must also establish criteria for the sports that require a registered testing pool and implement an effective number of in- and out-of-competition tests for athletes included in this pool. Registered testing pools are developed by both International Federations (IFs) and NADOs and consist of those athletes competing at the highest level. Athletes selected for respective registered testing pools are required to provide whereabouts information (see Chapter 4).

Furthermore, NADOs and IFs must comply with the Technical Document for Sport Specific Analysis (TDSSA). This technical document is intended to ensure that the Prohibited Substances within the scope of the TDSSA (i.e. erythropoiesis stimulating agents, growth hormone and growth hormone-releasing factors) are subject to an appropriate and consistent minimum level of analysis by all anti-doping organisations in those sports/disciplines that are deemed to be at risk of misuse (WADA, 2017a).

Sample provision

The key stages and procedures for sample provision are outlined in the International Standards for Testing and Investigations (WADA, 2016a). However, some variations will occur depending on the testing authority (i.e. NADO, IF or major event organiser). Key stages in sample provision include: selection, notification, chaperoning, reporting to the doping control station and sample collection. These stages are carried out by authorised individuals typically known as doping control officers (DCOs).

Selection

Where the test is random, a specific selection process must be performed. The selection draw will often involve a lead DCO in addition to an IF or national sports governing body representative or additional member of the doping control personnel. The draw may take several forms including assigning numbers to named athletes prior to a random number selection. Alternatively, selection maybe based on finishing position, for example, the winner, runner-up and fifth position.

Notification

Strict procedures are followed when an athlete is notified and vary slightly according to whether an athlete is considered an adult or a minor (i.e. under 18 years of age) or has a disability, such as a visual impairment. As soon as possible after a competition, a doping control staff member approaches selected athletes to notify them of their selection for a drugs test. At this stage the athletes will be informed of their rights and responsibilities, which include: the right to have a representative with them and an interpreter where available; their responsibility to report to the doping control station immediately; the need to be chaperoned at all times until the sample provision has been completed; and their responsibility to comply with doping control procedures including the provision of the first urine sample passed subsequent to notification (WADA, 2016a).

If an athlete selects to have a representative, it may be any individual they choose, such as a friend, training partner, family member, coach or team doctor. In the event that an athlete is a minor there is a requirement that notification, chaperoning and actual sample provision is performed under the supervision of an additional individual. Whilst at notification and up until the athlete reports to the doping control station (DCS) this might be a designated representative, once inside the DCS additional doping control staff may fulfil this role.

The same notification procedures are also followed during out-of-competition tests which normally occur at athlete homes or training venues.

Chaperoning

From the instant that an athlete is notified they must be chaperoned by a doping control staff member at all times until sample collection procedures are completed. The chaperoning process involves observation of the athlete in full view of a doping control staff member.

Reporting to the doping control station

Athletes are required to report to the DCS immediately after notification. The DCS is a designated facility that might ordinarily be a medical or physiotherapist treatment room, a hotel room or changing room. The DCS is a controlled environment with a strict policy for both entry and exit of specified individuals. A register is kept to record all those, other than doping control personnel, that enter and exit the DCS. It is essential that the facility allows for the privacy of an athlete to be maintained during sample collection; where possible, the DCS should be used solely for the purpose of sample provision. A lead DCO must ensure that a designated DCS is able to maintain sample integrity and that no part of the collection process is compromised.

A delay in reporting to the DCS is acceptable in specific circumstances, such as when an athlete is required to attend an awards ceremony, undertake media commitments, collect identification documents (e.g. passport), locate a representative or interpreter (where necessary), compete in further competitions, complete a cool-down or training session (in the case of an out-of-competition test), or receive medical treatment. Where medical treatment is required, the lead DCO will assess (through consultation with medical staff) whether the athlete is fit enough to continue with the test and determine whether it is appropriate to abort the test. Delayed reporting for other reasons must be approved by the lead DCO. Reasons typically deemed to be unacceptable include showering and meeting family and friends.

Sample collection

On arrival at the DCS, athletes will typically wait in a designated area until they are ready to provide a sample. Whilst formal notification has occurred, further details may be obtained from the athlete to complete the notification process. When blood collection is required, athletes are required to sit for a designated period (a minimum of 10 minutes) before a sample can be taken (to allow the cardiovascular system and the vascular volumes to equilibrate). For urine collection athletes are required to wait only as long as is necessary until they are able to provide a sample. If athletes are considered to be dehydrated, they might be encouraged to drink fluids (in moderation) to promote diuresis.

When athletes are ready, they will be asked to select a collection vessel and provide a sample under the supervision of a DCO of the same sex. Athletes are required to remove sufficient clothing to enable direct observation of sample provision by the supervising DCO. A minimum volume of 90ml of urine is required for analysis. Once collected this is divided into the A and B sample bottles. If less than 90ml is collected, additional samples are required. An additional sample is added to the previous sample(s) until the minimum volume is reached.

The concentration of the sample is determined through the assessment of specific gravity using a digital refractometer. In the event that specific gravity is less than 1.005, further samples will be collected until the specified range (i.e. ≥1.005) is met. This ensures that any potential substances (on the Prohibited List or part of the Monitoring Program) can be determined using current analytical technologies. In the event that further samples are required, athletes will be encouraged not to consume further fluids in an attempt to increase urine concentration.

In the cases where blood collection is required, a qualified phlebotomist (blood collection officer; BCO), will perform the procedure. Blood collection uses evacuated tubes that enables a specific amount of blood to be collected. If the BCO is unable to collect a sample or collects insufficient volume, a maximum of three attempts are performed before sampling is terminated. All samples collected are then sealed into a tamperproof transport vessel by the athlete, ready for shipment. Blood is transported refrigerated, ideally at a temperature of 4°C.

Following sample collection, athletes will be asked to declare on a doping control form (DCF) any medication and supplements that they have taken over the previous seven days. For blood passport samples, athletes are also asked to declare additional information such as blood transfusions received, blood losses sustained and their altitude exposure history. This information is essential in providing the necessary detail to supplement any potential adverse finding. Following a declaration of the athlete's approval (or not) for the sample to be used in anonymised anti-doping research, the DCF is checked and signed by the athlete and DCO to confirm that a satisfactory procedure has been followed and all necessary detail is present and correct. Athletes receive a duplicate copy of the form for their records; the NADO or organisation that authorised the test receives a copy and an anonymised version is stored with the sample for shipment to the WADA-accredited laboratory.

Athletes are directed throughout the whole process by the DCO including (in the case of urine samples) the apportioning of samples into A and B storage bottles and the packaging of those bottles ready for shipment. This is to ensure that the procedure and sample are not compromised and at no stage is there any possibility of anyone other than the athlete tampering with the sample.

Shipment of sample

Urine samples are stored in identical glass bottles (labelled A and B) with tamperproof lids. Similarly, blood samples are also sealed in tamperproof A and B bottles, but these must be stored temporarily in a cool storage container until despatched to the laboratory via a refrigerated courier. All sealed samples remain in the custody of the DCO until they are signed over to the courier responsible for delivering the samples to a WADA-accredited laboratory. A chain of custody form is transported along with the samples to ensure the integrity of the samples is not compromised. Guidelines are in place to ensure that samples arrive at the laboratory within set timeframes related to the type of analysis. Extended turnover time from the moment of sampling to analysis might alter certain types of samples, especially those made of active biological material such as blood. To ascertain that the results are reliable, measures are in place to guarantee sample stability. For blood passport samples for example, the accepted turnover time depends on the storage temperature of the sample and is assessed through the so-called blood stability score, which combines these two measures and provides an indication of expected sample quality (Robinson et al., 2016).

Sample analysis

On receipt of samples, laboratories endeavour to analyse samples and report the results in a timely manner – normally within ten working days unless there is agreement between the laboratory and Anti-Doping Organisation to extend this timeframe (WADA, 2016b). Initial analysis occurs to determine the presence of prohibited substances, metabolites of prohibited substances or markers of prohibited substances or methods. In the event of a potential adverse analytical finding (AAF) pertaining to a particular prohibited substance or method, further confirmatory analysis occurs.

This step confirms the identity of the substance present in the sample (Figure 5.4). The type of substance identified (i.e. a threshold or non-threshold substance) will then determine whether the quantity present in the sample can be reported to the testing authority as an adverse analytical finding (AAF).

It is a requirement of WADA that all laboratories have the capability to routinely detect and identify non-threshold substances at a defined concentration which is known as the minimum reported performance level (MRPL) (WADA, 2017b). A laboratory not able to detect non-threshold substances at the MRPL may have their accreditation suspended or even revoked by WADA. As the MRPL is not a threshold or a limit of detection, laboratories with more sensitive techniques can also report an AAF at a concentration below the established MRPL for that particular substance (WADA, 2017b).

MRPL values do not apply to threshold substances. The detection and identification of a threshold substance can only be reported as an AAF when the specific threshold limit for the substance is exceeded and the concentration quantified is greater than WADA's agreed decision limit. In reality, a laboratory can only report an AAF for the presence of a threshold substance when the threshold value for that substance has been exceeded with a statistical confidence of at least 95 per cent (WADA, 2017c). Decision limits for the reporting of AAFs for threshold substances are set to protect both the athlete and laboratory since a measure of uncertainty exists with the confirmation of any scientific measurement.

Laboratories use gas or liquid chromatography separation techniques coupled with mass spectrometry detection to identify the majority of substances on the WADA Prohibited List. Exceptions include the use of the following:

- Isoelectric focussing (IEF) and sarcosyl polyacrylamide gel electrophoresis (SAR-PAGE) or sodium dodecyl sulphate polyacrylamide gel electrophoresis (SDS-PAGE) to detect erythropoiesis stimulating agents (ESAs) (WADA, 2014).
- Immunoassays used to detect recombinant human growth hormone (WADA, 2015b).
- Isotope ratio mass spectrometry to detect synthetic forms of endogenous AAS (WADA, 2015c) and determine whether 19-norandrosterone is of endogenous origin (WADA, 2017d).

Alcohol testing

Breath analysis is performed in those sports where alcohol is prohibited in-competition (e.g. motor sports). Breath analysis may be performed immediately prior to a competition or after the competition has been completed. Whilst the protocol is similar to both blood and urine sample provision in terms of selection and notification, the actual analysis is performed using an alcometer and records breath alcohol content in milligrams per litre (mg.l^{-1}). If the reading is equal to or greater than the level stated by the NGB/IF rules then this is considered to be a positive result. A second reading is subsequently performed to confirm the positive result. Significant presence is generally considered to be greater than 0.05 mg.l^{-1}. Further detail with regards to alcohol can be found in Chapter 21.

Discussions are currently ongoing within the anti-doping community to decide on whether alcohol should remain on the Prohibited List. Many stakeholders believe that alcohol is primarily a safety or welfare issue within sport, rather than a doping issue. As such, individual sporting organisations may be handed responsibility in the future for addressing the issue of alcohol use where concerns arise within specific sports.

WADA laboratory accreditation system

Laboratories that undergo sample analysis for the purpose of doping control on behalf of WADA must adhere to strict operating procedures and undertake an accreditation process as set out in the International Standard for Laboratories and related technical documents. Any laboratory wishing to become accredited must follow the necessary steps:

- Express interest via an official letter to WADA;
- Submit an initial application to WADA;
- Provide letters of support which will guarantee that the laboratory will be in receipt of sufficient samples (i.e. 3000) on an annual basis, that it will receive sufficient financial support and that it has the required equipment to carry out its duties and that there is support for research and development;
- Complete a detailed questionnaire that enables the collection of information relating to staff and qualifications, facilities and security, method validation, reference materials, standards and validated biological sample reference collections, and the business plan including laboratory sponsors;
- Host an initial visit from WADA personnel;
- On receipt of the final report from WADA, ensure that all necessary recommendations or improvements are made in order to receive probationary accreditation status;
- Prior to granting probationary status make payment of accreditation fees to WADA;
- Ensure independence from anti-doping organisations and comply with the Laboratory Code of Ethics (WADA, 2016b).

The WADA laboratory accreditation programme is designed to continuously monitor the capabilities of the laboratories, to evaluate laboratory proficiency and to improve test result consistency between laboratories. Laboratories must demonstrate their compliance with the following two international standards: the International Organisation for Standardisation/International Electrotechnical Commission 17025:2005 (ISO/IEC 17025:2005) and the WADA International Standard for Laboratories and its related technical documents.

The ISO/IEC 17025:2005 contains all of the requirements that a laboratory has to meet in order to demonstrate that they operate a management system, are technically competent, and are able to generate technically valid results. In the UK, the UK Accreditation Service is the national accreditation body recognised by government to assess UK-based laboratories against this standard.

International Standard for Laboratories (ISL) and related Technical Documents

The ISL includes requirements for obtaining and maintaining WADA laboratory accreditation, and sets out the required operating standards that laboratories must achieve (WADA, 2016b). WADA also set mandatory performance requirements through a series of technical documents (WADA, 2017e). These technical documents provide direction to the laboratories on specific technical issues such as advances in methodology and prevent the need for the ISL to be updated every time this occurs.

WADA External Quality Assessment Scheme

The performance of WADA-accredited laboratories is monitored via an external quality assessment scheme (EQAS). Participation in the EQAS is mandatory and allows WADA to evaluate laboratory competency through continual assessment of their performance, and provides laboratories with opportunities to compare their results to improve test result consistency between laboratories.

Urine or blood samples are periodically distributed by WADA to accredited laboratories to be tested for the presence of prohibited substances and markers. These samples may be sent blind or double-blind, which means that the content is unknown to the laboratories. Laboratories receive points if they fail to correctly identify or fail to accurately measure the presence of the prohibited substance or marker within an EQAS sample. A false-positive EQAS result earns a laboratory 25 points and automatic suspension, whereas a false negative EQAS result earns a laboratory 10 points. If a laboratory receives 20 points or more in a single EQAS round its WADA accreditation will be suspended. When a laboratory receives 30 points or more over a 12-month period its accreditation will be either suspended or revoked (WADA, 2016b). In some cases the content of urine or blood samples may be made known to the recipient for educational purposes and in such cases the results are not incorporated into the performance monitoring process.

5.3 Athlete Biological Passport

As explained above, 'classical' doping testing is associated with the direct detection of forbidden substances in a biological sample of urine or blood. The key element in the detection is the fact that the forbidden substance is usually foreign to the human organism and can thus readily be isolated and identified by appropriate analytical methods. With the ever-accelerating technological progress, new treatments for many diseases and new therapeutic substances are emerging every day, many of which potentially enhance athletic performance. A large number of these new substances are identical to body components as they are aimed at replacing lacking production of these in the diseased human organism. Typical examples are hormones such as Insulin or Erythropoietin (EPO), which are nowadays produced through genetically modified cells that will provide molecules that are nearly identical to the endogenous hormones. Therefore, the detection of these substances in conventional doping tests is virtually impossible. For example, EPO was massively abused in all endurance sports and was therefore a major problem for anti-doping authorities.

A first attempt at indirect doping detection: threshold values for blood markers

To tackle the phenomenon of rampant, undetectable EPO abuse in the 1990s, sporting federations implemented a new approach of doping detection, the so-called 'indirect doping detection', where in contrast to conventional tests that aim at detecting the forbidden substance directly in a sample, the effects of the substance on the organism are investigated. Blood manipulation aims at increasing the number of oxygen carrying red cells in the human organism, the laboratory marker that describes the red cell mass of the organism is haemoglobin concentration, which can easily be measured in any blood sample. Thus, the first approach of indirect detection of blood manipulation through EPO abuse was, in 1997, the definition of threshold levels for haemoglobin concentration or haematocrit (a measure that describes the percentage of cellular elements in the blood, closely related to haemoglobin concentration). Male cyclists who presented with haemoglobin values above $17g.dl^{-1}$ or haematocrit readings above 50 per cent at pre-competition blood tests were not allowed to start the race, officially for health reasons, as this indirect approach could, at that time, not be defined as a doping test as no forbidden substance was detected.

Given that approximately 3 per cent of the healthy male population have haemoglobin values above $17g.dl^{-1}$ or haematocrit above 50 per cent, it quickly became clear that these measures were unsuitable to lead any further in the fight against doping, due to lacking specificity and poor sensitivity (Schumacher et al., 2000).

Second generation blood tests: a combination of markers

The 'second generation' of blood tests for the detection of blood manipulation in sports used combinations of several blood markers related to the red blood cell production. The most commonly used combination is the so called OFF score, which is calculated from the aforementioned haemoglobin concentration and the percentage of young red blood cells (reticulocytes) (Gore et al., 2003). The name 'OFF score' stems from the fact that this approach is most sensitive to discontinuation of erythropoietic substances, thus will flag individuals who have stopped taking EPO shortly before the test. The score can be related to a likelihood of finding such a result in a healthy, un-doped population of athletes. Threshold values of this 'OFF score' were soon established in addition to the existing simple haemoglobin or haematocrit cut-off values.

An individual approach: the longitudinal monitoring of biomarkers

One of the main points of criticism to the first and second generation approaches based on fixed thresholds was the fact that athletes with naturally low haemoglobin values could use EPO until they reach a level close to the defined thresholds without ever raising suspicion, whereas athletes with higher natural levels would have a much higher risk of being found falsely positive. This gave birth to the idea of individual, longitudinal monitoring of certain biological markers to identify doping specific patterns (Sharpe et al., 2006; Sottas et al., 2010). The ideal marker for a longitudinal monitoring is a marker with a small intra-individual but a large inter-individual variability. Another condition is a standardised analytical procedure to reduce the analytical variation, which might also impact any longitudinal monitoring.

Several mathematical approaches have been developed to formally evaluate longitudinal data. These algorithms compare the biological marker to a reference collective and the previous data from the athlete. To describe the variance of each marker, variance estimates from large reference collectives are used, assuming a universal individual variance, which is the same for each athlete. The mathematical algorithms thus define individual limits (upper and lower) for each variable taking into account the previous data of each athlete individually. The range of these individual limits is pre-defined by the desired specificity of the analysis: A typical specificity would be for example 99.9 per cent, which would define an individual range that is only exceeded in one in 1,000 cases of un-doped athletes. (The mathematically interested reader might be referred to Sharpe et al. (2006) and Sottas et al. (2006, 2010) for details of the calculations for the different approaches.) A typical profile

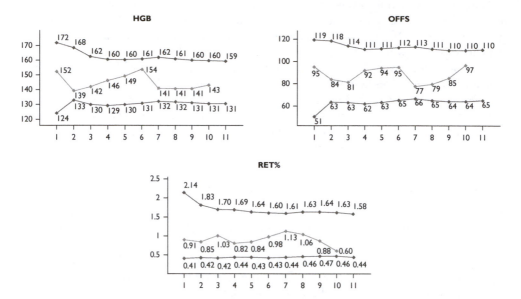

Figure 5.1 Normal haematological profile depicting the haematological markers

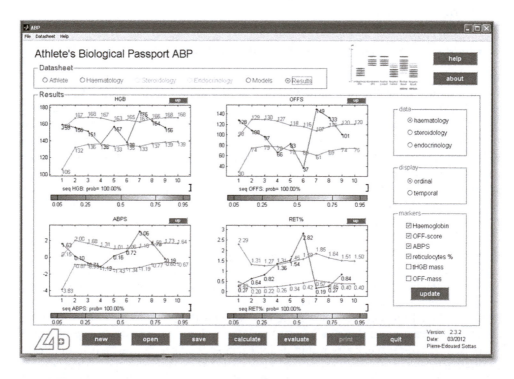

Figure 5.2 Example of a blood passport indicating the abuse of an erythropoietic stimulant such as EPO

analysis is illustrated in Figure 5.1, where the measured haemoglobin values of the athlete are shown in the centre and the individually calculated limits are presented on either side. Figure 5.2 shows an example of a profile indicative of the abuse of an erythropoiesis-stimulating substance.

The Athlete Biological Passport procedure

If a value is found outside the individually calculated reference ranges (a so-called 'atypical passport finding'), it must be emphasised that this does not automatically mean that it is caused by doping. To identify potential causes for such abnormalities, the profile is then examined by a dual-layer system of experts, who determine whether:

1   The observed abnormality is an extreme of natural variation and can therefore be considered as normal;
2   The observed abnormality is caused by a pathology;
3   The observed abnormality is indicative of doping but further testing is required to confirm the suspicion; or
4   The observed abnormality and the profile bear clear features of doping and do not need any further tests.

A first expert evaluates the profile and renders one of the four opinions mentioned above. If he deems the profile typical of doping, it is then independently evaluated by two further experts under the same criteria. For their evaluation, they can ask for additional information such as the athlete's whereabouts or competition schedule. One of the key elements in their evaluation is the identification of a doping scenario (i.e. a likely manipulation strategy), which is necessary to take legal action in order to prevail in court. If all three experts independently conclude from the available data that the profile is highly likely caused by doping and unlikely by any other cause, a so-called 'adverse passport finding' (corresponding to the 'adverse analytical finding' in conventional anti-doping testing) is declared. The athlete is contacted to provide explanations regarding their profile. These explanations are again anonymously evaluated by the expert panel that will reassess their previous opinion in light of the explanations by the athlete. If they confirm their suspicion, an ADRV disciplinary procedure will be lodged against the athlete. The process of evaluation of the data of the Athlete Biological Passport is illustrated in Figure 5.3.

Implementation

The first sporting federation to implement the Athlete Biological Passport was the International Cycling Union (UCI) in 2008. In their passport programme, approximately 800 athletes are followed on a regular basis. Since 2008, the programme has had significant success: as of 2017, close to 200 athletes have been charged with ADRV through passport data alone. Also, many other athletes were found positive for forbidden substances in targeted, traditional doping tests scheduled based on information from the athlete's blood passport. For example, the number of 'traditional' anti-doping tests positive for EPO has increased by 300 per cent due to improved target testing guided by passport information. Epidemiological data also shows that the prevalence of abnormal blood values in the collective of cyclists submitted to the longitudinal monitoring has heavily decreased since

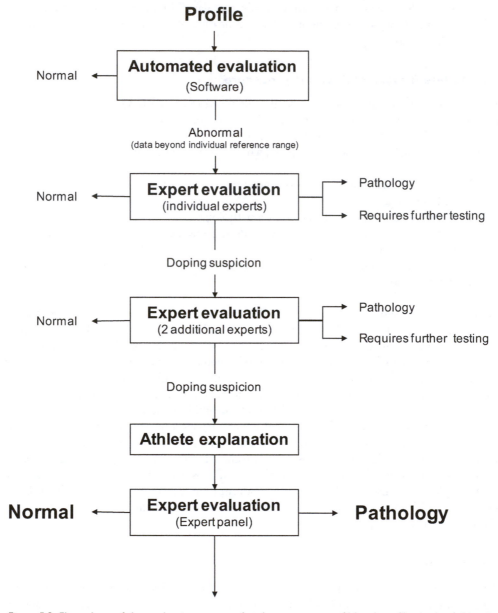

Figure 5.3 Flow chart of the evaluation process for the assessment of blood profiles in the Athlete´s
Biological Passport (adapted from Schumacher and d'Onofrio, 2012)

the introduction of the Athlete Biological Passport (Zorzoli and Rossi, 2010). Since then, a large number of national and international anti-doping stakeholders have implemented the Athlete Biological Passport Programme under the supervision of WADA. The organisation publishes and updates the guidelines for the Athlete Biological Passport on a regular basis (WADA, 2016c).

Other applications

Unlike conventional anti-doping samples, data from the tests conducted for the Athlete Biological Passport contain valuable information that can be used for a multitude of purposes in the fight against doping. Firstly, testing a large number of competitors at a given race allows the calculation of the prevalence of doping in the examined collective at the given race. Through comparison of the distribution of the passport markers in the tested collective with the data of an un-doped reference group, the prevalence can be estimated (Sottas et al., 2011). As mentioned above, the scrutiny of passport data also allows the identification of new doping trends through changes of athletes' profiles for certain variables (Zorzoli and Rossi, 2010). Lastly, the Athlete Biological Passport and its targeted testing has a considerable deterrent effect, as athletes that are tested will know that – unlike in conventional doping tests with a borderline result – the data from the Athlete Biological Passport will remain with them over their entire career.

Future developments

The current passport application with its haematological module aims at detecting blood doping with erythropoietic stimulants or blood transfusions. A module for the detection of steroid hormone abuse has recently been introduced and a similar system for growth hormone abuse is under development. For the steroidal module, several metabolites in testosterone metabolism are analysed and traced over time, adhering to the same principles as described for the haematological variables: Testosterone/Epitestosterone (T/E) ratio, Testosterone/Androsterone (T/A) ratio, Androsterone/Atiocholanolone (A/Etio) ratio and the 5a-androstane-3a,17b-diol/5b-androstane-3a,17b-diol (a-diol/b-diol) ratio (Sottas et al., 2010).

The endocrinological module for growth hormone detection is currently under development and will likely include the main mediators of growth hormone in the body, namely Insulin-like growth factor 1 (IGF 1) and procollagen type III (P-III-P) as primary markers.

5.4 Non-analytical investigations

Whilst drug detection will always remain an integral part of the anti-doping effort, many ADRVs identified in the Code (e.g. possession, administration, trafficking) can only be identified and pursued through the gathering and investigation of 'non-analytical' anti-doping intelligence. Anti-doping intelligence is mainly used by anti-doping organisations to assist test distribution planning and inform target testing and to provide the basis for further investigation to determine potential ADRVs (WADA, 2015a). It is the responsibility of anti-doping organisations to ensure that they have an effective system in place to enable intelligence gathering from a wide range of sources. Possible sources of intelligence include athletes, athlete support personnel, doping control personnel and members of the public as well as organisations including national sports governing bodies, laboratories, pharmaceutical companies, law enforcement agencies and the media (WADA, 2016a).

Many high-profile ADRVs have only been uncovered by anti-doping organisations following the receipt of information from public authorities such as law enforcement agencies, Customs and Borders, and other sport regulatory agencies. Examples of seminal cases, taken from WADA's guidelines on coordinating investigations (WADA, 2011), include:

1   The 2003 federal investigation into the trafficking of doping substances by BALCO, which led to the uncovering of information that was used by the United States Anti-Doping Agency to sanction track and field athletes Michelle Collins, Tim Montgomery and Chrystie Gaines, as well as coaches Trevor Graham and Remi Korchemny;

2   The Italian police raid which caught Austrian cross-country ski athletes and team officials in possession of blood doping paraphernalia at the Turin Olympic Games; this provided the IOC and International Ski Federation with evidence to bring proceedings against those involved; and

3   The sanction imposed by the International Tennis Federation on American tennis player Wayne Odesnik in 2010 for the possession of human growth hormone; this was the result of Australian customs officials alerting the Australian Anti-Doping Agency to their search findings.

These cases demonstrate the need for NADOs to establish effective partnerships and information sharing protocols with law enforcement agencies so that intelligence uncovered during public authority investigations can be shared to enable doping sanctions to be pursued under the Code. Such relationships also allow for anti-doping organisations to share intelligence in the other direction to tackle the manufacture, distribution and supply of certain prohibited substances that are also considered to be public health issues. Tackling upstream perpetrators normally falls outside of the jurisdiction of sport, which means that anti-doping regulators are often reliant on the prosecution of these individuals under national laws.

Obtaining information about new medicines from the pharmaceutical industry is another key strategy used to minimise the misuse of these compounds in sport. WADA have established an active cooperation agreement with the International Federation of Pharmaceutical Manufacturers and Associations (IFPMA) and its member pharmaceutical companies that alerts WADA when medicinal compounds have been identified through clinical trials to have doping potential (IFPMA, 2014). Receiving this information from the pharmaceutical industry enables WADA to develop detection methods far sooner than would occur if WADA only found out about them on launch to market.

5.5 Sanctions

Sanctions are an essential element of doping control not only as retribution/punishment to those that commit an ADRV but also in deterring others from doping. Sanctions are determined by the severity of the ADRV and any previous convictions within a ten-year period. In most cases the sanction is determined by a hearing whereby an athlete will put forward a reasoned defence towards the accusations placed in front of them. The hearing will determine whether an ADRV has occurred and establish the degree of liability and the intention to dope. Sanctions usually include a period of ineligibility from sport or at the very least a warning and reprimand (Figure 5.4). Sanctions can also include disqualification from an event and forfeiture of points, medals and prizes.

An ADRV involving the possession or use or attempted use of a prohibited substance or method will typically involve a standard sanction of four years ineligibility. A deviation from the standard sanction might occur in response to a varied set of circumstances

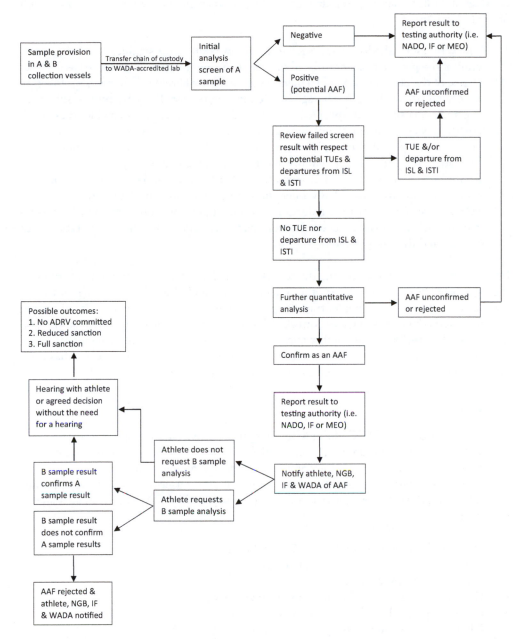

Figure 5.4 A flow diagram illustrating the chain of events with respect to sample provision, analysis and potential sanctioning following the confirmation of an adverse analytical finding

considered during a hearing. A reduction in the period of ineligibility may occur as a result of the following:

1   It may be established that the athlete bears no fault or no significant negligence in terms of the presence of a prohibited substance in their sample. This may be as a consequence of the contamination of a dietary supplement where due care has been taken to avoid such risk or through sabotage by a fellow competitor. If the prohibited substance detected is classified as a 'specified substance' then an athlete may be able to establish that there was no intent to enhance performance by administering the substance. In such cases the period of ineligibility may be reduced to two years or in exceptional circumstances the period of ineligibility may be eliminated completely.

2   If an athlete admits to an ADRV voluntarily without a case being called to answer, or having committed an ADRV offers substantial assistance in determining a further ADRV by another athlete, a reduction in their suspension from sport may be considered. In such cases any reduced sanction may only occur following consultation with WADA and their respective IF.

In addition to a reduced sanction, athletes may receive an increased sanction according to the type of ADRV committed or other circumstances including their previous history of doping convictions. For example, trafficking (or attempted trafficking) and administration (or attempted administration) are both ADRVs that currently carry a four-year suspension from sport. The period of ineligibility may also be increased if aggravated circumstances are believed to have occurred where an athlete has doped using multiple substances or has committed multiple ADRVs (e.g. use or attempted use and possession).

5.6 Education

A key element of the WADC is the promotion of preventative measures in an attempt to limit both intentional and unintentional ADRVs. In the Code education is highlighted as a key preventative measure that all signatories are expected to engage in.

Education programmes should be viewed as an important aspect of an anti-doping strategy and as such the Code outlines the following key topics (WADA, 2015a) that should be included:

*   The List of Prohibited Substances and Methods;
*   Anti-doping rule violations and sanctions;
*   Doping control procedures;
*   The potential health and social consequences of doping;
*   The Therapeutic Use Exemption process;
*   Whereabouts requirements;
*   The risks associated with supplement use and how to minimise them;
*   The rights and responsibilities of athletes and athlete support personnel; and
*   The impact of doping on the spirit of sport;

In addition to information-based programmes, WADA promote values-based education and have developed resources directed not only at elite athletes, but also at aspiring athletes via school-based education. In an attempt to foster an environment that is conducive to drug-free sport, athlete support personnel are an essential audience and, as such, resources have been developed for coaches and sports physicians as well. Although deemed to be a key strategy in doping prevention, it would seem strange that no International Standard for education exists to raise the quality and standardise education programmes across the world.

5.7 Summary

In view of the varied ADRVs that constitute doping, the strategies and procedures involved in its control are diverse. The major goal of such strategies is the prevention of doping through both education and drug testing. Drug testing serves two purposes in that it enables the implementation of an effective sanctioning system which provides culpability to those who dope but most importantly it acts as a deterrent to those who might be tempted to dope in the future. The challenge to the anti-doping movement is the implementation of drug testing that is both cost effective and a real deterrent to athletes. New strategies in doping control involve a non-analytical approach that uses intelligence amassed from a wide range of sources through the development of key partnerships including law enforcement agencies, the pharmaceutical industry and other sport regulatory agencies. Such evidence is proving fruitful in the conviction of individuals and organisations that fall foul of the wide range of ADRVs not involving sample analysis.

5.8 References

Gore, C.J., Parisotto, R., Ashenden, M.J. et al. (2003). Second-generation blood tests to detect erythropoietin abuse by athletes. *Haematologica* 88(3): 333–344.

de Hon, O., Kuipers, H., van Bottenburg, M. (2015) Prevalence of doping use in elite sports: A review of numbers and methods. *Sports Medicine* 45: 57–69

IFPMA (2014) 2 Fields 1 Goal: Protecting the Integrity of Science and Sport. Available at: https://www.wada-ama.org/en/resources/science-medicine/2-fields-1-goal-points-to-consider (Accessed on 26 June 2017).

Robinson, N., Kirchbichler, A., Banuls, O., Mader, M., Aikin, R., Sottas, P.-E. and D'Onofrio, G. (2016). Validation of a Blood Stability Score as an easy-to-use blood sample quality index. *International Journal of Laboratory Hematology* 38(6): 685–693.

Schumacher, Y.O., and d'Onofrio, G. (2012). Scientific expertise and the Athlete's Biological Passport: 3 years of experience. *Clinical Chemistry* 58(6): 979–985.

Schumacher, Y.O., Grathwohl, D., Barturen, J.M. et al. (2000). Haemoglobin, haematocrit and red blood cell indices in elite cyclists: Are the control values for blood testing valid? *International Journal of Sports Medicine* 21(5): 380–385.

Sharpe, K., Ashenden, M.J., and Schumacher, Y.O. (2006). A third generation approach to detect erythropoietin abuse in athletes. *Haematologica* 91(3): 356.

Sottas, P.-E., Robinson, N., Fischetto, G. et al. (2011). Prevalence of blood doping in samples collected from elite track and field athletes. *Clinical Chemistry* 57(5): 762–769.

Sottas, P.E., Robinson, N., Giraud, S. et al. (2006). Statistical classification of abnormal blood profiles in athletes. *The International Journal of Biostatistics* 2(1): 3.

Sottas, P.-E., Robinson, N. and Saugy, M. (2010). The athlete's biological passport and indirect markers of blood doping. *Handbook of Experimental Pharmacology* 195: 305–326.

WADA (2011) WADA Guidelines Document: Coordinating Investigations and Sharing Anti-Doping Information and Evidence. Available at: https://www.wada-ama.org/en/resources/world-anti-doping-program/coordinating-investigations-and-sharing-anti-doping-information (Accessed on 26 June 2017).

WADA (2014) WADA Technical Document: TD2014EPO. Harmonization of analysis and reporting of erythropoiesis stimulating agents (ESAs) by electrophoretic techniques. Available at: https://www.wada-ama.org/en/resources/science-medicine/td2014-epo (Accessed on 26 June 2017).

WADA (2015a) World Anti-Doping Code. Available at: https://www.wada-ama.org/en/resources/the-code/world-anti-doping-code (Accessed on 26 June 2017).

WADA (2015b) WADA Technical Document: TD2015GH. Technical document on Human Growth Hormone (hGH) isoform differential immunoassays for doping control analyses. Available at: https://www.wada-ama.org/en/resources/science-medicine/td2015-gh (Accessed on 26 June 2017).

WADA (2015c) WADA Technical Document: TD2016IRMS. Detection of synthetic forms of endogenous anabolic androgenic steroids by GC/C/IRMS. Available at: https://www.wada-ama.org/en/resources/science-medicine/td2016-irms (Accessed on 26 June 2017).

WADA (2016a) International Standard for Testing and Investigations. Available at: https://www.wada-ama.org/en/resources/world-anti-doping-program/international-standard-for-testing-and-investigations-isti-0 (Accessed on 26 June 2017).

WADA (2016b) International Standard for Laboratories. Available at: https://www.wada-ama.org/en/resources/laboratories/international-standard-for-laboratories-isl (Accessed on 26 June 2017).

WADA (2016c) Athlete Biological Passport Operating Guidelines. Available at: https://www.wada-ama.org/en/resources/athlete-biological-passport/athlete-biological-passport-abp-operating-guidelines (Accessed on 26 June 2017).

WADA (2017a) Technical Document for Sport Specific Analysis. Available at: https://www.wada-ama.org/en/resources/the-code/tdssa-technical-document-for-sport-specific-analysis (Accessed on 29 July 2017).

WADA (2017b) WADA Technical Document: TD2017MRPL. Minimum required performance levels for detection and identification of non-threshold substances. Available at: https://www.wada-ama.org/en/resources/science-medicine/td2017-mrpl (Accessed on 30 July 2017).

WADA (2017c) WADA Technical Document: TD2017DL. Decision limits for the confirmatory quantification of threshold substances. Available at: https://www.wada-ama.org/en/resources/science-medicine/td2017-dl-version-2 (Accessed on 30 July 2017).

WADA (2017d) WADA Technical Document: TD2017NA. Harmonization of analysis and reporting of 19-norsteroids related to nandrolone. Available at: https://www.wada-ama.org/en/resources/science-medicine/td2017-na (Accessed on 30 July 2017).

WADA (2017e) List of WADA Technical Documents. Available at: https://www.wada-ama.org/en/what-we-do/science-medical/laboratories (Accessed on 30 July 2017).

Zorzoli, M. and Rossi, F. (2010). Implementation of the biological passport: The experience of the International Cycling Union. *Drug Testing and Analysis* 2(11–12): 542–547.

Zorzoli, M. and Rossi, F. (2012). Case studies on ESA-doping as revealed by the Biological Passport. *Drug Testing and Analysis* 4(11): 854–858.

Chapter 6

Inadvertent use of prohibited substances in sport

David R. Mottram and Neil Chester

6.1 Introduction

Recent statistics from World Anti-Doping Agency (WADA) accredited laboratories show that over 300,000 tests are conducted, worldwide, annually, with 1–2 per cent showing an adverse analytical finding (AAF) (WADA 2016a). Amongst these doping violations, athletes frequently claim that the prohibited substance had been taken inadvertently, with contaminated supplements often being cited as the cause.

Whether taken deliberately or inadvertently, a strict liability rule applies within doping regulations. Strict liability is defined in the World Anti-Doping Code (WADA, 2015; Article 2.1.1) as "it is not necessary that intent, fault, negligence, or knowing use on the athlete's part be demonstrated by the Anti-Doping Organization in order to establish an anti-doping rule violation". Inadvertent doping therefore leaves the athlete liable to sanctions.

This chapter will explore the circumstances under which athletes may take prohibited substances inadvertently, review the WADA rules and regulations regarding inadvertent use of prohibited substances and provide suggestions as to how athletes and their support staff have a role in preventing inadvertent use.

6.2 Why athletes may take prohibited substances inadvertently

Definition of inadvertent

Inadvertent may be defined as "Not resulting from or achieved through deliberate planning".

Some athletes may put themselves at greater risk of inadvertent doping through ill-advised consumption of products that may contain prohibited substances. In addition, athletes may put themselves at risk of unintended doping through other means, including passive inhalation (in environments where individuals are smoking illicit drugs) and intimate contact with an individual who has recently consumed prohibited substances. Sabotage is also a suspected cause of inadvertent doping where athletes are deliberately targeted and their food, supplements and massage oils might be spiked with prohibited substances. Several athletes who have failed a drugs test have cited sabotage as a likely cause; this is, however, difficult to verify.

Products that may contain prohibited substances

Prohibited substances may be a component of:

- Foodstuffs;
- Medicines (prescribed or taken through self-medication);
- Recreational drugs; or
- Dietary and sports supplements.

Examples of prohibited substances that may be taken inadvertently together with their methods of ingestion are shown in Table 6.1.

6.3 Risk levels for inadvertent prohibited substance use in sport

The risk of taking a prohibited substance inadvertently varies according to the behaviour of the athlete and their support staff. Whilst athletes and their entourage should be aware of the risks and how to minimise them it is clear that those risks cannot be removed entirely. Risks of inadvertent doping may vary according to the type and quantity of products consumed (i.e. foodstuff, medicine, recreational drugs and supplements) and the degree of caution used in selecting the most appropriate source of product.

Risks associated with foodstuffs

A number of doping cases have involved the consumption of foodstuffs that unknowingly contained prohibited substances. A notable example is that of contaminated meat, whereby prohibited substances are administered to livestock as growth promoters in an attempt to increase yield. Examples of such growth promoters include the anabolic agents clenbuterol and zeranol. Whilst use of such growth promotors in livestock rearing is not permitted in the EU there is evidence of use outside of the EU, thus increasing the risk of inadvertent doping from meat consumption.

Table 6.1 Examples of prohibited substances that may be taken inadvertently

Prohibited substance	Potential route(s) of ingestion
Clenbuterol	Medicine
	Food
	Supplement
Anabolic androgenic steroids/Prohormones	Supplement
Cocaine	Recreational
	Intimate contact
Amphetamine	Recreational
Ephedrine	Medicine
	Supplement
Methylhexaneamine and other stimulants	Supplement
Cannabinoids	Recreational
	Food
	Passive inhalation

Box 6.1   Alberto Contador (2010)

Contador tested positive for clenbuterol at the 2010 Tour de France. He claimed it was through eating contaminated meat. The Court of Arbitration for Sport (CAS) concluded that the presence of clenbuterol was more likely caused by the ingestion of a contaminated food supplement. Contador was given a two-year backdated suspension and a fine.

A number of similar cases relating to inadvertent use of clenbuterol have subsequently been reported (Guddat et al., 2012; Thevis et al., 2013a). The ability to differentiate between the intentional use of clenbuterol or its consumption through food contamination during anti-doping testing is challenging, however, analytical procedures are being investigated (Thevis et al., 2013b). Cases involving foodstuffs contaminated with other growth promoting agents, which have resulted in an AAF during routine anti-doping tests, have been described (Geyer et al., 2014).

Other types of foodstuff that have the potential to produce inadvertent doping include products containing hemp, derived from *Cannabis sativa*. Brownies, cookies and cakes prepared with hemp could result in excretion of the metabolites of tetrahydrocannabinol within the urine (Yonamine et al., 2004). An example of this involved the US judo athlete Nick Delpopolo.

Box 6.2   Nick Delpopolo (2012)

Delpopolo tested positive for Cannabinoids at the London 2012 Olympic Games. He claimed it was through eating food baked with marijuana prior to the Games. He was disqualified and expelled from the Games with a subsequent three-month ban.

Similarly, the consumption of poppy seeds in bread or cakes could give rise to morphine excretion within the urine and trigger an AAF (ElSohly et al., 1990). However, the level of morphine found in poppy seeds has reduced due to a number of factors including the baking process itself, making it less likely for inadvertent doping to occur (Anderson, 2011).

Risks associated with medicines

Prescribed medicines

Many of the classes of drugs that appear on the WADA Prohibited List are prescribed for the treatment of medical conditions, such as asthma, Type 1 diabetes, cardiovascular disorders and sports injuries. Inadvertent use of these drugs by an athlete and a subsequent anti-doping rule violation should not occur provided the medical practitioner prescribing such drugs is conversant with and complies with the WADA regulations appertaining to Therapeutic Use Exemption (TUE) (WADA, 2016b).

The effective use of the TUE procedure is reliant on accurate and effective advice by medical practitioners. However, it is clear that many practitioners have limited knowledge and understanding of the anti-doping rules and regulations (Backhouse and McKenna, 2011; Auersperger et al., 2012; Dikic et al., 2013; Mazanov et al., 2014; Momaya et al., 2015). The case of Andreea Raducan illustrates the danger to athletes of ill-advised support from medical practitioners.

Box 6.3   Andreea Raducan (2000)

The gymnast Andreea Raducan tested positive for pseudoephedrine at the Sydney 2000 Olympic Games. She was prescribed the drug by her team physician. Strict liability rules were applied and she was stripped of her gold medal. Her physician was sanctioned for his action.

WADA acknowledges the need for better education for Athlete Support Personnel, such as healthcare professionals, a call that has been addressed by the US Anti-Doping Agency (USADA, 2015; Tandon et al., 2015).

A significant case of inadvertent doping through contamination of a prescribed medicine was reported in 2016 (Helmlin, 2016). A 23-year old Swiss athlete took the non-steroidal anti-inflammatory drug, ibuprofen, prior to competing and was selected for an in-competition doping control urine test. The medicine had been purchased by the athlete's medical support personnel from a German pharmacy. Subsequent analysis of the medicine showed contamination with the prohibited diuretic, hydrochlorothiazide. As a result, the sanctioning body ruled that the athlete bore no fault or negligence and sanctions were removed. This case illustrates the importance of athletes declaring all medicines taken at the time of testing and of retaining samples of the product for subsequent analysis, if required.

Self- medication

As a consequence of the increasing burden on health services, self-medication or self-care is often encouraged for non-critical, self-treatable ailments. Such a move, whilst reducing the burden on general medical practitioners, requires the support of other primary healthcare services, such as pharmacies for success. There is also the need to educate the general public and empower them to make sound decisions regarding their health. Despite this move towards self-care, there is a need to understand the pitfalls, particularly from an athlete's perspective.

It would seem that self-medication, without any health professional's advice, is a widespread behaviour by athletes. For example, analgesics, such as non-steroidal anti-inflammatory drugs (NSAIDs), have been reported to be used extensively prior to and during competition in triathlon events, where 25.5 per cent, 17.9 per cent and 47.4 per cent of competitors consumed NSAIDs the day before, immediately before and during the race, respectively (Gorski et al., 2011). Among the NSAID users, 48.5 per cent consumed them without medical prescriptions. In a study of female runners, 34.6 per cent reported self-administration of medicines during the period immediately preceding competition, with non-opioid analgesics and NSAIDs the therapeutic agents most often cited (Locquet et al., 2016).

Other drugs used commonly for self-medication include preparations to treat conditions such as hay fever, the common cold or coughs. Such over-the-counter medicines contain a wide variety of substances but which frequently include stimulants, some of which (cathine, ephedrine and pseudoephedrine) appear on the WADA Prohibited List. The landmark doping case of Alain Baxter, who was deprived of an Olympic bronze medal through using a nasal decongestant that contained the prohibited substance levmetamfetamine (see Chapter 2), clearly illustrated the risks that athletes run by using self-medication without seeking professional advice. More recent cases involved the German boxer Timo Hoffmann and Nicklas Backstrom, both of whom had claimed to have sought approval for use of their medication from medical practitioners.

Box 6.4   Timo Hoffmann (2013)

Hoffmann tested positive for ephedrine during a test conducted at a heavyweight prize fighter event in London in February 2013. He claimed it was a result of purchasing Vicks MediNaid and Aspirin complex from an airport pharmacy. He further claimed that he had informed an official doctor at the event who had said it was "OK". The investigating panel stated that the burden of establishing how the prohibited substance entered the athlete's body rests upon the athlete and he had failed to discharge it in this case. He was therefore given a two-year ban.

Box 6.5   Nicklas Backstrom (2014)

Backstrom was a member of the Swedish ice-hockey team at 2014 Sochi Winter Olympics. He presented a urine sample containing pseudoephedrine which exceeded the WADA decision limit of 170 micrograms/ml. He had sought advice from his Olympic Team Physician as to whether it was safe to take a medicine containing pseudoephedrine.

The IOC found he had committed an ADRV but allowed him to keep his team silver medal. Subsequently appeals to CAS were submitted by both Backstrom and WADA. However, both withdrew their appeals and it was agreed that a reprimand was sufficient sanction.

Another potential route for inadvertent doping is through the use of OTC "natural" medicines that include animal tissues containing endogenous anabolic androgenic steroids such as extracts from deer musk pods, detected during the FIFA Women's World Cup in 2011 (Geyer et al., 2014).

Risks associated with recreational drugs

"Recreational" use of drugs is an increasingly common aspect of social behaviour in many countries. Published research evidence concerning the extent to which athletes use recreational drugs is scarce. However, it is reasonable to assume that a proportion of athletes use drugs recreationally. Indeed, a study on self-admitted behaviour among competitive Hungarian athletes indicated that 31.7 per cent used recreational drugs (Uvacsek et al., 2011). Other evidence relates to enquiries made by athletes via the Drug Information Database, which revealed that 10.4 per cent of enquiries related to recreational drugs (Petróczi and Naughton, 2009).

The more frequently used recreational drugs that are included in the WADA Prohibited List and which may therefore result in inadvertent doping are amphetamines, narcotics, cocaine and cannabinoids. These classes of drugs, with the possible exception of cannabinoids, have the potential to significantly enhance sport performance and are liable to be used deliberately as doping agents. However, it is argued by some athletes that using such drugs in a recreational context, some period of time prior to competing then testing positive during competition, could be deemed to be inadvertent doping. Such cases invariably result in a submaximal period of suspension for the athlete.

A case in which the drug cocaine was claimed to have been taken for a specific reason other than deliberate doping is illustrated by the jockey Frankie Dettori.

Box 6.6   Frankie Dettori (2012)

Dettori was given a six-month ban by the French racing authority France Galop, after testing positive for cocaine following a test at Longchamp. He claimed that he had taken the drug in a "moment of weakness".

With specific regard to cannabis, its use may reduce anxiety and produce a feeling of euphoria. These properties could be beneficial in alleviating the stress induced through competition, either pre- or post-event. However, cannabis smoking impairs cognition and psychomotor and exercise performance (Saugy et al., 2006). The balance of evidence suggests that cannabinoids, in most sports, are ergolytic rather than ergogenic (Eichner, 1993). Nonetheless, the annual statistics from WADA Accredited Laboratories show that cannabinoids are a class of drugs that is frequently detected (WADA, 2016a).

It is worth noting that cannabinoids are only tested in-competition, therefore, any positive results found in urine samples taken out-of-competition are not reported by laboratories. The extent of cannabis use by athletes could therefore be significantly higher than that indicated by these WADA statistics.

Cannabinoids accumulate in fatty tissue from where they are slowly released over extended periods of time. Complete elimination from the body may take as long as 30 days (Huestis et al., 1995). A further reason for the extended period of elimination for cannabinoids is that the metabolites are only partially excreted in the urine whereas most (65 per cent) are excreted into the gastrointestinal tract from where they are re-absorbed into the body, a process that continues over a considerable period of time (Ashton, 2001). This delayed elimination is likely to be associated with non-performance related use of cannabinoids by athletes.

One such case involved the cricketer Abdur Rehman.

Box 6.7   Abdur Rehman (2012)

The cricketer Abdur Rehman tested positive for cannabinoids during a county championship match in August 2012. He asserted that he attended a party, about a week before he flew to England to play cricket for Somerset, at which he inadvertently smoked part of a roll-up cigarette which he wrongly assumed to be a tobacco cigarette. His admission and explanation of how the prohibited substance entered his system was accepted by the English Cricket Board. He was given a three-month ban.

Unsurprisingly, some athletes who have recorded an AAF for cannabinoids have claimed that it was through the passive inhalation of cannabis smoke from other users. However, WADA regulations now state that urinary levels of tetrahydrocannabinol (Carboxy-THC) must exceed a urinary threshold of 180ng/mL in order to trigger an AAF (WADA 2016c), a situation which is unlikely to occur through passive inhalation (Yonamine et al., 2004).

Several reports of inadvertent doping have been attributed to the transfer of drugs via intimate contact with an individual who has consumed a prohibited substance. Several athletes have claimed the transfer of cocaine via kissing, the most notable being the French tennis player Richard Gasquet. A recent case concerning kissing involved the US athlete Gil Richards, who tested positive for the drug probenecid.

Box 6.8   Richard Gasquet (2009)

The French professional tennis player tested positive for cocaine following a drugs test at the Miami Masters tournament in 2009. He was provisionally suspended for 12 months, however CAS cleared him of any wrongdoing. His defence was that he had inadvertently tested positive for cocaine after kissing a woman in a nightclub.

Box 6.9   Gil Richards (2016)

The US track and field athlete, who was part of the US 4x400m winning squad at the Rio Olympics in 2016, tested positive for probenecid following an out-of-competition test in March 2017. He was cleared of any wrongdoing following a hearing, where his defence was that it had entered his body after kissing his girlfriend, who had been administering the drug to treat a sinus infection.

The appropriateness of including recreational drugs on the WADA Prohibited List has been questioned by some, on the basis that resources should be focused on enforcing sporting values related to doping rather than policing athletes' lifestyles (Waddington et al., 2013).

Risks associated with supplements

Supplement use by high performance athletes has been estimated to be between 65 and 95 per cent (Vernac et al., 2013). In support of this estimate, some recent reports relating to the extent of supplement use by elite athletes are shown in Table 6.2.

A meta-analysis of 159 research studies on the use of dietary supplements by athletes showed that around 60 per cent of athletes used dietary supplements, with vitamins/minerals, multivitamins/multiminerals, Vitamin C, proteins, sports drinks and sports bars among the most commonly used (Knapik et al., 2016).

Evidence shows that supplements are used extensively by elite athletes, however this practice is imitated by sportsmen and sportswomen at all levels of performance. The critical question is: *are supplements safe to use?* A thorough review of supplement use and the doping risks attributed to their use is provided in Chapter 24 of this book.

Since 2003, a significant number of nutritional supplements have appeared on the market, with claims that they can produce remarkable increases in muscle growth and improved strength. In some cases, these claims were attributable to ingredients with unapproved names

Table 6.2 Reports on the extent of supplement use by elite athletes

Brief details on the extent of use	Most frequently used supplements within the study	Reference
97% of elite Australian swimmers reported taking supplements or sports foods over the preceding 12 months	Vitamins; minerals; sports foods	Shaw et al., 2016
34.5% of elite athletes in Bosnia Herzegovina used dietary supplements, with 62.3% of users taking more than one product (average 2.9±2.8 products)	Amino acids; proteins; vitamins; minerals	Omeragic et al., 2015
55% of young German elite athletes had used supplements, of which 74% were regular users	Minerals; vitamins; protein; carbohydrate	Dietz et al., 2014
87% of high performance Canadian athletes had taken 3 or more dietary supplements within the previous 6 months	Sports drinks; multivitamins and mineral preparations; carbohydrate sports bars; protein powder	Lun et al., 2012
77% Croatian elite sailors consume dietary supplements	Vitamins; minerals; proteins (amino acids); isotonics	Rodek et al., 2012
82% female and 79% male Korean Olympic athletes used supplements at the Beijing Olympic Games	Vitamins; oriental supplements; amino acids; creatine	Kim et al., 2011
61.2% Serbian elite athletes use dietary supplements (average 3.17 per person)	Vitamins; minerals; amino acids; herbal supplements	Suzic Lazic et al., 2011
87.5% elite athletes within a state-based sporting institute used supplements	Minerals; vitamins; iron; caffeine	Dascombe et al., 2010
66.8% of track and field athletes competing at IAAF World Championships used supplements (average 1.7 per athlete)	Not stated	Tscholl et al., 2010

which have been analysed as containing anabolic steroids such as metandienone, stanazolol, oxandrolone and dehydrochloromethyltestosterone (Geyer et al., 2014). Supplements that contain "designer steroids" have produced positive doping results with serious consequences for the athletes' concerned (Parr et al., 2011). Other supplements, advertised as fat burners or mood enhancers, may contain prohibited stimulants such as ephedrine, sibutramine or methylhexaneamine, undeclared on the product label (Geyer et al., 2011). A typical case involved the skier Evi Sachenbacker-Stehle.

Box 6.10   Evi Sachenbacker-Stehle (2014)

Sachenbacker-Stehle tested positive for methylhexaneamine at the Sochi 2014 Winter Olympic Games. She took a supplement reputed to be "clean". She was disqualified and expelled from the Games with a subsequent two-year ban reduced, on appeal, to six months by the Court of Arbitration for Sport.

It has been reported that a significant percentage (5–20 per cent) of supplements contain prohibited substances, which are present either through inadvertent contamination or through deliberate adulteration during the production process (Vernac et al., 2013). In another review, the percentage of doping cases that might be attributed to supplement use was found to be between 6.4 per cent and 8.8 per cent (Outram and Stewart, 2015).

The risk of sabotage

Since the stakes are particularly high in elite sport there is a need to appreciate the hypothetical risk of sabotage. The possibility that foodstuffs, supplements, massage oils and so on might be spiked with prohibited substances in an attempt to trigger a positive drugs test of a competitor cannot be overlooked. Whilst sabotage is difficult to prove there are a number of incidences, whereby athletes have attributed their positive drug test to sabotage.

Box 6.11   Dieter Baumann (1999)

The German long-distance runner, who won gold in the 5,000-metres at the Barcelona Olympics tested positive for nandrolone in 1999. Baumann received a two-year ban from the sport but continued to plead his innocence. He attributed his positive test to sabotage, specifically to the adulteration of his toothpaste by a third party.

Box 6.12   Justin Gatlin (2006)

The US track and field athlete, who won gold in the 100m at the Athens Olympics and the 2017 World Athletics Championships in London, tested positive for testosterone in 2006. Gatlin subsequently received a four-year ban from sport since it was his second doping offence. Gatlin pleaded his innocence, attributing his positive test to his massage therapist who had allegedly administered testosterone topically during a massage therapy session.

Whilst the likelihood of sabotage is particularly difficult to determine there is clearly a need for the athlete and their support staff to be vigilant.

6.4 WADA rules and regulations regarding inadvertent use of prohibited substances

The 2015 World Anti-Doping Code (Article 2.1.1) states that: "It is each Athlete's personal duty to ensure that no prohibited substance enters his or her body. Athletes are responsible for any prohibited substance or its metabolites or markers found to be present in their samples. Accordingly, it is not necessary that intent, fault, negligence or knowing use on the athlete's part be demonstrated in order to establish an anti-doping rule violation".

WADA sanctions

Athletes who commit one or more Anti-Doping Rule Violation are subject to two types of sanction:

- Disqualification of results if the violation occurred during or in connection with an event; and
- A period of ineligibility from competing.

With regard to ineligibility, the period depends on a number of factors which include the type of prohibited substance misused (i.e. specified or non-specified substance) and the degree of intention to dope. For inadvertent doping the athlete may claim "No Fault or Negligence" or "No Significant Fault or Negligence". The definition of these terms is shown in Table 6.3.

In both definitions, a key statement is "The athlete must also establish how the Prohibited Substance entered his or her system". It is this evidence that the athlete must present in order to be considered for a reduced sanction. The type of evidence that must be presented includes:

- The need for the supplement was discussed with an appropriate healthcare provider;
- A thorough internet search was conducted regarding the product taken;
- Evidence of these searches was recorded, with reference numbers, where appropriate; and
- The use of the supplement was declared at the time of testing.

Table 6.3 Definition of "No fault or negligence" and "No significant fault or negligence"

No fault or negligence	No significant fault or negligence
The athlete or other person's establishing that he or she did not know or suspect, and could not reasonably have known or suspected even with the exercise of utmost caution, that he or she had used or been administered the prohibited substance or prohibited method or otherwise violated an anti-doping rule.	The athlete or other person's establishing that his or her fault or negligence, when viewed in the totality of the circumstances and taking into account the criteria for no fault or negligence, was not significant in relationship to the anti-doping rule violation.
The athlete must also establish how the prohibited substance entered his or her system.	The athlete must also establish how the prohibited substance entered his or her system.

Table 6.4 Summary of WADA's ineligibility sanctions

Type of doping	Period of ineligibility
Intentional	Four years – lifetime
No significant fault or negligence	Reprimand – two years
	(Depending on the degree of fault)
No fault or negligence	0 years

The ineligibility sanctions that WADA apply are summarised in Table 6.4.

The complete set of regulations regarding sanctions can be found in Article 10 of the World Anti-Doping Code (WADA, 2015).

On the basis that prevention offers a more rational approach to this problem, athletes would benefit from expert advice and support in order to avoid inadvertent prohibited drug use.

6.5 The role of Athlete Support Personnel in preventing deliberate and inadvertent use of prohibited substances

Athlete Support Personnel (ASP) include many groups, all of whom can play a role in preventing both the deliberate and inadvertent use of prohibited substances in sport. Chapter 7 of this book provides a thorough review of the roles and responsibilities of ASP from an anti-doping perspective. Parents of athletes can have a significant influence, although their knowledge and attitudes on the issue of doping is often limited, leaving athletes vulnerable to inadvertent doping from the earliest stages in their sporting career (Blank et al., 2015).

The risk of inadvertent use of prohibited substances in sport can be minimised. There are a number of ways in which healthcare professionals can advise and support athletes to reduce the incidence of inadvertent use of prohibited substances.

Advice on the use of medicines

In cases where medicines are being prescribed by healthcare professionals, the prescriber should be fully conversant, with the current WADA Prohibited List and understand and apply TUE regulations when prescribing medicines containing prohibited drugs. WADA provide advice for athletes on medication use (WADA, 2016d). The prescriber should advise the athlete to declare any prescribed medicines that have been taken in the previous seven days if called for a drugs test.

Where possible, ASP should be aware of any self-medication undertaken by athletes they are involved with. In such cases, the athlete should be advised to get their medication checked by a doctor or pharmacist. Again, declaration of any medicines taken in the previous seven days should be made at the time of testing.

In any cases involving the use of medicines by athletes, advice and help in checking the prohibited status of the drugs within the medicines being taken can be made using Global Drug Reference Online (Global DRO) or other equivalent validated online checking systems. Information that is required includes the country of purchase of the medicine (since the active ingredients may vary between countries) and the sport in which competing as some drugs are only prohibited in certain sports. The reference number of any enquiry made via Global DRO (or any alternate online database), or emails of enquiry to NADOs should be logged as proof that due diligence has being exercised. Checks should be made regularly as manufacturers may change the formulation of a medicine.

Advice on the use of recreational drugs

It should be made clear that many recreational drugs appear on the WADA Prohibited List. Although they are prohibited in-competition only, if used within hours or even days prior to competing these drugs may appear in test results as they may take significant time to be metabolised and excreted from the body. In addition to advising athletes about reducing the risk of inadvertent prohibited drug use, ASP who are healthcare providers should adopt a harm minimisation approach to recreational drug use and, where appropriate, offer additional support and drug rehabilitation services to athletes.

Advice on the use of supplements

Athletes should be advised to assess the need, the risk and the consequences of taking supplements. Consultation with appropriate ASP, such as appropriately qualified sports nutritionists, should be recommended. The risks of supplement use has been summarised by WADA as:

> The use of dietary supplements by athletes is a concern because in many countries the manufacturing and labelling of supplements may not follow strict rules, which may lead to a supplement containing an undeclared substance that is prohibited under anti-doping regulations. A significant number of positive tests have been attributed to the misuse of supplements and taking a poorly labelled dietary supplement is not an adequate defence in a doping hearing.
>
> (WADA, 2016e)

Whilst avoiding the use of supplements might be an obvious way to evade the risks associated with contamination and adulteration, this might not always be practical and may place an athlete at a disadvantage over their competitors who may continue to use supplements. Specific supplement testing programmes have therefore been established to help minimise the risk of a tested supplement containing a prohibited substance, thus protecting athletes against inadvertent doping. Such testing programmes test batches of supplements for prohibited substances and supply certification that helps the athlete and ASP to make informed choices regarding the safety of the supplements they use. Athletes should therefore be advised to seek supplements which have undergone batch testing, programmes such as Informed Sport (2016), Cologne List (2016) and NZVT (2016) can be accessed online.

In summary, the risk associated with supplement use may be minimised in a number of ways:

- Consulting with appropriate ASP;
- Undertaking a thorough internet search on products and their ingredients;
- Using only batch-tested products;
- Keeping evidence of research on products; and
- Declaring any supplements used in the previous seven days when tested.

Professional responsibilities

As ASP, roles and responsibilities include:

- To understand and comply with all anti-doping policies and rules applicable to the athletes they support;
- To influence the athletes they care for to foster anti-doping attitudes; and
- To cooperate with NADOs and IFs investigating anti-doping rule violations.

Continuing professional development is a necessary requirement to keep up-to-date.

In particular, physicians have been identified as a group of ASP who must educate themselves about drug use in sport and who, in turn, can educate athletes at all levels to prevent the use of potentially dangerous performance enhancing substances (Momaya et al., 2015).

In recognition of the influence that ASP have on athletes and their intent to dope, they are being more closely monitored by WADA. The 2015 World Anti-Doping Code introduced two new Anti-Doping Rule Violations (ADRV) specifically aimed at ASP:

- **Complicity** – If involved in an ADRV committed by another person (e.g. helping to cover up an ADRV) you can be sanctioned in the same manner as the person who has committed that ADRV.
- **Prohibited Association** – Athletes associating with ASP, such as a healthcare professional, who has been found guilty of either an ADRV or a criminal or disciplinary offence equivalent to an ADRV can be sanctioned.

By April 2017, 148 ASP were recorded as suspended on the WADA Prohibited Association List (WADA, 2016f).

6.6 Summary

1   Athletes who record an adverse analytical finding, arising from an anti-doping test, frequently claim that the drug had been taken inadvertently.
2   Inadvertent use of prohibited substances in sport may arise through drug treatment for medical conditions, taking drugs recreationally, using nutritional supplements or consuming contaminated food.
3   Sanctions for inadvertent doping can be severe where athletes bear fault and negligence.
4   Although the potential for inadvertent use of prohibited substances is recognised by anti-doping agencies, the onus to prove no fault or negligence rests with the athlete.
5   There are a number of ways in which Athlete Support Personnel can advise and support athletes in order to reduce the incidence of inadvertent use of prohibited substances in sport.

6.7 References

Anderson, J.M. (2011) Evaluating the athlete's claim of an unintentional positive urine drug test. *Current Sports Medicine Reports* 10(4): 191–196.

Ashton, C.H. (2001) Pharmacology and effects of cannabis: A brief review. *British Journal of Psychiatry* 178: 101–106.

Auersperger, I., Topic, M.D., Maver, P., Pusnik, V.K., Osredkar, J. and Lainscak, M. (2012) Doping awareness, views and experience: A comparison between general practitioners and pharmacists. *Wener Klinische Wachenschrift* 124(1-2): 32–38.

Backhouse, S.H. and McKenna, J. (2011) Doping in sport: A review of medical practitioners' knowledge, attitudes and beliefs. *International Journal of Drug Policy* 22: 198–202.

Blank, C., Leichtfried, V., Schaiter, R. et al. (2015) Doping in sports: Knowledge and attitudes among parents of Austrian junior athletes. *Scandinavian Journal of Medicine and Science in Sports* 25: 116–124.

Cologne List (2016) Available online at: http://www.koelnerliste.com/en/cologne-list.html (Accessed on 12 December 2016).

Dascombe, B.J., Karunaratna, M., Carloon, J. et al. (2010) Nutritional supplementation habits and perceptions of elite athletes within a state-based sporting institute. *Journal of Science and Medicine and Sport* 13(2): 274–280.

Dietz, P., Ulrich, R., Niess, A. et al. (2014) Prediction profiles for nutritional supplement use among young German elite athletes. *International Journal of Sport Nutrition and Exercise Metabolism* 24: 623–631.

Dikic, N., McNamee, M. Gunter, H. et al. (2013) Sports physicians, ethics and anti-doping governance: Between assistance and negligence. *British Journal of Sports Medicine* 47: 701–704.

Eichner, E.R. (1993) Ergolytic drugs in medicine and sport. *American Journal of Medicine* 94(2): 205–211.

ElSohly, H.N., ElSohly, M.A. and Stanford, D.F. (1990) Poppy seed ingestion and opiates urinalysis: A closer look. *Journal of Analysis and Toxicology* 14: 308–310

Geyer, H., Braun, H., Burke, L.M. et al. (2011) A-Z of nutritional supplements: Dietary supplements, sports nutrition foods and ergogenic aids for health and performance: Part 22. *British Journal of Sports Medicine* 45: 752–754.

Geyer, H., Schänzer, W. and Thevis, M. (2014) Anabolic agents: Recent strategies for their detection and protection from inadvertent doping. *British Journal of Sports Medicine* 48: 820–826.

Gorski, T., Cadore, E.L., Pinto, S.S. et al. (2011) Use of NSAIDs in triathletes: Prevalence, level of awareness and reasons for use. *British Journal of Sports Medicine* 45: 85–90.

Guddat, S., Fusshöller, G., Geyer, H. et al. (2012) Clenbuterol: Regional food contamination a possible source for inadvertent doping in sport. *Drug testing Analysis* 4: 534–538.

Helmlin, H-J., Murner, A., Steiner, S. et al. (2016) Detection of the diuretic hydrochlorothiazide in a doping control urine sample as a result of a non-steroidal anti-inflammatory drug (NSAID) tablet contamination. *Forensic Science International* 267: 166–172.

Huestis, M.A., Mitchell, J.M. and Cone, E.J. (1995) Detection times of marijuana metabolites in urine by immunoassay and GC-MS. *Journal of Analytical Toxicology* 19(6): 443–449.

Informed Sport (2016) Informed Sport. Available at: http://www.informed-sport.com/ (Accessed on 12 December 2016).

Kim, J., Kang, S., Jung, H. et al. (2011) Dietary supplementation patterns of Korean Olympic athletes participating in the Beijing 2008 Summer Olympic Games. *International Journal of Sport Nutrition and Exercise Metabolism* 21: 166–174.

Knapik, J.J., Steelman, R.A., Hoedebecke, S.S. et al. (2016) Prevalence of dietary supplement use by athletes: Systemic review and meat analysis. *Sports Medicine* 46: 103–123.

Locquet, M., Beaudart, C., Labbuisson, R. et al. (2016) Self-administration of medicines and dietary supplements among female amateur runners: A cross-sectional analysis. *Advances in Therapy* 33(12): 2,257–2,268.

Lun, V., Erdman, K.A., Fung, T.S. et al. (2012) Dietary supplementation practices in Canadian high-performance athletes. *International Journal of Sport Nutrition and Exercise Metabolism* 22: 31–37.

Mazanov, J., Backhouse, S., Conner, J. et al (2014) Athlete support personnel and anti-doping: Knowledge, attitudes and ethical stance. *Scandinavian Journal of Medicine and Science in Sports* 24: 846–856.

Momaya, A., Fawal, M., Estes, R. et al. (2015) Performance enhancing substances in sports: A review of the literature. *Sports Medicine* 45: 517–531.

NZVT (2016) Available online at: http://www.dopingautoriteit.nl/nzvt/nzvt-english (Accessed on 12 December 2016).

Omeragic, E., Dedibergovic, J., Sober, M. et al. (2015) Use of dietary supplements among elite athletes. *SportLogia* 11(1): 49–56.

Outram, S. and Stewart, B. (2015) Doping through supplement use: A review of the available empirical data. *International Journal of Sport Nutrition and Exercise Metabolism* 25: 54–59.

Parr, M.K., Pokrywka, A., Kwiatkowska, D. et al. (2011) Ingestion of designer supplements produced positive doping cases unexpected by the athletes. *Biology of Sport* 28(3): 153–157.

Petróczi, A. and Naughton, D.P. (2009) Popular drugs in sport: Descriptive analysis of the enquiries made via the Drug Information Database (DID). *British Journal of Sports Medicine* 43: 811–817.

Rodek, J., Sekulic, D. and Kondric, M. (2012) Dietary supplementation and doping-related factors in high level sailing. *Journal of the International Society of Sports Nutrition* 9: 51–61.

Saugy, M., Avois, L., Saudan, C. et al. (2006) Cannabis and sport. *British Journal of Sports Medicine* 40(Suppl 1): i13–i15.

Shaw, G., Slater, G. and Burke, L.M. (2016) Supplement use in elite Australian swimmers. *International Journal of Sport Nutrition and Exercise Metabolism* 26: 249–258.

Suzic Lazic, J., Dikie, N., Radivojevic, N. et al. (2011) Dietary supplements and medications in elite sport: Polypharmacy or real need? *Scandinavian Journal of Medicine and Science in Sports* 21: 260–267.

Tandon, S., Bowers, L.D. and Fedoruk, M.N. (2015) Treating the elite athlete: Anti-doping information for the health professional. *Missouri Medicine* 112(2): 122–128.

Thevis, M., Gayer, L., Geyer, H. et al. (2013a) Adverse analytical findings with clenbuterol among U-17 soccer players attributed to food contamination issues. *Drug Test Analysis* 5: 372–376.

Thevis, M., Thomas, A., Beuck, S. et al. (2013b) Does the analysis of the enantiomeric composition of clenbuterol in human urine enable the differentiation of illicit clenbuterol administration from food contamination in sports drug testing? *Rapid Communications in Mass Spectrometry* 27(4): 507–512.

Tscholl, P., Alonso, J.M., Dollé, G. et al. (2010) The use of drugs and nutritional supplements in top-level track and field athletes. *American Journal of Sports Medicine* 38: 133–140.

USADA (2015) USADA's Science Team addresses anti-doping information for health professionals. Available online at: http://www.usada.org/usadas-science-team-addresses-anti-doping-information-for-health-professionals/ (Accessed on 23 November 2016).

Uvacsek, M., Nepusz, T., Naughton, D.P. et al. (2011) Self-admitted behaviour and perceived use of performance-enhancing vs psychoactive drugs among competitive athletes. *Scandinavian Journal of Medicine and Science in Sports* 21: 224–234.

Vernac, A., Stear, S.J., Burke, L.M. et al. (2013) A-Z of nutritional supplements: dietary supplements, sports nutrition foods and ergogenic aids for health and performance: Part 48. *British Journal of Sports Medicine* 47: 998–1000.

Waddington, I., Christiansen, A.V., Gleaves, J. et al. (2013) Recreational drug use and sport: Time for a WADA rethink? *Performance Enhancement and Health* 2: 41–47.

WADA (2015) World Anti-Doping Code. Available online at: https://wada-main-prod.s3.amazonaws.com/resources/files/wada-2015-world-anti-doping-code.pdf (Accessed on 23 November 2016).

WADA (2016a) Anti-doping testing figures. Available online at: https://www.wada-ama.org/en/resources/laboratories/anti-doping-testing-figures (Accessed on 23 November 2016).

WADA (2016b) Therapeutic Use Exemption regulations. Available online at: https://www.wada-ama.org/en/what-we-do/science-medical/therapeutic-use-exemptions. (Accessed on 23 November 2016).

WADA (2016c) Technical Document on Thresholds. Available online at: https://www.wada-ama.org/en/resources/science-medicine/td2014-dl-summary-of-modifications. (Accessed on 23 November 2016).

WADA (2016d) Athletes and medications. Available online at: https://www.wada-ama.org/en/questions-answers/athletes-and-medications (Accessed on 12 December 2016).

WADA (2016e) Dietary and nutritional supplements. Available online at: https://www.wada-ama.org/en/questions-answers/dietary-and-nutritional-supplements (Accessed on 12 December 2016).

WADA (2016f) Prohibited Association List. Available online at: https://wada-main-prod.s3.amazonaws.com/resources/files/2016-11-11-asp_disclaimer_and_list_in_full_0.pdf) (Accessed on 12 December 2016).

Yonamine, M., Garcia, P.R. and de Moraes Moreau, R.L. (2004) Non-intentional doping in sports. *Sports Medicine* 34(11): 697–704.

Chapter 7

The role of Athlete Support Personnel in drug use in sport

Neil Chester, Mark Stuart and David R. Mottram

7.1 Introduction

A wide range of individuals each with specific roles form a key network for the support and development of the athlete. Each individual has a critical role in not only ensuring performance goals are met but first and foremost in safeguarding the welfare of the athlete. Welfare includes a range of provisions for the safety and wellbeing of individuals; however, in competitive sport protection from an anti-doping perspective is particularly important. The roles of Athlete Support Personnel, related to education, ethical medical treatment, and the rational and safe use of drugs in sport is presented in this chapter.

Recognition of the important role Athlete Support Personnel (ASP) have with respect to anti-doping is evident in the third revision of the World Anti-Doping Code (WADC). The 2015 WADC outlines anti-doping rules and responsibilities that acknowledge the influence of ASP on athletes with respect to doping infractions; the anti-doping movement recognises that individual support staff are critical in developing a 'clean sport' ethos amongst their athletes.

Like athletes, ASP can unfortunately be implicated in anti-doping rule violations, and sometimes have direct involvement in facilitating doping offences. Their role in athlete development may also directly or indirectly influence athletes towards external performance aids, including doping, through the fostering of a 'win at all costs' philosophy.

7.2 Athlete Support Personnel

'Athlete Support Personnel' is a broad term that includes a wide range of individuals who together make up an important network that helps to develop and maintain the performance and wellbeing of an athlete or team. Supporting roles may be focused on a specific element of performance but should operate in a complimentary manner. The range of individuals that provide such support is illustrated in Figure 7.1. It is clear that the roles represented in Figure 7.1 have varying functions from a sports performance perspective but all have a responsibility to ensure athletes abide by the spirit of sport and in doing so comply with anti-doping rules. Nevertheless, it is clear that many traditional support roles (e.g. coaches), as well as those roles that have evolved relatively recently (e.g. sport scientists) are primarily focused on optimising performance.

Parental support

Parents and guardians play an essential role particularly in the young, developing athlete. It is generally recognised that the values held by parents are particularly influential during

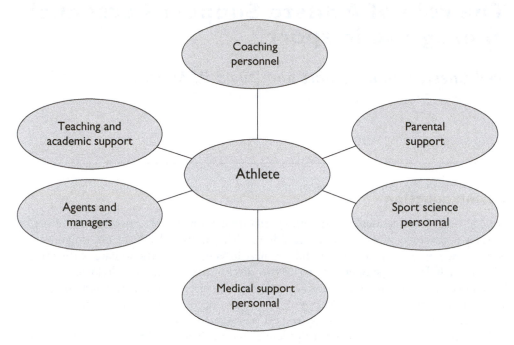

Figure 7.1 The various roles that individuals fulfil to support the athlete

childhood. There is, however, some conjecture as to the extent of the role parents play in children's attitudes, beliefs and behaviour, with some believing that peers have greater influence from ten years old (Chan et al., 2012) and others identifying the parental role as remaining a strong influence throughout adolescence (Steinberg, 2001). There is evidence to show a supportive personal network has influence on sporting success (Baker et al., 2003). Indeed the role of parents in providing both financial and emotional support has been recognised amongst other influential factors in the development of elite athletes (Cote, 1999). However, there is less research in support of the notion that parents/guardians have a key part to play developing anti-doping behaviour. Nevertheless, it understood that parents can provide a protective role against doping in sport and studies report that fathers are seen to be the most influential in preventing doping behaviour (Blank et al., 2015).

Coaching support

Coaches are deemed an integral part of an athlete's development and the athlete–coach relationship is recognised as a particularly critical one in the performance pathway. Much emphasis is placed upon the abilities of a coach and if athlete performances dip it is often the coach that is held ultimately responsible. In the high-pressured field of professional sport this responsibility is particularly evident.

Whilst in elite sport, performance is viewed as the primary goal, the importance of the health and welfare of the athlete can sometimes be overlooked. From an anti-doping perspective there is a clear appreciation of the essential role a coach plays in fostering an anti-doping attitude and influencing the athlete in terms of following an ethical, clean sport path. Coaches therefore require both the knowledge and appropriate belief and attitude to provide such a role effectively. According to research by Laure et al. (2001), 98.1 per cent of coaches were in agreement with the notion that they had a preventative role to play regarding doping but lacked the necessary skills to provide this.

Possibly one of the most famous coaches implicated in a doping scandal was Charlie Francis, who testified that he had introduced the Canadian sprinter, Ben Johnson to ana-bolic androgenic steroids (AAS) in the early 1980s. Johnson later won the 100m sprint at the Seoul Olympics in 1988 but subsequently tested positive for the AAS stanozolol and was disqualified. In more recent times coaches have continued to be linked with ath-letes doping infractions. An independent commission investigation by WADA in 2015 of the Russian anti-doping system confirmed the existence of widespread and systematic cheating through the use of doping substances and methods to ensure, or enhance the likelihood of, victory for athletes and teams. The cheating was done by the athletes' entourages, officials and the athletes themselves, with involvement by doctors, coaches and laboratory personnel (Pound et al., 2015).

Strength and conditioning coaches have evolved in recent years as particularly important support staff. Many athletes and sports teams make use of experts who specialise in strength and conditioning in appreciation of the importance of this key element within athletes training. Despite the recognition of strength and conditioning coaches, individuals occupy-ing such positions may take on extended responsibilities including athlete nutrition and supplementation. If teams do not have designated medical or dietary experts closely and regularly working with the athletes, the level of support in terms of medication and supple-ment advice may be less than those with regular medical support or supervision.

Medical support

Medical practitioners have particular responsibility for the health of the individual and those with specialism in sports medicine typically fulfil important roles within sport. Whilst most athletes might have access to general practitioners only those competing at a high level generally have regular contact with expert sport physicians. Sports physicians occupy an interesting position within the athlete support network. Whilst physicians' roles are cen-tred primarily on the health of an individual a sports physician's role is also focused on performance. In some situations, these roles might be viewed as conflicting and as such may compromise the professional ethics of the physician (Testoni et al., 2013; Vernec, 2013). In addition, there may be incongruence between a physician's medical code of ethics and the WADC in situations where they are presented with an athlete who is known to be dop-ing. As a healthcare professional, a physician has a duty of confidentiality to their patients, however according to the WADC (WADA, 2015a) they would be expected to break con-fidentiality and disclose doping practices. This may impose significant pressures on doctors who serve their athlete patients (Griffith et al., 2011; McNamee and Phillips, 2011). Some experts have suggested that anti-doping agencies need to do more to engage with ASP, such as medical practitioners, to support and resolve contradictions between anti-doping policies and the realities of medical practice, and the ethical principles that govern them (Mazanov et al., 2015).

From an anti-doping perspective sports physicians play a central role in providing per-mitted healthcare to the athlete and providing advice around the safe use of medication. Strategies for the prevention of doping in sport can be improved by sharing the experiences

Sports nutritionists

Sports nutritionists have a key role to play not least in ensuring that athletes do not dope inadvertently. Establishing effective risk management strategies is critical in not only limiting the occurrence of inadvertent doping but also providing the evidence of due diligence in the event of a case of inadvertent doping. The role of supplements in an athlete's diet has become particularly important but is fraught with risk in terms of doping and health (see Chapter 24). Instilling responsible dietary approaches in athletes to complement their training and competitive performance is essential to limit the over-reliance on supplements.

Professional associations representing Athlete Support Personnel

Professional bodies that represent practitioners working with athletes in a supporting role serve particularly important functions. Not least, these organisations help to support their members through training, accreditation and providing ethical codes of conduct. Such documents provide an ethical framework that practitioners/members are required to follow and outline the support channels available when problems arise. Anti-doping should be a key component within any code of conduct set out for practitioners providing support to athletes. In addition specific training needs with regards to anti-doping should be addressed in light of the important role ASP have in educating athletes (WADC Article 18.2; WADA, 2015a). Indeed close relationships between professional associations and their respective NADO should be encouraged.

Manager and agents

Managers and agents have both an important and varied role in elite sport. Whilst such roles may vary according to the sport and the level of competition they tend to be of particular importance amongst the most successful athletes. Their role in particular is concerned with ensuring the best possible competition and the best financial deals for the athlete. As sport has become more lucrative so has the need to manage athletes' sporting and non-sporting financial interests.

Teachers and academic support

Recognition of the importance of teaching fair play and traditional sporting values within formal education is demonstrated by the focus that WADA places on its support for teachers. A teaching resource (WADA, 2015b) including lessons plans has recently been introduced by WADA to support anti-doping education within the age range of 10 to 16 years. WADA also published the Sports Physician Toolkit, which is an education resource specifically aimed at healthcare professionals and covers anti-doping information.

The role of teachers in the development of the young athlete is particularly important. In addition to parents, sports teachers are often cited as the key individuals that introduce athletes to a particular sport. They play a significant and important role in developing a healthy attitude to sport and fair play.

Within higher education there is an appreciation that education relating to the ethics of sport and anti-doping are important, specifically in sport-related programmes where future ASP are likely to come from. The development of partnerships between NADOs and universities not only provides strong links from a research perspective but also ensures that anti-doping education might be embedded into the curriculum and that an anti-doping ethos may be fostered across collegiate sport.

7.3 Medical support personnel and athlete therapy

The primary role of medical support personnel is to maintain the health of athletes. Whilst athletes experience the same ailments as the wider society there is evidence that the practice of competitive sport offers additional risk to health in terms of injury and illness. Indeed, the prevalence of particular conditions such as asthma and exercise-induced bronchoconstriction (see Chapter 11) and upper respiratory tract infection (see Chapter 17) is believed to be higher in athletes compared to the general population. Many sports also offer additional risks to acute injury by virtue of the specific demands of training and competition. Contact sports are particularly risky in terms of musculoskeletal injury, and the prevention and treatment of concussion in contact sports such as rugby has received attention in recent years from the scientific and medical community. The need to ensure effective treatment of athletes is essential, and sometimes use of otherwise prohibited substances is legitimately required for the treatment of particular medical conditions. There is a mechanism whereby exemption can be applied for to use prohibited substances for emergency or legitimate purposes. This process is referred to as 'Therapeutic Use Exemption' and the framework for applying to use prohibited medications is detailed in the WADC (see Chapter 4).

The WADA International Standards document for Therapeutic Use Exemption outlines clearly the process to which athletes, ASP and their respective NADOs, sports governing bodies and major event organisers must adhere in order to use prohibited substances where there is an important therapeutic need.

According to the International Standard for Therapeutic Use Exemption (WADA, 2015c) an athlete may be granted if the following criteria are met:

1   The absence of treatment would incur a detrimental effect on health;
2   The use of the prohibited substance or method would not enhance performance above that of 'normal' levels;
3   There is no permitted alternative therapy available for use; and
4   The necessity for the use of the prohibited substance or method is not a consequence of the prior use of a substance or method which was prohibited at the time of such use.

The effectiveness of the TUE process is in part down to the quality of the supporting evidence, which includes diagnostic results and notes carried out by adequately qualified individuals namely medical personnel and experts in particular fields of health. A sound diagnosis is essential to support the need for therapy. Further evidence is required to justify the proposed mode of therapy. A committee comprised of medical practitioners and experts in the fields of sports medicine and the condition under consideration is assembled to review the TUE application and provide a decision on whether to grant the TUE.

7.4 The World Anti-Doping Code and Athlete Support Personnel

Whilst it is clear that all those individuals represented in Figure 7.1 have a role in ensuring the athlete complies with anti-doping rules the WADC recognises that particular ASP may play a significant role in whether an athlete commits an anti-doping rule violation (ADRV). The WADC therefore enables ASP to be sanctioned if they commit ADRVs as a consequence of the following (WADA, 2015d):

- Administering or attempted administration of a prohibited substance or method to an athlete;
- Possession of a prohibited substance or method without an acceptable justification;
- Trafficking or attempted trafficking of a prohibited substance or method; or
- Assisting, aiding, abetting, covering up or any other type of complicity involving an anti-doping rule violation

Whilst not all anti-doping rules outlined in the WADC apply directly to ASP, further issues are considered elsewhere under the 'Roles and responsibilities of athlete support personnel' (Article 21.2; WADA, 2015a). The 2015 WADC clearly states that ASP have the following responsibilities:

- To be knowledgeable of and comply with all anti-doping policy and rules applicable to ASP and the athlete;
- To cooperate with the athlete testing programme;
- To use their influence on athlete values and behaviour to foster anti-doping attitudes;
- To disclose to their NADO and International Federation any ADRV committed within the previous ten years;
- To cooperate with anti-doping organisations investigating any ADRVs; and
- ASP should not use any prohibited substance or method without valid justification.

Whilst there is an appreciation that ASP who fail to honour these responsibilities are not liable for disciplinary action under the WADC they may be sanctioned under sport disciplinary rules. The WADC requires International Federations, National Sports Federations and National Olympic and Paralympic Committees to put in place rules that ensure that individuals who use prohibited substances and methods without valid justification are unable to work with athletes (Articles 20.3.15 and 20.4.13; WADA, 2015a).

Athlete Support Personnel and Anti-Doping Rule Violations

Since 2013, WADA have published Anti-Doping Rule Violation Reports in which analysis has been made of the anti-doping testing figures produced, annually, by WADA-accredited laboratories (WADA, 2013; WADA, 2014; WADA, 2015e). These reports include the decisions made of all adverse analytical findings (AAFs) arising from analysis of athletes' urine and blood samples in WADA-accredited laboratories. In addition, the reports review cases of non-analytical ADRVs committed by both athletes and ASP.

A non-analytical ADRV is where an athlete or ASP commits an ADRV that does not involve the detection of a prohibited substance in a urine or blood sample, as outlined in the WADC (Articles 2.2 to 2.10; WADA, 2015a). Table 7.1 shows the profile of the non-analytical ADRVs reported by WADA from 2013 to 2015.

Table 7.1 Profile of non-analytical Anti-Doping Rule Violations (ADRVs) (including athletes and Athlete Support Personnel)

	2013	2014	2015
Total number of non-analytical ADRVs	266	231	280
Type of violator:			
Athlete	Not specified	185	252
Athlete Support Personnel (ASP)	Not specified	46	28
Nationalities involved	44	59	61
Sports involved	37	30	38

It is clear that significant numbers of non-analytical ADRVs are committed by both athletes and by ASP across a number of sports and nationalities. The occurrence of these violations has been classified according to the specific type of ADRVs, listed in Articles 2.2 to 2.10 of the WADC (Table 7.2).

It can be seen that the total number of ADRVs committed are higher than the totals shown in Table 7.1, reflecting the fact that many cases included multiple violations committed by individuals.

With respect to ASP, the highest number of violations related to Article 2.8 involved the administration, assisting, encouraging, aiding, abetting or covering up of doping by athletes, although occurrences of trafficking and possession of prohibited substances by ASP were also significant.

The nationality of ASP who committed non-analytical ADRVs in 2014 and 2015 were presented in the respective reports for these years (WADA, 2014; WADA, 2015e), as shown in Table 7.3.

Table 7.2 Profile of non-analytical Anti-Doping Rule Violations (ADRVs) by type of violation

Type of violation according to code article	Occurrences [+]				
	2013	2014		2015	
		Athletes	ASP	Athletes	ASP
Article 2.2 – Use or attempted use	69	61	4	106	2
Article 2.3 – Refusing, failing without compelling justification, evading	128	79	0	97	0
Article 2.4 – Whereabouts violation	25	21	0	31	0
Article 2.5 –Tampering or attempted tampering	13	7	2	6	2
Article 2.6 – Possession	42	35	12	70	7
Article 2.7 – Trafficking or attempted trafficking	6	13	25	18	6
Article 2.8 – Administration, attempted administration or assisting, encouraging, aiding, abetting, covering up	18	7	37	3	19
Article 2.9 – Complicity	4				3
Article 2.10 – Prohibited association	0				1
Grand total	301	162	80	335	40

+ Cases that are classified under multiple code article violations are calculated as single occurrences for each type of violation. Therefore the total occurrences is larger than the number of violations.

Table 7.3 Non-analytical ADRV cases committed by Athlete Support Personnel classified according to the nationality of the ASP

Nationality	Athlete Support Personnel	
	2014	*2015*
Austria	1	1
Belgium	1	1
Brazil	1	
Bulgaria	1	
China	1	
France	1	
Iran, Islamic Republic of	1	3
Iraq	1	
Italy	14	7
Jamaica	1	
Mexico		2
Morocco		1
Netherlands	1	
Nigeria	1	
Panama		1
Qatar	1	
Romania	1	1
Russian Federation	1	3
Saudi Arabia		1
Spain	1	1
Switzerland		1
Turkey	11	3
Ukraine		1
United Kingdom	2	
United States	2	
Uruguay	2	
Grand total	46	28

The limited number of countries listed probably reflects the inconsistent approach to the investigation of non-analytical ADRVs committed by ASP by ADOs, worldwide. For comparison, the number of countries listed for non-analytical ADRVs for athletes were 39 (2014) and 46 (2015).

WADA suspension of Athlete Support Personnel

As a further measure to control the doping-related activities by ASP, in September 2015, WADA published a list of 114 Athlete Support Personnel (ASP) who were suspended from working with athletes or other persons under the 2015 WADC Prohibited Association rule (Article 2.10). Under this rule, athletes and other persons are prohibited from working with ASP who are currently sanctioned for an ADRV or have been sanctioned within the previous six years.

The list of sanctioned ASP was created, based on case decisions and information presented to WADA by Anti-Doping Organisations (ADOs). Consequently, WADA makes no representations or warranties of any kind, express or implied, about the completeness, accuracy or reliability of the Prohibited Association List. However, WADA encourage all ADOs to communicate with the Agency should they become aware of any individuals who should be included on the Prohibited Association List.

The majority of suspended ASP have been coaches but the list also included medical services personnel and sport administrators. The list provides details on the names of the suspended ASP, their nationality and their period of suspension. The Prohibited Association List is updated by WADA on a quarterly basis, or more frequently if necessary (WADA, 2015f).

In November 2016, WADA published an updated list of 151 suspended ASP in which those ASP who had served their suspension were removed from the list and in which 57 new ASP suspensions were added.

Table 7.4 Country of origin for the 148 Athlete Support Personnel listed as suspended by WADA on 10 April 2017 (WADA, 2017)

Country	Number of ASP suspended
Italy	70
Russia	11
Turkey	
Romania	6
Spain	5
USA	
Iran	4
Canada	3
Kazakhstan	
Austria	2
Great Britain	
Mexico	
Panama	
Ukraine	
Belarus	1
Belgium	
Bulgaria	
Brazil	
China	
Egypt	
Estonia	
Hungary	
Iraq	
Jamaica	
Liechtenstein	
Malaysia	
Morocco	
Netherlands	
New Zealand	
Nigeria	
North Korea	
Serbia	
South Africa	
Switzerland	

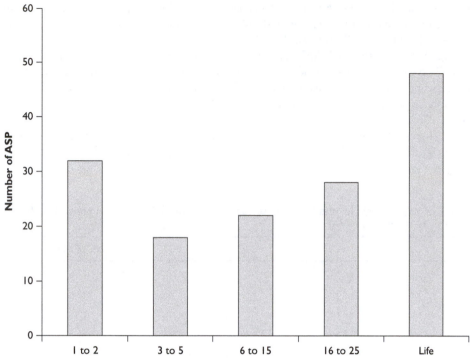

Figure 7.2 Range of suspension periods (in years) for the Athlete Support Personnel listed as suspended by WADA on 10 April 2017 (WADA, 2017)

In April 2017, WADA published a further, updated list of 148 suspended ASP including nine new ASP suspensions. Data from the list updated on 10 April 2017 (WADA, 2017) are shown in Table 7.4 and Figure 7.2, which reveal the number of ASP serving a suspension on that date, according to their country (Table 7.1) and the range of suspensions imposed (Figure 7.2).

These data clearly show that ASP are being closely scrutinised by certain ADOs. The high number of suspended ASP from Italy could reflect the thoroughness by which anti-doping organisations within this country have conducted their investigations on ASP.

Sanctions for anti-doping rule violations can be severe (Figure 7.2). Clearly, the periods of suspension applied to ASP greatly exceed those applied to athletes who commit an ADRV. This would seem to be an appropriate action by WADA considering the potential wide-ranging adverse influence that ASP may exert on one or more athletes under their supervision and influence.

Despite the clear role that ASP play in anti-doping there is evidence, albeit limited, to suggest that many are unaware of their responsibilities and are in fact ill-equipped to carry out their duties. Research examining physicians in particular suggests that they had limited knowledge and awareness of anti-doping rules (Backhouse and McKenna, 2011).

7.5 Education and support for Athlete Support Personnel

A key aspect of the support that ASP provide with respect to anti-doping is associated with education. It is essential that those that surround the athlete are, themselves, knowledgeable regarding anti-doping rules, responsibilities and procedures. Whilst much of the research associated with anti-doping knowledge is centred on the athletes there is some research that has examined the knowledge of various groups of ASP, namely medical personnel (Laure et al., 2003; Blank et al., 2014), football coaches and technical staff (Barghi et al., 2015; Morente-Sanchez and Zabala, 2015), and a range of ASP including family (Mazanov et al., 2014).

Education must not only focus on those currently in support positions but also on those aspiring to work in sport, in roles supporting the athlete. The integration of anti-doping education within coaching courses and other professional education programmes is essential. The partnership of such organisations with their respective NADOs is a key relationship helping to orchestrate effective education. Higher education also has a key role to play with the need for all sport-related HE programmes to ensure that the area of drugs in sport is included and anti-doping is seen as a key element.

WADA produce a number of resources aimed at key individuals that support athletes through their career pathway. Specifically, WADA produce educational resources (e.g. WADA Sports Physician Toolkit), to support coaches, teachers and sports physicians. Similar resources are developed by NADOs to help support ASP locally and provide specific information centred on a particular nation (Tandon et al., 2015). Nevertheless, there is some suggestion that the impact of such resources may be limited. According to research by Patterson et al. (2014) there is a lack of engagement with resources centred on coaches and therefore their effectiveness in reaching their target audience might be questioned (Patterson et al., 2014). Whilst education is recognised as a key preventative measure in anti-doping there remains a discrepancy in the focus and financial resources it receives when compared to those provided to run an effective testing programme. Recognition of the importance of education directed at ASP, in addition to athletes, is an important step forward; however, there is a need to ensure both the quality and delivery are enhanced if it is to be an effective preventative strategy.

7.6 Summary

It is clear that a wide range of individuals have a significant role to play in the development of an athlete. This role is an essential one; not only to optimise performance and achieve targets but also to protect and safeguard the athlete throughout their career. One role, recognised as particularly important, is that of a mentor who adopts the ideals of fair play and anti-doping. The part that ASP play in anti-doping has been formally recognised by WADA not only through the educational support that it provides but also by including them as potential perpetrators of anti-doping rule violations. Whilst there is an appreciation that athletes do not associate with individuals who have committed a doping offence there are also sanctions in place to ensure that ASP who violate anti-doping rules are disciplined accordingly. Nevertheless, in recognition of their critical role there is a need to ensure the provision of effective anti-doping education to all ASP. The challenge remains to ensure that ASP not only recognise their need to abide by the anti-doping rules but also that they perform a fundamental part themselves in education by ensuring athletes abide by anti-doping principles.

7.7 References

Ambrose, P.J. (2011) Educational opportunities and anti-doping roles and responsibilities for pharmacists. *Yakugaku Zasshi* 131: 1,761–1,764.

Auersperger, I., Topic, M.D., Maver, P. et al. (2012) Doping awareness, views and experience: A comparison between general practitioners and pharmacists. *Wiener Klinische Wochenschrift* 124(1-2): 32–38.

Backhouse, S.H. and McKenna, J. (2011) Doping in sport: A review of medical practitioners' knowledge, attitudes and beliefs. *International Journal of Drug Policy* 22: 198–202.

Baker, J., Horton, S., Robertson-Wilson, J. and Wall, M. (2003) Nurturing sport expertise: factors influencing the development of elite athletes. *Journal of Sport Science and Medicine* 2: 1–9.

Barghi, T.S., Halabchi, F., Dvorak, J. and Hosseinnejad, H. (2015) How the Iranian football coaches and players know about doping? *Asian Journal of Sports Medicine* 6(2): e24392.

Blank, C., Leichtfried, V., Muller, D. and Schobersberger, W. (2015) Role of parents as a protective factor against adolescent athletes' doping susceptibility. *South African Journal of Sports Medicine* 27(3): 87–91.

Blank, C., Muller, D. and Schobersberger, W. (2014) Discrepancy between knowledge and interest of Austrian sports physicians with respect to doping and doping prevention in sports. *International Sports Medicine Journal* 15(2): 136–146.

Chan, D.K., Lonsdale, C. and Fung, H.H. (2012) Influences of coaches, parents and peers on the motivational patterns of child and adolescent athletes. *Scandanavian Journal of Medicine and Science in Sports* 22(4): 558–568.

Cote, J. (1999) The influence of the family in the development of talent in sports. *Sport Psychology* 13: 395–417.

D'Ath, P.J., Thomson, D.W. and Wilson, C.M. (2013) Seeing you through London 2012: Eye care at the Olympics. *British Journal of Sports Medicine* 47(7): 463–466.

Dikic, N., McNamee, M., Gunter, H., Makovic, S.S. and Vajgic, B. (2013) Sports physicians, ethics and anti-doping governance: Between assistance and negligence. *British Journal of Sports Medicine* 47: 701–704.

Dvorak, J., Saugy, M. and Pitsiladis, Y.P. (2014) Challenges and threats to implementing the fight against doping in sport. *British Journal of Sports Medicine* 48: 807–809.

FDI (2017) FDI policy statement on sports dentistry. *International Dental Journal* 67: 18–19.

Griffith, R., McNamee, M. and Phillips, N. (2011) On the duty of the doctor not to disclose athlete doping data without consent. *International Journal of Sports Policy* 3(2): 191–204.

Kato, T. (2014) The role of pharmacists and student pharmacists in education and providing advice about over the counter (OTC) medications. *Yakugaku Zasshi* 134: 223–235.

Laure, P., Binsinger, C. and Lecerf, T. (2003) General practitioners and doping in sport: Attitudes and experience. *British Journal of Sports Medicine* 37: 335–338.

Laure, P., Thouvenin, F. and Lecerf, T. (2001) Attitudes of coaches toward doping. *Journal of Sports Medicine and Physical Fitness* 41(1): 132–136.

Malek, S., Taylor, J. and Mansell, K. (2014) A questionnaire examining attitudes of collegiate athletes towards doping and pharmacists as information providers. *Canadian Pharmaceutical Journal* 147: 352–358.

Mazanov, J., Backhouse, S., Connor, D., Hemphill, F. and Quirk, F. (2014) Athlete support personnel: Knowledge, attitudes and ethical stance. *Scandanavian Journal of Medicine and Science in Sports* 24: 846–856.

Mazanov, J., Hemphill, F., Connor, J. et al. (2015) Australian athlete support personnel lived experience of anti-doping. *Sport Management Review* 18: 218–230.

McNamee, M. and Phillips, N. (2011) Confidentiality, disclosure and doping in sports medicine. *British Journal of Sports Medicine* 45: 174–177.

Morente-Sanchez, J. and Zabala, M. (2015) Knowledge, attitudes and beliefs of technical staff towards doping in Spanish football. *Journal of Sport Science* 33(12): 1,267–1,275

Mottram, D., Khalifa, S., Alemrayat, B. et al. (2016) Perspectives of pharmacists in Qatar regarding doping and anti-doping in sports. *Journal of Sports Medicine and Physical Fitness* 56(6): 817–824.

Needleman, I., Ashley, P., Petrie, A. et al. (2013) Oral health and impact on performance of athletes participating in the London 2012 Olympic Games: A cross-sectional study. *British Journal of Sports Medicine* 47(16): 1,054–1,058.

Nicholson, R.G.H., Thomas, G.P.L., Potter, M.J. et al. (2012) London 2012: Prescribing for athletes in ophthalmology. *Eye* 26: 1,036–1,038.

Patterson, L.B., Duffy, P.J. and Backhouse, S. (2014) Are coaches anti-doping? Exploring issues of engagement with education and research. *Substance Use and Misuse* 49(9): 1,182–1,185.

Pound, R.W., McLaren, R.H. and Robertson, J. (2015) Independent Commission Investigation. Available at: https://www.wada-ama.org/sites/default/files/resources/files/wada_independent_commission_report_1_en.pdf (Accessed on 1 July 2017).

Steinberg, I. (2001) We know some things: Parent–adolescent relationships in retrospect and prospect. *Journal of Research of Adolescence* 11(1): 1–19.

Stuart, M., Mottram, D., Erskine, D. et al. (2013) Development and delivery of pharmacy services for the London 2012 Olympic and Paralympic Games. *European Journal of Hospital Pharmacy.* 20: 42–45.

Tandon, S., Bowers, L.D. and Fedoruk, M.N. (2015) Treating the elite athlete: Anti-doping information of the health professional. *Missouri Medicine* 112(2): 122–128.

Testoni, D., Hornik, C.P., Smith, P.B. et al. (2013) Sports medicine and ethics. *American Journal of Bioethics* 13(10): 4–12.

Vernec, A.R. (2013) Doping ethics and the sport physician. *Current Sports Medicine Report* 12(5): 283–284.

WADA (2013) 2013 Anti-Doping Rule Violations (ADVRs) Report. Available at: https://www.wada-ama.org/sites/default/files/resources/files/wada-2013-adrv-report-en.pdf (Accessed on 16 June 2017).

WADA (2014) 2014 Anti-Doping Rule Violations (ADVRs) Report. Available at: https://www.wada-ama.org/sites/default/files/resources/files/wada-2014-adrv-report-en_0.pdf (Accessed on 16 June 2017).

WADA (2015a) 2015 World Anti-Doping Code. Available at: http://www.wada-ama.org/en/resources/the-code/world-anti-doping-code (Accessed on 7 May 2017).

WADA (2015b) Teacher's Tool Kit. Available at: https://www.wada-ama.org/sites/default/files/resources/files/wada_teachers_toolkit_v4_2015_eng.pdf (Accessed on 7 May 2017).

WADA (2015c) International Standard Therapeutic Use Exemptions. Available at: https://www.wada-ama.org/sites/default/files/resources/files/wada-2016-istue-final-en_0.pdf (Accessed on 12 May 2017).

WADA (2015d) Significant changes between the 2009 Code and the 2015 Code, Version 4.0. Available at: https://www.wada-ama.org/sites/default/files/wadc-2015-draft-version-4.0-significant-changes-to-2009-en.pdf (Accessed on 7 May 2017).

WADA (2015e) 2015 Anti-Doping Rule Violations (ADRVs) Report. Available at: https://www.wada-ama.org/sites/default/files/resources/files/2015_adrvs_report_web_release_0.pdf. (Accessed on 16 June 2017).

WADA (2015f) WADA publishes global list of suspended athlete support personnel. Available at: https://www.wada-ama.org/en/media/news/2015-09/wada-publishes-global-list-of-suspended-athlete-support-personnel (Accessed on 13 June 2017).

WADA (2017) Prohibited association list. Available at: (https://www.wada-ama.org/en/resources/the-code/prohibited-association-list (Accessed on 13 June 2017).

Wilson, C.M., Thomson, D.W. and D'Ath, P.J. (2013) Seeing you through London 2012: Eye care at the Paralympics. *British Journal of Sports Medicine* 47(13): 869–871.

Woods, C.B., Moynihan, A. (2009) General practitioners knowledge, practice and training requirements in relation to doping in sport. *Irish Medical Journal* 102(1): 8–10.

Yamaguchi, T, Horio, I, Aoki, R. et al. (2013) Identification of the role of the sports pharmacist with a model for the prediction of athletes' actions to cope with sickness. *Yakugaku Zasshi* 133: 1,249–1,259.

Chapter 8

Medical and pharmacy services for international games

Mark Stuart

8.1 Introduction

Providing a medical service at international multi-sport events such as Olympic, Paralympic, European and Commonwealth Games is a truly unique challenge on a scale unrivalled by any other sporting event. Not only must the medical services cater to the highly specialised therapeutic needs of up to 15,000 athletes during the course of these events, but they must also supply the needs of accredited support staff, team officials and medical units, press and broadcast teams, volunteer workforce, and spectators. Issues around drug use by athletes in sport are of key importance to medical and pharmacy services.

For both the London 2012 and Rio 2016 Olympic and Paralympic Games around 250,000 accredited people were under the care of the games medical services and could access free treatment if required. In addition, first-aid and emergency medical support was available for an estimated nine million spectators while they were at the competition venues. Over 53,000 medical encounters for 32,000 people were recorded during the period of both the Olympic and Paralympic Games for London 2012, which occurred across all of the medical facilities provided by the Organising Committee. Around 30 per cent of these medical encounters were athletes.

In terms of drug use and medicines management in the games environment, pharmacy services are an integral part of delivering this care to athletes. Pharmacists are at the front-line when it comes to drug use and supply to athletes at international games. In this special-ist environment, pharmacists require an advanced level of sport-specific pharmacological and clinical knowledge in order to effectively contribute to the healthcare of the athlete. They are also responsible for supporting anti-doping during the games by implementing robust systems of supply of drugs to athletes and by the provision of expert information to athletes on drugs banned in sport and their permitted alternatives.

An extensive array of complex clinical, professional, legal and regulatory issues related to medicines use must be considered by organising committees, as medicines are stocked across all healthcare rooms and stations at the games. As part of the games medical depart-ment, pharmacy services are responsible for ensuring that the necessary medicines manage-ment and clinical governance frameworks are in place to ensure medicines are administered closely within the rules of the World Anti-Doping Code and excellent standards of health-care provision for athletes.

8.2 Medical services at sporting venues

At every Olympic sporting venue, specific medical facilities are provided for athletes and spectators. At the main Olympic stadium, there may be two main athlete medical rooms near the field of play stocked with equipment and medicines for sports injuries and emergency situations. There will also be a number of spectator medical rooms on each tier or level of the stadium, and additional medical stations in the public areas immediately outside the venue. For both the Rio 2016 and London 2012 Olympic Games, medical services were provided at 35 spectator competition venues, 41 training venues and 55 non-competition venues (such as official hotels).

The nature of the sporting event also determines how the medical services are delivered and the types of drugs that are available for athlete use. For sailing and rowing, medical boats closely follow the competition, and motorbikes will carry supplies for the road cycling and marathon events. During the Olympic Games, the equestrian events carry the most risk of serious trauma injuries; along the 5.7 km route for the Olympic cross-country events in Hong Kong in 2008, 24 medical teams were stationed at any one time. Each medical team was equipped with a drug suitcase containing over 30 emergency drugs and a variety of medical equipment suitable for trauma.

8.3 The games polyclinic

Within the athlete village at every Olympic, Paralympic, European and Commonwealth Games is a purpose built medical centre known as the polyclinic – this is the main medical facility for athletes and team officials.

Medical services offered in the polyclinic are comprehensive and include: emergency medical services, sports medicine, general practice, medical imaging, dentistry, eye services (ophthalmologists, opticians, and optometrists), physiotherapy, massage therapy, hydrotherapy, podiatry, pathology, medical records, interpreter services, doping control, gender verification and pharmacy. Medical services are provided free to the athletes and team officials for the duration of the games and the polyclinic is usually staffed by a dedicated team of expert volunteers.

The games polyclinic provides an environment unlike any other regular medical practice. On admission, an athlete has immediate access to state-of-the-art diagnostic and treatment equipment and a multidisciplinary team with expertise in sports medicine. It is a unique environment where fast and comprehensive care can be provided. For example, with a single visit an athlete might have a specialist sports medicine consultation, ultrasound or MRI scan interpreted by a radiographer, physiotherapy or nursing intervention, and counseling on their prescribed medicine by the polyclinic pharmacists. At the Rio 2016 Olympic Games, there were 12,300 medical encounters recorded from the Olympic Village polyclinic alone.

At all games, the polyclinic has close connections with nearby hospitals where patients are referred if they require longer-term or intensive care. At the London 2012 Games, three designated hospitals were appointed in central London for this purpose if required, and 532 referrals to designated hospitals were made over the period of the Olympic and Paralympic Games from the games medical services. For the Rio 2016 Olympic Games, a number of hospitals across Rio formed a network which provided medical capacity for the events held across the city. There were 305 hospital transfers made to these hospitals throughout the duration of the Rio Olympic Games, involving athletes, officials and spectators.

In Beijing there were 21 official Olympic hospitals. If an athlete, official or Olympic Family member was admitted, their care was coordinated through a 'green passage' process, which meant a speedy and priority service was provided. The designated Olympic hospitals were also able to provide the Olympic pharmacies with any medicines not stocked in the village as needed.

8.4 Polyclinic services

Pharmacy

Each village at an Olympic Games will contain a fully stocked pharmacy to provide the medicine requirements of accredited athletes, team officials, Olympic and Paralympic Family. Polyclinic pharmacies operate in a similar style to a hospital outpatient dispensary and are the coordinating points of medicines supply for the athlete and spectator medical facilities at all venues. During the course of the London 2012 Olympic and Paralympic games, a total of 5,200 prescriptions were dispensed through the three polyclinic pharmacies. During the Rio 2016 Olympic Games, 2,446 prescriptions were dispensed during the operational period of the Olympic and Paralympic Games.

Imaging

One of the most complex installations in the polyclinic is the imaging equipment. At both Rio 2016 and London 2012 there were two magnetic resonance imaging (MRI) scanners, one X-ray commuted tomography scanner (CT), one digital X-ray and two ultrasound machines (US). Given the size and sensitivity of the machines, the MRI and CT scanners were positioned in demountable buildings outside the front entrance of the polyclinic. During the Rio 2016 Olympic Games, there were 745 MRI scans, 410 X-rays and 167 ultrasound scans made for the athletes and officials in the Olympic Village.

Physical therapies

The physical therapy area of the polyclinic requires a large area because the high volume of consultations and the amount of equipment it contains, including a full rehabilitation gymnasium, ice bath area and hydrotherapy pool. This department is often the busiest service during the games with thousands of athletes accessing these services. During the Rio 2016 Olympic Games there were 7,147 separate medical encounters involving physical therapies including physiotherapy and sports massage. The London 2012 Games were the first to introduce chiropractors and osteopathy to the range of medical services available, which proved to successfully complement the physiotherapy and sport massage services.

Dentistry

Dental services are always in high demand at international games. The dental services for the Rio 2016 Olympic Games undertook 2,832 separate treatments for 1,700 athletes and officials, with 420 mouth guards being supplied and fitted. The polyclinic services provide an opportunity for athletes from countries with limited access to medical resources to access routine and screening services for dental and optical treatment; the provision of these services is considered an obligation of the host city.

Optometry

Optometry services are similarly busy: For the Rio 2016 Olympic Games, 2,293 separate optometry consultations were conducted, with 1,904 eyeglasses distributed. At London 2012,

2,258 pairs of spectacles were issued over the period of both the Olympic and Paralympic Games, mainly to athletes and team officials.

8.5 Role of healthcare professionals in anti-doping

As well as looking after the athletes' therapeutic sports-medicine requirements, the doctors, pharmacists and other healthcare professionals are also responsible for ensuring that the athletes do not inadvertently take a prohibited substance. In the international games environment, athletes rely heavily on the knowledge and advice of healthcare professionals for information on drugs banned in sport, particularly for drugs that are prescribed for the first time in the polyclinic at the games.

Healthcare professionals must be familiar with the list of prohibited substances, and the regulations for the provision of drugs that have a restricted status. They must also be aware of drugs that require prior notification through the Therapeutic Use Exemption (TUE) procedure in order to advise athletes appropriately.

There are very tight procedures, and a specific Olympic prescription form to ensure that the athletes do not fall foul of a doping offence. Strict systems of dispensing prohibited drugs are in place to ensure that drugs issued to athletes comply with the World Anti-Doping Agency (WADA) regulations. This involves meticulous scrutiny of prescribing new drugs to athletes that require TUEs.

8.6 Medical workforce and training

Staffing Olympic and Paralympic medical services is a huge logistical operation, and planning usually starts five years prior to any games.

For the London 2012 Olympic and Paralympic Games, around 4,500 medical volunteers provided specialist care at 35 Olympic venues – similar numbers ran the Sydney 2000 medical service. For the Atlanta 1996 Olympics, 4,000 medical volunteers were recruited, and in Athens 2004, 400 specialist doctors, 400 nurses and 400 physiotherapists made up the core of the local medical team.

In addition to the local medical workforce, over 1,000 doctors and hundreds of visiting medical professionals who travel with the teams will also reside in the athlete village and will access the games medical services to treat members of their own team.

The provision of games medical services requires healthcare professional volunteers to have knowledge and skills in a variety of areas beyond normal professional duties, particularly with respect to the provision of medicines to athletes, including knowledge of prohibited drugs and the pharmacology of specific drugs used routinely in sports medicine. Intensive and specialist training on drugs in sport is provided for all doctors, pharmacists and other healthcare professionals working in the games environment, which is usually in the year before the start of the games.

For the Rio 2016 Olympic Games, an enhanced level of training was provided by the International Olympic Committee and the World Anti-Doping Agency around issues relating to drugs in sport and the specific measures in place to prevent doping and to encourage safe and best medical practice by healthcare professionals during the Games.

In early 2016, prior to the Rio Olympics, the WADA Sports Physician Toolkit was launched, and is accessed through the WADA website at www.wada-ama.org. Completion of a number of games-specific modules was a compulsory requirement of practicing as a team physician at the Rio Games. The games-specific training included learning modules for team doctors on:

1   How to identify prohibited drugs in sport;
2   Applying for TUEs in the Olympic environment;
3   How to prescribe prohibited drugs for therapeutic use at the Games;
4   The IOC Needle Policy and how to comply with it; and
5   The process for importing medicines to the Games host country for their own team use.

Prior to the Rio 2016 Olympics, the games-specific modules were completed by a total of 944 team physicians. The impact of this training initiative was particularly evident with the success of the IOC Needle Policy, where 367 declarations for injections for legitimate therapeutic reasons were made over the course of the Games, which indicated a significant increase in compliance by team doctors from the Sochi 2014 Games, where 90 declarations were submitted for therapeutic injections.

8.7 Drug administration to athletes

Prescribing and dispensing of drugs in the games polyclinic is undertaken with great caution to ensure that the prescription falls within the WADA rules. If a prohibited drug is prescribed, approval for a TUE must be obtained and shown to the pharmacy at the time of dispensing – the signatures from the athlete, doctor, and pharmacist are obtained to indicate the informed consent of the athlete.

As an additional precaution, the pharmacy in the polyclinic will have a bespoke dispensing system, which alerts the pharmacist if a prohibited substance is being supplied – the pharmacist can then ensure that the athlete completes the necessary documentation and obtains the appropriate authorisation from the games medical commission to use the drug.

If a WADA-prohibited drug is considered necessary for the treatment of an athlete, the doctor and pharmacist informs the athlete about the consequence of taking the drug. The athlete must then sign the prescription to acknowledge understanding of the treatment being prescribed. Prohibited drugs require notification to the games medical commission, using a TUE form, before the athlete competes.

Failing to submit a TUE form declaring the therapeutic use of a prohibited drug could result in a doping violation should the athlete test positive for these substances. However, any drug is permitted to be administered to an athlete for treatment in an emergency or life-threatening situation.

8.8 Prescribing prohibited substances to athletes

Prohibited substances are drugs that, according to the World Anti-Doping Code or International Sports Federation's (IF) rules, cannot be used by athletes who will be competing in the Olympic or Paralympic Games, unless a TUE has been obtained from the relevant Therapeutic Use Exemption Committee (TUEC). Every major international games will appoint a TUEC to consider new TUEs that arise during the games. In addition, athletes are required to submit existing TUEs to the games medical commission before the start of the games.

Prescriptions for drugs which are prohibited according to the World Anti-Doping Agency List of Prohibited substances are often made for genuine therapeutic reasons. During the Rio 2016 Olympic Games, a total of ten prescriptions for prohibited drugs were made for athletes, who all had appropriate TUEs in place prior to receiving the medication from the pharmacy.

In general, prescribing prohibited substances for athletes should be avoided unless a TUE is obtained in advance or in a medical emergency when an athlete's health takes absolute priority and a retrospective TUE should be obtained (e.g. for opiates or intravenous fluids).

If a TUE has already been obtained from the TUEC prior to the prescription being written, a copy of the TUE documentation should be presented to the dispensing pharmacist who would then proceed to dispense the medicine for the athlete. If a copy of the TUE cannot be presented the athlete needs to sign to confirm that a valid TUE is in place.

Box 8.1   Prescription procedure for prohibited substances at international games

- In an emergency a doctor must treat an athlete, including using prohibited substances and methods, if clinically necessary and apply for a TUE afterwards.
- If it is not an emergency situation the prescribing doctor must explain to the athlete that a 'prohibited' substance is being prescribed and explain the consequences if a TUE is not obtained in advance. A TUE should normally be submitted to the TUEC before treatment.
- The prescribing doctor and the athlete who is receiving the medication are to sign the prescription to confirm that they are aware of the status of the substance, and the pharmacist should sign the prescription to verify that they have informed the prescribing doctor and the athlete that the substance is prohibited.
- The dispensing pharmacist should stamp the prescription as 'prohibited' and label the dispensed medicine as 'prohibited' before giving the medication to the athlete.
- Full understanding and consent by the athlete is essential throughout this process, as according to the World Anti-Doping Code rule of strict liability, ultimately it is the athletes' responsibility for all substances that are put into their body.

8.9 Medicines governance

Comprehensive policies and standard operating procedures are required at international games around the use and management of medicines, with a particular focus on their use within the rules of the World Anti-Doping Code. These are to ensure a safe and standardised approach to medicines management by all members of the medical and pharmacy team; also to comply with drug laws of the host country and the recommendations of governing organisations such as the International Olympic Committee.

For the London 2012 Games, these policies and procedures were developed in collaboration with national pharmacy organisations and professional and regulatory bodies. The policies and procedures covered all aspects of services involving medicines provision such as:

- The storage and supply of medicines at competition venues;
- Prescribing and dispensing procedures;
- Issuing WADA prohibited drugs; and
- Accessing international medicines information.

8.10 Selection of medicines for athlete treatment at games

The main focus of medical treatment at international games is to provide care for newly acquired injuries or disease rather than treating or diagnosing existing complaints – this is reflected in the list of drugs available for prescribing in the polyclinic. The range of medicines stocked in the pharmacy needs to reflect those known and used by the global medical community as well as those frequently used in the host country.

The medicines formulary is compiled to reflect the specific drug needs of all the medical specialties including sports medicine, dentistry, physiotherapy, podiatry and ophthalmology. A consultation process is usually undertaken with experts in sports medicine and with clinical representatives of the various polyclinic medical departments.

For events such as Commonwealth or Olympic Games a list of around 200 different drugs is available for prescribing within the athlete village by local and visiting team doctors. A smaller list of essential medicines for urgent care is also available for doctors to administer from the medical rooms at competition venues.

At every games, a medicines handbook is published which contains the list of drugs on the formulary and also lists the status of each drug according to the WADA list of prohibited substances. This handbook serves as a primary reference for both local and international prescribing doctors. It also contains specific advice to team doctors about how they access medicines for their team and the prescribing procedures specific to the host country.

Drugs for winter versus summer games

Planning for a pharmacy at a Winter Olympic Games must take into account unique environmental factors such as freezing temperatures and high altitude, and the medical conditions that can result.

At the 2002 Salt Lake City Winter Olympics there were around 11,000 people including spectators treated at 35 medical stations located throughout the venues. There were around 2,000 medical encounters in the Olympic Village polyclinic. The majority of cases were influenza and respiratory infections, but 43 cases of altitude sickness, and 16 cases of frostbite were treated. The relatively moderate altitude of the mountain venues for the Turin 2006 and Sochi 2014 Winter Olympic Games meant that drugs to treat altitude-related conditions were not considered as essential to include.

Tropical and international medicine

With athletes and support staff from over 200 countries living in close proximity in the athlete village, the risk of intercontinental disease transmission exists. The medical services must consider having access to drugs for conditions that may not necessarily be endemic or common in the host country.

At the 1996 Atlanta Games, eight cases of malaria were reported, and there was one case of an athlete with malaria and thrombocytopenia who required hospitalisation. There were also three cases of hepatitis and one case of filariasis. Several athletes requested HIV tests with no positive results. At the 2002 Manchester Commonwealth Games, a purpose-built observation ward in the polyclinic was used for overnight observation of an athlete with malaria, with the pharmacy promptly obtaining the appropriate anti-malarial treatment. This four-bed ward in the polyclinic would be used to quarantine the athlete from the rest of the team should an infectious disease be diagnosed. At the Melbourne 2006 Commonwealth Games, there was one case of malaria, a condition which is rarely seen in Australia.

Rigorous reporting systems are in place to notify public health authorities of suspected medical conditions that might pose a threat to public health. During the Rio 2016 Olympic Games, a dedicated team of public health experts worked closely with the medical services to carefully consider all public health issues during the Games.

Public health issues were of a particular focus of the Rio 2016 Olympic Games, especially relating to the prevalence of the Zika virus in Brazil at the time of the Games. Health advice for athletes, officials, volunteer workforce and other people travelling to Rio for the Games was communicated by the IOC, which provided information on preventative measures and specific cautions relating to pregnant women or couples planning a pregnancy. Additional mosquito eradication measures were undertaken prior to the Games by the Brazil Government health authorities around the Olympic Village and Olympic venue sites across the city to mitigate the potential public health risk posed.

8.11 Patterns of drug use

Elite athletes at international games are in peak physical condition, and are possibly the fittest and healthiest people on Earth. The patterns of therapeutic drug use at these events are therefore very different to those seen in the average community.

The athletes are most focused in the days before the start of competition. For most, participation at the event will be the culmination of years of intense training and the highlight of their sporting career. Their anxiety about maintaining perfect health in the days before competition is understandably high, and obsession for perfect physical state is reflected in the initial demands of the medical services.

At Olympic Games, medical services begin about two weeks before the opening ceremony when the athlete village opens and the athletes start arriving, until a few days after the closing ceremony. Drug usage commonly peaks just before the opening ceremony and continues until the end of the first week of competition. After this time there is typically a gradual decline in dispensed prescriptions until the closing ceremony, then a dramatic drop in drug usage occurs as the athletes start to leave the village. Conversely, the demand for physiotherapy, MRI and ultrasound imaging services increase over the course of the games as injuries in athletes become more prevalent.

During the London 2012 Games a total of 5,200 prescriptions representing 6,849 individual items were dispensed from the polyclinic pharmacies over the Olympic and Paralympic period. Similar to previous Games, the vast majority of items prescribed were for acute conditions. The most commonly prescribed drugs during the 2012 Games are shown in Table 8.1

At the Manchester Commonwealth Games in 2002, antibiotic prescriptions accounted for the majority of the prescriptions dispensed before the start of the competition period. But after the opening ceremony, the daily number of antibiotic prescriptions dropped considerably. This trend might be explained by the possible inappropriate over-prescribing of antibiotics for either prophylactic measures, or very mild respiratory symptoms. The high level of antibiotic prescribing very early at these games illustrates the immediate focus of sports medicine at this level – there can be pressure on prescribers from athletes and coaches to act in some way on the most minor of symptoms to ensure they do not hinder performance. In addition, athletes may be less likely to seek medical attention before their event than after competition.

Table 8.1 Most commonly prescribed medicines during the London 2012 Olympic Games period

Medicine	No. of prescriptions	% of total prescriptions dispensed
Paracetamol (Acetaminophen) 500mg tablets	456	10.95%
Ibuprofen 400mg tablets	162	3.89%
Diclofenac sodium 50mg gastro-resistant tablets	132	3.17%
Ibuprofen 200mg tablets	96	2.30%
Antiseptic throat lozenges	96	2.30%
Amoxicillin 500mg capsules	87	2.09%
Hydrocortisone 1% cream	79	1.90%
Amoxicillin 250mg capsules	78	1.87%
Xylometazoline 0.1% nasal spray	77	1.85%
Cetirizine 10mg tablets	73	1.75%
Loratadine 10mg tablets	72	1.73%
Omeprazole 20mg gastro-resistant capsules	63	1.51%
Diclofenac 1% gel	60	1.44%
Diclofenac sodium 75mg modified-release tablets	57	1.37%

Anti-inflammatory drugs are by far the most commonly prescribed class of drugs for athletes over the course of the games. Diclofenac has long been the drug most prescribed to athletes at Olympic Games, accounting for about half of all the prescriptions for anti-inflammatory drugs.

The use of injectable local anaesthetics and corticosteroids is common for the treatment of sporting injuries affecting the joints. Prescriptions for drugs such as lignocaine and methylprednisolone are commonly dispensed for severe injuries, where they are injected intra-articularly for treatment of acute pain and inflammation. These drugs can be subject to abuse because of their ability to enable an otherwise injury-free athlete to exert themselves past natural pain limits. Such use contravenes sporting ethics and can put the athlete at risk of more serious injury.

Antifungal drugs usually account for a significant number of prescriptions at international sporting events. The use of shared training and changing facilities accounts for a high rate of fungal infections such as 'athlete's foot'. The incidence of fungal infections varies with the seasons and games held in warmer, tropical climates would typically see a higher demand for antifungal drugs. There were a greater proportion of antifungal drugs prescribed at the Sydney 2000 Games than at the much cooler Manchester 2002 Commonwealth Games.

Monitoring illness and injury surveillance

The protection of athletes' health is a key priority at international games and is a fundamental principle of the work of the International Olympic Committee's Medical and Scientific Commission. At recent summer and winter Olympic Games, the IOC has conducted an extensive surveillance study, collecting games-time information about newly acquired injuries and illnesses of athletes, spanning a number of Olympic Games.

Table 8.2 Some results of sports injuries and illnesses at London 2012 Olympic Games (from L. Engebretsen et al. (2013) Sports injuries and illnesses during the London Summer Olympics. *British Journal of Sports Medicine*, 47: 407–414)

Number of athletes competing in the Games = 10,568	
Injuries: 13% of all athletes	
Highest incidences	**%**
Taekwondo	39.1
Football	35.2
BMX	31.3
Handball	21.8
Mountain bike	21.1
Athletics	17.7
Weightlifting	17.5
Illnesses: 7% of all athletes	
Highest incidences	**%**
Beach volley ball	18.8
Synchro swimming	12.5
Football	12.2
Taekwondo	10.9
Athletics	10.5
Sailing	10.0

The injury and illness surveillance data is collected from both the organising committee medical services, and participating team physicians relating to the medical conditions of the athletes they treat.

Selected results from the IOC surveillance of injuries and illnesses at the London 2012 Olympic games are shown in Table 8.2

Of the illnesses, the main bodily systems affected were respiratory (41%), gastro-intestinal (16%) and dermatological (11%), with 46 per cent of all illnesses due to infections.

This data is used to assess safety and risk factors in particular sports and to establish recommendations for prevention strategies to prevent injury. These recommendations may include technical modifications to sporting equipment or improvements to the field-of-play environment for specific sports in order to improve the safety of the athletes that compete in them.

8.12 Importation of drugs for team use

Most teams will bring complete medical kits with them, which will include significant amounts of medicines and injury rehabilitation equipment. All teams will have allocated space within the athlete village to set up their own medical clinics and are provided with secure storage for medicines. Around 80 per cent of all teams at the Sydney 2000 Games bought their own medical teams and drug supplies with them.

Guidance is always given to the participating countries by the games organisers about the legal procedures for importing large quantities of drugs for therapeutic use. The team doctors are usually required to submit detailed lists of imported medicines to the medical services at the games, and to government customs and importation authorities. The importation of performance enhancing drugs and other controlled substances such as narcotics, psychotropics, growth hormones, anabolic steroids and erythropoietin is illegal and is monitored closely during the Olympic period.

8.13 Anti-doping support for local healthcare services

An additional responsibility of the games medical and pharmacy services is to ensure that healthcare professionals in the host city have the necessary information to hand should an athlete seek advice or treatment outside of the athlete village environment.

For the Manchester 2002 Commonwealth Games, an education program containing information about drugs in sport was delivered to pharmacies and emergency departments within the vicinity of the games. For the Beijing 2008 Games, all medical staff working in the city received training to equip them with knowledge about the drugs restricted in sport. Similarly, for the London 2012 Games, local and national pharmacy organisations worked together to distribute information for community and hospital pharmacies to support them during the games should they need to provide care to a competing athlete.

8.14 Summary

In summary, medical and pharmacy services for international games are a complex and integral part of delivering these huge events safely. The design and planning of these services is undertaken many years prior to the games and involves creating new facilities and coordinating local and national healthcare services across the host country. These events present unique professional challenges for healthcare professionals, requiring specialist attention to the safe and effective use of drugs in sport, anti-doping issues and the specific requirements of sports medicine for elite athletes. Games medical and pharmacy services are at the forefront of promoting safe and effective medicines use in sport, and have a key role in the education of athletes and other healthcare professionals in preventing doping in sport.

8.15 Bibliography

Anon. (2002) *Thousands Treated for Medical Needs*. Salt Lake City, Utah, KSL Television & Radio. 15 November 2004; Available at: http://2002.ksl.com/news-6801i.php?p=1

Brennan, R.J., Keim, M.E., Sharp, T.W., Wetterhall, S.F., Williams, R.J., Baker, E.L. et al. (1997) Medical and public health services at the 1996 Atlanta Olympic Games: An overview. *Medical Journal of Australia* 167: 595–598.

Clements A. (2003) Medical support for the greatest show on earth. *The British Travel Health Association Journal* 5: 52–54.

Eaton, S.B., Woodfin, B.A., Askew, J.L., Morrisey, B.M., Elsas, L.J., Shoop, J.L. et al. (1997) The polyclinic at the 1996 Atlanta Olympic Village *Medical Journal of Australia*, 167: 599–602.

Mottram, D. and Stuart M. (2011) Pharmacy planning gains momentum for the Olympic and Paralympic Games. *Pharmaceutical Journal* 286: 77–78.

NSW Health Department (2000) *NSW Health Services for the Sydney 2000 Olympic and Paralympic Games*. Sydney, NSW Health Department.

Stiel D., Trethowan P., Vance N. (1997) Medical planning for the Sydney 2000 Olympic and Paralympic Games. *Medical Journal of Australia* 167: 593–594.

Stuart M. (2012) Delivering pharmacy services for the London 2012 games is no easy task. *Pharmaceutical Journal* 289: 61.

Stuart M. and Mottram D. (2012) The final preparations of pharmacy services for the London 2012 games. *Pharmaceutical Journal* 289: 60.

Stuart, M. and Mottram, D. (2013) The emerging specialty of sports pharmacy. *Aspetar Sports Medicine Journal* 2(1): 66–71.

Stuart, M., Mottram, D., Erskine, D., Simbler, S. and Thomas, T. (2013) Development and delivery of pharmacy services for the London 2012 Olympic and Paralympic Games. *European Journal of Hospital Pharmacy* 20: 42–45.

Stuart, M., Mottram, D. and Thomas, T. (2013) Innovations in Olympic and Paralympic pharmacy services. *British Journal of Sports Medicine* 47: 404–406.

Stuart, M.C. (2005) Pharmacy for elite athletes at international games. In: S.B. Kayne (ed.) *Sport and Exercise Medicine for Pharmacists*. London, Pharmaceutical Press, 269–296.

Sydney Organising Committee of the Olympic Games, Olympic Co-ordination Authority, 2001. *Official Report of the XXVII Olympiad*. Sydney, SOCOG.

Substances and methods prohibited in sport

Chapter 9

Anabolic agents

Neil Chester

9.1 Introduction

Anabolic agents are a classification of substances on the WADA Prohibited List comprising of largely anabolic androgenic steroids (AAS). These substances have become synonymous with the term performance enhancing drugs and remain one of the most prevalent groups of doping agents in sport. In addition, they are widely used by those involved in sport and exercise at a recreational level due to their image-enhancing properties.

Despite the fact that these substances were first developed over 70 years ago, their efficacy is such that they remain a popular choice of doping agent. Whilst research over recent decades has confirmed the anecdotal evidence and belief that many users held in terms of their efficacy, there remains some conjecture regarding their purported side effects. Clearly, research conducted to mirror their use by athletes and recreational users alike is difficult as a consequence of the extremely high, supra-physiological doses administered in practice. However, the availability of sub-standard preparations via the internet has led to much wider public health concerns.

Whilst methods of detection for such substances have developed throughout the years athletes have attempted to circumvent such methods by turning to 'designer steroids'. Such substances are designed to combat current detection methods simply as a consequence of the fact that their existence from a doping control perspective is unknown. In addition the use of endogenous AAS, such as testosterone, androstenedione and dehydroepiandrosterone (DHEA) pose their own specific problems with regards to detection as a consequence of their natural occurrence in the body.

As therapeutic agents AAS use is limited but tends to centre on their anabolic properties. Indeed potential clinical uses include combating cachexia associated with post-operational recovery and conditions such as HIV/AIDS, renal failure, chronic obstructive pulmonary disease (COPD) and burns. In addition, AAS have been used to treat osteoporosis in post-menopausal women and to treat aplastic anaemia.

In addition to AAS, under the classification of anabolic agents on the Prohibited List there are β_2-agonists, including clenbuterol and zilpaterol, selective androgen receptor modulators (SARMs), and tibolone and zeranol (Table 9.1). The selective androgen receptor modulators are a class of pharmacological agents that currently remain under development and offer the advantage over AAS in being selective to specific tissue types.

Table 9.1 Class S1 of the 2017 WADA list of prohibited substances and methods (WADA, 2016a)

S1. Anabolic agents

- Anabolic Androgenic Steroids (AAS)
  - ○ Exogenous AAS
  - ○ Endogenous AAS when administered exogenously
- Other anabolic agents, including but not limited to:

Clenbuterol, selective androgen receptor modulators (SARMs), Tibolone, Zeranol, Zilpaterol.

9.2 Anabolic androgenic steroids

Anabolic androgenic steroids are typically defined as compounds structurally and functionally related to the hormone testosterone. They may be categorised according to whether they exist endogenously or whether they are synthetically derived.

Whilst testosterone was first isolated in 1935 it was soon realised that when administered orally or parentally testosterone was broken down rapidly by the liver by first pass metabolism. This would clearly hamper its use as a therapeutic agent and consequently there was a determination to develop an exogenous AAS that would resist first pass metabolism.

Since the effects of testosterone were believed to be extensive both from an androgenic and anabolic perspective there was great interest in its potential as a therapeutic agent. However, as a non-therapeutic agent its use as an anabolic agent was to be exploited in sport.

Testosterone

Testosterone is the primary male androgenic hormone, responsible for the control of a wide range of processes, most notably the development and maintenance of male characteristics. Such characteristics include those that develop during puberty, such as growth of the penis and testes and the development of secondary sex characteristics, such as body hair growth particularly that of facial, pubic and axillary hair and deepening of the voice, as a consequence of vocal cord thickening and enlargement of the larynx. Testosterone is produced largely in the testes by the Leydig cells (95%) but also by the adrenal glands and via conversion from weaker androgens such as androstenedione (also produced by the adrenal glands) in the periphery. It is also present in females and is produced in much smaller amounts by the ovaries, the adrenal glands and via the conversion of androstenedione produced by the adrenal glands. After puberty, plasma testosterone levels are approximately 250 to 1,045ng. dl^{-1} in males and 1 to 44ng.dl^{-1} in women with levels declining steadily in males over the age of 60 years (Salameh et al., 2010). As with males, testosterone has an important role in the development and maintenance of lean body mass (i.e. muscle and bone) in females. Testosterone also affects the central nervous system (CNS) and has a significant role to play in human behaviour, particularly sexual behaviour, namely libido.

Whilst testosterone is considered the primary androgen, it is by no means the only one, with a number of androgens serving important roles in both the development and maintenance of sex determining characteristics. Several weak androgens are synthesised by the adrenal cortex, most notably dehydroepiandrosterone (DHEA) and androstenedione (Andro).

In females these act as an important circulating pool of more potent androgen precursors and their conversion is via several intracellular enzymes (Figure 9.1). After testosterone, 5α-dihydrotestosterone (DHT) is probably the most notable androgen and with a greater affinity to the androgen receptor (AR) it has a direct role in the development of secondary sex characteristics. Indeed testosterone typically acts as a precursor to DHT in reproductive tissue and the skin where the presence of 5α-reductase mediates its conversion, promoting prostate gland and hair growth respectively.

The presence of androgens at a cellular level is determined by enzyme action. In addition to the intracellular enzyme, 5α-reductase in the skin and reproductive tissue the presence of aromatase converts testosterone into oestradiol (Figure 9.1) in adipose tissue. In skeletal muscle, however, 5α-reductase is undetectable (Thigpen et al., 1993) and therefore testosterone exerts its effect directly via ARs. Thus, not only is the presence of ARs important in determining the effects of androgens, but so too is the expression of specific enzymes.

The immediate precursor of testosterone in the biosynthetic sequence is androstenedione, which is converted to testosterone via the action of 17β hydroxysteroid dehydrogenase (Figure 9.1). This enzyme also acts on other steroids with similar structures, including 19-norandrostenedione, to form 19-nor testosterone otherwise known as nandrolone (Figure 9.1).

Testosterone production is controlled by the hypothalamic-pituitary-gonadal axis. Specifically, testosterone is produced in response to luteinising hormone (LH) and follicle-stimulating hormone (FSH) secreted by the pituitary gland. Gonadotropin-releasing hormone (GnRH) produced by the hypothalamus stimulates the release of LH and FSH from the pituitary gland. This integrated system enables regulatory feedback control, whereby increased levels of circulating testosterone inhibit the release of GnRH, LH and FSH. Androgen production from the adrenal gland is, however, less clear. Control, nevertheless involves adrenocorticotropin (ACTH) as well as other factors including gonadal sex steroids, insulin, growth hormone and other signalling molecules (Alesci et al., 2001).

Testosterone circulates in the bloodstream either freely (approximately 2 to 3%) or bound to proteins such as sex hormone-binding globulin (SHBG) or albumin. Testosterone bound to SHBG (approximately 44%; Dunn et al., 1981) is essentially inactive due to the high binding affinity of these molecules and the fact that in this state testosterone is unable to penetrate the cell walls of target cells. However, free testosterone and that which is weakly bound to albumin is deemed to be bioavailable since in its free form it may penetrate the cell wall and bind with the AR.

9.3 Pharmacology of anabolic androgenic steroids

The structural modifications of testosterone to create synthetic AAS have been introduced in order to achieve one or more of the following: maximise anabolic effects; minimise androgenic effects; increase metabolic half-life; limit first pass metabolism; and reduce absorption rate from an intramuscular depot. Clearly, such modifications aim to improve both the efficacy of testosterone as an anabolic agent and its mode of administration. Whilst the anabolic potency, compared to testosterone, may have been increased in some AAS, the disassociation from androgenic effects has not been achieved and therefore as performance and image enhancing drugs (PIED) they all carry potential androgenic side-effects.

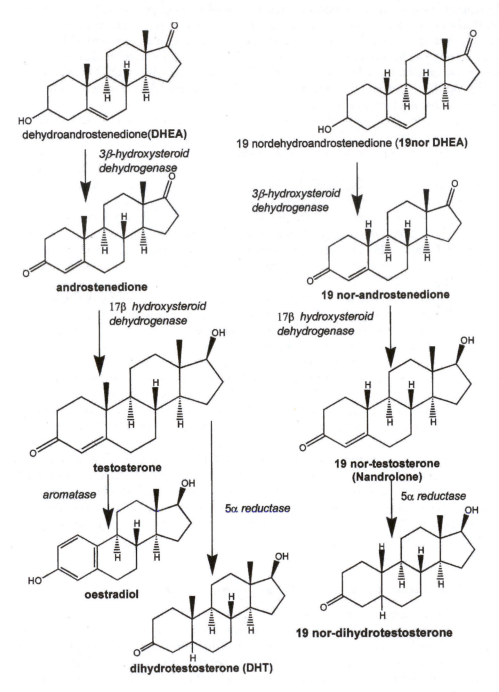

Figure 9.1 The formation of testosterone and its derivatives (George and Mottram, 2011; p. 52)

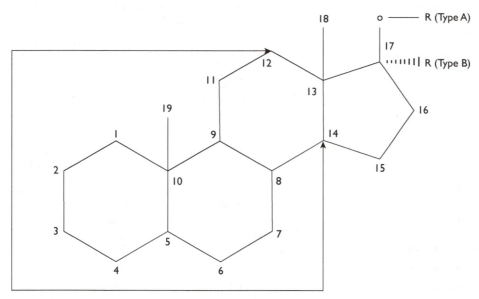

Type C substitution at any point

Figure 9.2 The molecular structure of testosterone illustrating the major sites of modification in the formation of synthetic anabolic androgenic steroids (adapted from Wilson, 1988)

Testosterone has a 19-carbon skeleton consisting of four fused rings, which may be commonly modified at three positions to create synthetic AAS (Figure 9.2; positions A, B and C). Such modifications include esterification of the 17-β-hydroxyl group (A) to form a group of AAS collectively known as testosterone esters. Testosterone esters have enhanced lipid solubility and when administered intramuscularly they are released slowly into the circulation thus enabling prolonged activity and reduced hepatotoxicity. Alkylation at the 17-α position (B) produces 17α-alkylated AAS, which are orally active due to their ability to limit first-pass metabolism. Structural modifications to other positions on the testosterone skeleton (C) will tend to increase anabolic potency. Examples of AAS categorised according to their modification and route of administration are provided in Table 9.2.

Besides oral or parenteral administration via injection, AAS may also be administered topically as gels or creams. Unmodified testosterone is available as a dermal gel or patch, which must be administered daily due to its short half-life (Table 9.2).

In addition to testosterone, the naturally occurring 18-carbon AAS, 19-nortestosterone (otherwise known as nandrolone) is considered a doping agent and so too are its modifications particularly its decanoate ester known as Deca-durabolin (Table 9.2). As a PIED nandrolone is attractive since it has less androgenic effects in comparison to other AAS as it is not converted to DHT and its 5α-reductase metabolite, 19 nor-dihydrotestosterone, has a low binding affinity to the AR (Toth and Zakar, 1982).

Table 9.2 Categorisation of AAS according to their route of administration and their structural modification from testosterone (adapted from Clark, 2009)

AAS	Trade name	Route of administration
Unmodified testosterone		
Testosterone	Androgel, Testim	Topical gel
Testosterone	Androderm, Testoderm	Dermal patch
Testosterone esters		
Testosterone enanthate	Delatetryl	Intramuscular injection
Testosterone cypionate	Depo-Testosterone	Intramuscular injection
Testosterone propionate	–	Intramuscular injection
17α-alkylated AAS		
Methyltestosterone	Android, Virilon	Oral
Fluoxymesterone	Halostestin	Oral
Stanozolol	Winstrol	Oral
Methandrostenelone	Dianabol	Oral
19-nor testosterone esters		
Nandrolone deconate	Deca-durabolin	Intramuscular injection
Nandrolone phenylproprionate	Durabolin	Intramuscular injection

9.4 Clinical uses of anabolic androgenic steroids

Despite the wide-ranging effects of AAS in terms of stimulating not only muscle growth but also bone and red blood cell production their current use in clinical settings is limited. Whilst the traditional use of AAS was to promote muscle growth in those with degenerative conditions their effectiveness has been questioned. Indeed, since the late 1980s the licence of many AAS has been removed. Remaining AAS are typically used in hormone replacement therapy in males with hypogonadism. However, the use of AAS to combat muscle atrophy has been reconsidered. Both testosterone esters and 17α-alkylated steroids may now be considered useful therapeutic agents for the treatment of muscle wastage associated with HIV/AIDS, severe burns and renal failure (Basaria et al., 2001). Nevertheless, although evidence exists to support AAS use in post-operative recovery and in those with chronic conditions such as HIV/AIDS, further research is needed to establish the effects of sustained use on health and wellbeing before clear recommendations can be made (Woerdeman and de Ronde, 2011).

9.5 Anabolic androgenic steroids as performance- and image-enhancing agents

Despite the wealth of anecdotal evidence supporting the efficacy of AAS as performance enhancers, it has only been in recent decades that the scientific community has provided confirmation. Indeed, until the landmark study by Bhasin et al. (1996), research involving AAS had significant shortcomings, which limited its potential for making a significant impact on the field. Work by Bhasin et al. (1996) was able to clearly demonstrate that individuals who were not deficient in testosterone could increase both muscle mass and function following the administration of supraphysiological doses of testosterone enanthate. Their work was also able to shed light on the likely mechanisms involved in such enhancement. Whilst exercise training was shown to have an additive effect on muscle growth and function, significant increases were still demonstrated in those who did not perform exercise training. These findings suggested that AAS were able to exert their effects by traditional genomic action via the AR without the need for anti-catabolic effects.

As regards genomic action, AAS bind with the AR and through interaction with the DNA mediate transcription thus leading to protein synthesis. AAS passively diffuse into the cell of target tissues and bind to the AR and translocate into the nucleus and link with additional AAS-AR complexes to form homo-dimers. DNA binding domains on the AR then bind with steroid response elements on the DNA and, with the addition of co-regulators, gene activation is initiated. Gene activation then leads to gene transcription, translation and ultimately the production of contractile protein and muscle hypertrophy.

The potential anti-catabolic effect relates to the fact that the release of cortisol in response to heavy exercise has a catabolic effect as regards skeletal muscle. Cortisol is released from the adrenal cortex in response to stress to aid energy provision. This is achieved by promoting gluconeogenesis in the liver and the provision of gluconeogenic substrate in the form of protein through the breakdown of skeletal muscle. Clearly, the ability of AAS to limit the effects of cortisol might have a profound effect on skeletal muscle growth and function. It has been suggested that AAS act as antagonists to glucocorticoid receptors thus reducing the effects of cortisol. However, by and large AAS are considered to have a low binding affinity to glucocorticoid receptors (Hickson et al., 1990). It is now thought that AAS might affect gene expression of glucocorticoid receptors (Kicman, 2008).

Clearly, hypertrophy through genomic pathways is reliant on the apparatus within myonuclei. Muscle fibres contain hundreds of myonuclei however, there is thought to be a ceiling in terms of the level of skeletal muscle hypertrophy, supported by a finite number of myonuclei. It is therefore suggested that by increasing myonuclei number, AAS are able to enhance hypertrophy (Kadi, 2008).

Research recently has provided evidence in support of the view held by many that the performance enhancing effects of AAS last for much longer than the period of administration. Egner et al. (2013) demonstrated, in an animal model, that increased myonuclei numbers following the administration of AAS are not lost during atrophy in response to AAS abstinence and that following subsequent training there was significant hypertrophy compared to a control group. This research suggests that the increased myonuclei are an important reserve that directly relate to hypertrophic potential, which is much greater in those that have used AAS. Further research is clearly needed to determine whether these findings might be transferable to humans. If this is found to be the case then it would be particularly significant from an anti-doping perspective in terms of the consideration of appropriate sanctions imposed on those caught misusing AAS (i.e. challenging the length of ban from competition).

Whilst the work by Bhasin and colleagues (1996) was able to show unequivocally that AAS were effective as a PIED, the mechanisms by which this result is achieved are complex. It is likely that positive results in terms of muscle hypertrophy and improvements in function are as a consequence of a combination of both physiological and behavioural responses. In addition to the mechanisms directly within skeletal muscle, activation of the CNS via AR and non-genomic actions to promote psychological effects may be particularly useful as an indirect mechanism by increasing exercise train-ing intensity and volume (Kicman, 2008).

AAS, known to play an important role in sexual behaviour in both male and females, are also believed to be important in elevating mood and reducing depression. Conversely, reports of increased aggression in those misusing AAS (Yates et al., 1992) might be useful to promote increased exercise tolerance and competitiveness in the sporting arena.

9.6 Adverse effects following anabolic androgenic steroid use

As the mismatch between anecdotal and scientific evidence in support of AAS as effective ergogenic aids fuelled the mistrust between users and the scientific and medical community so has the limited scientific evidence with regards to potential serious adverse health effects. The general acceptance by the medical community that AAS are indeed hazardous is a clear attempt to discourage non-therapeutic use of AAS.

Nevertheless, whilst the paucity of conclusive evidence to link AAS use directly with serious health effects remains, scientific evidence appears to be growing in support of many of the initial claims. However, a difficulty remains, in terms of good scientific evidence, due to the constraints relating to ethics and controlling many of the confounding variables that exist including concomitant supplement use and the practice of polypharmacy amongst users, and the difficulty in establishing the authenticity of products used.

The adverse effects associated with AAS use in humans have been reported in a number of ways, including: surveys, case studies and placebo-controlled trials involving subjects with hypogonadism. Despite the obvious shortcomings of such research, evidence surround-ing the effects of AAS is building as their use becomes more widespread. Nevertheless, pro-spective, longitudinal studies are required to address the possible development of pathology following long-term AAS use.

The main reported side effects of AAS use are widespread and may be categorised accordingly.

Liver effects

The 17 α-alkylated AAS would appear to offer the largest threat to liver damage as a con-sequence of first pass metabolism. Hepatotoxicity attributed to AAS use may take several forms including transient elevations in liver enzyme concentrations, cholestasis, vascular injury and hepatic tumours. Numerous studies have reported increased concentrations of liver enzymes amongst AAS users (Sanchez-Osorio et al., 2008; Nasr and Ahmad, 2009). Whilst raised hepatic enzymes may signal toxicity they may fall over time and hide the real extent of injury during prolonged AAS exposure. Alternatively, raised hepatic enzymes may simply reflect muscle damage as a consequence of heavy training (Hoffman and Ratamess, 2006). However, in those with liver damage other symptoms may predominate such as jaun-dice and pruritus (itchiness) (Sanchez-Osorio et al., 2008; Elsharkawy et al., 2012). Such symptoms are typical of cholestasis, a condition where there is retention of bile in the biliary capillaries of the hepatic lobules. Whilst there are reports of vascular injury in individuals using AAS these tend to be rare. The condition of peliosis hepatis is a vascular condition, which is characterised by the development of blood filled cysts throughout the liver and has been reported in numerous cases involving AAS use (Cabasso, 1994). Reports of carcinomas attributed to AAS use are uncommon and only the result of prolonged use (Shahidi, 2001).

Cardiovascular effects

Numerous reports have shown that the use of AAS has a diverse effect on the cardiovascular system. The most severe effects include death, as a consequence of cardiovascular disease (CD), and there is a developing body of evidence to link such events with chronic AAS use (Angell et al., 2012a; Montisci et al., 2012). Evidence of CD is based upon incidence of acute myocardial infarction, heart failure, coronary disease or cerebrovascular accidents (i.e. stroke) all reported via case studies.

There is a growing body of research that links AAS use with CD and the prevalence of numerous CD risk factors however the mechanisms behind such effects are unclear (Angell et al., 2012b). Reports of the incidence of hypertension (Freed et al., 1975; Kuipers et al., 1991; Riebe et al., 1992), adverse blood lipid profiles (Lenders et al., 1988; Lane et al., 2006), cardiac hypertrophy (Sachtleben et al., 1993; Angell et al., 2012c) and ECG abnormalities (Maior et al., 2013) amongst AAS users are numerous; however, there is a distinct lack of more controlled prospective cohort studies which are necessary to establish possible causal mechanisms.

Reproductive system effects

Hypogonadotrophic hypogonadism is a side effect of AAS use as a consequence of the hypothalamic negative feedback loop responding to increased circulating androgens. Testicular atrophy and impaired spermatogenesis are symptomatic of reduced release of gonadotrophins. In females, suppressed secretion of gonadotrophins leads to menstrual irregularities and increased circulating androgens leads to clitoral hypertrophy following long-term AAS use. The inhibition of spermatogenesis may persist for many months after AAS withdrawal; however, such side effects are deemed to be reversible. Similarly, in females the menstrual cycle will recommence soon after AAS use is discontinued. However, side effects such as clitoral hypertrophy appear to be less reversible (Clark, 2009).

Cosmetic effects

Cosmetic effects are most pronounced in females as AAS result in an overall masculinising effect, which may be irreversible following the discontinuation of the drugs (Clark, 2009). These effects include hirsuitism and deepening of the voice. Chronic use of AAS may produce male pattern baldness, which has been reported in both males and females. Acne is a common condition reported by many AAS users due to androgenic stimulation of the sebaceous gland.

High dose AAS regimes practised by males may ironically result in high levels of circulating oestrogens as a consequence of aromatisation of androgens. High levels of oestrogen may result in gynecomastia, which is the development of breast tissue. Consequently, users will often co-administer Tamoxifen, a selective oestrogen receptor modulator (SERM), to combat such side effects (see Chapter 12).

Psychological effects

One of the most reported side effects attributed to AAS misuse is that relating to the CNS. Increased aggression may be regarded as a positive effect in terms of facilitating increased training load. However, numerous reports have cited episodes of aggression, violence and mania as common amongst AAS users (Pope and Katz, 1988). During abstinence from AAS, users have been reported to exhibit anxiety and depression (Kanayama et al., 2009), deemed to be attributed to the low circulating levels of endogenous AAS as a consequence of reduced production occurring in light of prior sustained circulating exogenous AAS. Opposing views are that those exhibiting marked changes in mood and behaviour are predisposed to such psychological effects, which are only heightened with AAS use (van Amsterdam et al., 2010).

Additional side effects

Amongst adolescents the administration of AAS can result in the premature closure of epiphyseal growth plates and thus lead to stunted growth (Johnson, 1990). Other musculo-skeletal issues relate to the potential for AAS to inflict problems associated with ligament and tendon damage (Giannotti et al., 2014). This is thought to be associated with the development of dysplasia of collagen fibrils, thus decreasing the tensile strength of tendons (Laseter and Russell, 1991) and the disproportionate loading related with increases in muscle strength (Wood et al., 1988).

Side effects that are prevalent amongst AAS users that are not directly related to the doping agent per se include those associated with inappropriate drug administration. Needle sharing and use of non-sterile equipment is a particular issue amongst AAS users, which poses serious risks in terms of infection and the acquisition of blood-borne diseases such as hepatitis and HIV/AIDS (Hope et al., 2013).

Possibly the greatest risk to AAS users are the unknown health risks associated with the use of products obtained from the illicit market. The illicit market contains drugs that are no longer licenced, those that are marketed as veterinary products, new drugs that have not been fully tested and AAS that have not been authorised but developed as part of pharmaceutical research projects (Evans-Brown et al., 2012). In addition to a wide range of AAS that do not carry with them the required safety checks and information that exists with licenced products there are real concerns relating to the sterility and authenticity of such products.

9.7 Use of anabolic androgenic steroids in sport

Whilst there is uncertainty as to who were the first to use AAS in sports competition it is suggested that the 1950s heralded the beginnings of their use in sport (Dimeo, 2007). In 1954 it is alleged that Russian athletes under the influence of AAS won numerous gold medals in the World Weightlifting Championships in Vienna. Throughout the 1950s and 1960s AAS use escalated and whilst the IOC introduced the first list of prohibited substances in 1967 it was not until 1976 that AAS were added to the list following the development of a reliable test for their detection in urine in 1974.

Following the reunification of Germany in 1990 it was revealed that the German Democratic Republic (GDR; the former state of East Germany) had run a systematic doping programme as part of their state-run sports programme. This programme, which was supported and financed by the state, ran from the mid-1960s, throughout the 1970s and 1980s and was instrumental in the success of GDR in international sports competitions throughout this period. Hundreds of scientists and physicians were involved in both

research and administering AAS and other doping agents to athletes with the sole purpose of improving sports performance and raising the profile of the nation on a world
stage (Franke and Berondonk, 1997). Particular emphasis was placed on females and their
performance where the effects of AAS are more pronounced. The real impact of such a
programme is, however, illustrated by the incidence of serious doping-related side effects,
many of which are irreversible.

Probably one of the most well-known cases of AAS use in sport is that of the Canadian
track and field athlete Ben Johnson at the 1988 Olympics in Seoul. Having been crowned
champion of the 100m he was subsequently stripped of his medal after failing a routine post-
competition drugs test. He tested positive for the AAS, stanozolol and put the issue of drug
use in sport firmly in the spotlight. As a consequence Charles Dubin, a Canadian lawyer,
was charged with leading a Canadian inquiry into the use of drugs in sport, otherwise known
as the Dubin Inquiry. The inquiry was to last one year and included the admission of AAS
use by 48 athletes (including Johnson) and recommendations that would help to improve
doping control globally through increased and improved drug testing and stricter penalties
for those who violate the rules (Moriarty et al., 1992).

In more recent times designer steroids have become a particular issue in elite sport. They
are designed specifically to circumvent routine anti-doping tests as their existence as doping agents is unknown. Indeed such is the covert nature of their manufacture and use that
they only become 'detectable' when the particular substance falls into the hands of anti-
doping personnel. In the early part of this century several international athletes, including
sprinters Marion Jones, Dwain Chambers and Kellie White, were convicted for the use of
tetrahydrogestrinone (THG), a designer steroid. This case was part of what became known
as the BALCO affair whereby a newly developed AAS was manufactured and distributed to
numerous athletes from the Bay Area Laboratory Cooperative (BALCO) in California, led
by its founder, Victor Conte (see Section 9.9).

Other than use by elite athletes and in competitive sport there is evidence of growing,
widespread use of AAS at a recreational level including among those engaged in gym
exercise and bodybuilding. Clearly a large extent of the bodybuilding culture is based
upon the use of and experimentation with drugs, particularly AAS. Indeed much of the
information we know regarding efficacy and adverse health effects is centred upon the
anecdotal evidence obtained from the gym community. The growth in the use of AAS
within the bodybuilding fraternity would appear to have followed a similar path to the
one we see in elite sport. However, with increased media focus on image and the ideal
body, coupled with increased accessibility to illicit products, via the internet, it would
seem that the market amongst recreational users is burgeoning (Evans-Brown et al., 2012;
see Chapter 26).

Sources, supply and control of Anabolic Androgenic Steroids

Clearly use of AAS is directly associated with supply and their control from a legal perspective. In the UK AAS are controlled as class C drugs under the Misuse of Drugs Act 1971.
Whilst it is illegal to possess these drugs with the intent to supply, it is not an offence to
possess for personal use. The control measures for AAS varies between different countries,
with some legislating specifically against the use of doping agents in sport. Nevertheless, the
supply of such drugs has never been greater, with the internet opening up a global market in
the trade of illicit products.

The illicit market consists of products that may come from several sources. Products that are deemed to be legitimate may be manufactured in countries where the purchase of such non-prescription drugs is legal or where products have entered the market as a result of theft. Alternatively, products may be manufactured in clandestine laboratories outside of any regulatory system (Evans-Brown et al., 2009).

The trade in substandard and counterfeit products is a particular problem. Such products are a significant health concern since their quality and thus safety cannot be guaranteed. In addition to the sub-standard manufacturing of many products there is a real issue concerning counterfeiting, that is deliberately mislabelling products so there are no assurances that the alleged ingredients are present and in the correct quantity. This issue has been highlighted extensively in the research literature (Graham et al., 2009; Evans-Brown et al., 2009) and appears to be a particular issue with respect to nutritional supplements (see Chapter 24).

In a report by the UK Advisory Council on the Misuse of Drugs (ACMD) recommendations were put forward to maintain the current legal classification whereby criminal prosecution is limited to those dealing, supplying, manufacturing and trafficking AAS. In addition improved education and harm reduction programmes should be introduced to support those engaged in non-therapeutic AAS use (ACMD, 2010).

Patterns of administration

Anabolic steroids are broadly available as three types of preparation, oral, oil-based or water-based injections and also available as topical gels or patches. Oral preparations have a structure resistant to breakdown by stomach acid, can be absorbed by the gastrointestinal tract and tend to withstand total breakdown by liver enzymes, however they have a short half-life and require frequent dosing. Injectable oil-based preparations have a longer half-life but produce a degree of pain at the injection site, have a slow absorption rate into the blood stream, so that lower concentrations pass through the liver, thereby reducing liver toxicity. Injectable water-based steroids have a long half-life, though normally less than oil-based preparations, produce less discomfort at the site of injection and can be mixed with other water-based steroids or other drugs (George and Mottram, 2011). Topical gels (or creams) or patches result in low dose administration of un-modified testosterone which has a short half-life requiring daily application.

There are a number of administration regimes in use, known as 'cycling', 'pyramiding' and 'stacking'. Experienced users will typically follow a combination of these regimes concurrently. Each regime is reputed to offer a particular advantage in terms of heightening the effect of a particular drug (or drugs) or limiting the potential side effects experienced. However, there is no scientific evidence to support such regimes.

Cycling is the administration of a particular drug over a period of time followed by a period of abstinence before the administration is recommenced. Cycling patterns are typically short (i.e. six to eight weeks of administration followed by six to eight weeks of abstinence) or long (i.e. six to eighteen weeks of administration followed by up to 12 months of abstinence). The rationale behind cycling is that the periods of abstinence may reduce the incidence of side effects.

Pyramiding is a variation of cycling whereby the dose is gradually increased during the cycle to a peak and then gradually reduced towards the end of the cycle. This regime allegedly results in fewer behavioural side effects caused by rapid withdrawal of the drug, such as lowered mood.

Stacking is a word used to describe the use of more than one AAS at a time. In its simplest form, this regime might involve the simultaneous use of both an orally administered steroid and an injectable one. More sophisticated regimes involve intricate schedules of administration using many different AAS, each with supposedly different pharmacological profiles. The aim of this technique is to avoid the development of tolerance to a particular drug (George and Mottram, 2011). In addition to AAS, common ancillary drugs include growth hormone, clenbuterol, insulin, insulin-like growth factor-1 (IGF-1), human chorionic gonadotrophin (HCG), ephedrine and tamoxifen, of which some will be taken for their alleged synergistic action whilst others because of their ability to combat unwanted side effects.

9.8 Prevalence of anabolic androgenic steroid use

As with all illicit drug use, it is difficult to establish an accurate indication of how prevalent AAS use is within sport. Most evidence in elite sport comes from data obtained from WADA-accredited laboratories, which highlights on a yearly basis the number of positive drug tests, according to the specific anabolic agent (Table 9.3). Whilst such data cannot provide an accurate estimate of absolute numbers administering AAS, they do reveal quite clearly that AAS remain an important choice for those looking to enhance sports performance illegally. Recent data suggests that AAS comprise half of all adverse analytical findings and atypical findings reported by WADA-accredited laboratories (WADA 2016b).

Table 9.3 Prohibited anabolic agents identified by WADA-accredited laboratories in 2015 (WADA, 2016b)

Anabolic agent	Occurrences	Per cent within class
• Anabolic Androgenic Steroids (AAS)		
Stanozalol	296	21.5%
Nandrolone metabolites	176	12.8%
Methandienone	143	10.4%
Drostanolone	124	9.0%
Dehydrochloromethyl-testosterone	91	6.6%
Metenolone	82	6.0%
Trenbolone	74	5.4%
Boldenone	60	4.4%
Oxandrolone	47	3.4%
Mesterolone	29	2.1%
Clostebol	14	1.0%
Others	238	17.3%
• Other anabolic agents, including but not limited to:		
Clenbuterol	314	88.7%
SARM (Ostarine or S-22)	28	7.9%
Tibolone	7	2.0%
SARM (Andarine)	2	0.6%
SARM (LGD-4033)	2	0.6%
Ractopamine	1	0.3%

Clearly, these figures do not reflect the true extent of AAS use in sport, particularly that at a sub-elite and recreational level. Use of AAS appears to be a significant problem in collegiate sport in the United States (Buckley et al., 1988; Berning et al., 2004; McCabe et al., 2007). Buckley et al. (1988) reported that 6.6 per cent of male high school seniors (aged 17 to 19 years old) had used AAS, however approximately 30 per cent of users did not participate in organised sport. Nevertheless, McCabe et al. (2007) were able to demonstrate that those who participated in collegiate sport were more likely to use AAS compared to their non-athletic counterparts. The structure of sport in the United States, in comparison with Europe, is such that collegiate sport is extremely popular for participants and spectators alike. Indeed collegiate sport regularly features on US television and the importance placed on success clearly heightens the pressure on young athletes and the likelihood that they may turn to performance-enhancing drugs (Calfee and Fadale, 2006).

Anecdotal evidence would suggest that AAS use is widespread amongst those engaged in recreational sport, and numerous reports suggest that it is a developing public health issue (Evans-Brown et al., 2012). Indeed, with the increased media attention on body image there is a burgeoning market for products aimed at developing musculature and reducing body fat (see Chapter 26). This growth is also reflected amongst children with 0.6 per cent of boys and 0.3 per cent of girls reporting having used AAS according to a survey administered to 7,242 English school children (boys: n = 3,646 and girls: n = 3,596; Omole, 2011). In the United States prevalence rates would appear to be higher, with 2.7 per cent of children attending middle schools (aged 9 to 13 years old) indicating that they had used AAS (Faigenbaum et al., 1998).

The first study to examine the extent of AAS use in the UK was by Korkia (1994). Of 21 gymnasia that were surveyed across five regions throughout the UK, including London, Merseyside, Edinburgh, Glasgow and Swansea, 1,669 questionnaires were returned and used in the study. Use of AAS was reported in all regions, with a total of 7.7 per cent of gym users admitting to taking AAS, of which 5 per cent were current users (6% males and 1.4% females). In a more recent study in Germany, Striegel et al. (2006) found that from a sample of 621 fitness centre visitors 13.5 per cent reported the use of 'anabolic ergogenic substances' (of which 83.6% were AAS), comprising 19.2 per cent males and 3.9 per cent females.

Over recent years there appears to have been an increase in the 'drive for muscularity' amongst adolescents (McCreary and Sasse, 2000) but also the general population. This would seem to be as a consequence of the way in which the media portray health and attractiveness particularly from the perspective of the male body form. Indeed, there is evidence of increased prevalence of body dissatisfaction and low self-esteem amongst males with respect to the level of musculature, which has been termed muscle dysmorphia (Pope et al., 1997). The focus on enhanced musculature is coupled with an increase in the use of image-enhancing drugs such as AAS (Kanayama et al., 2006), particularly amongst gym users. Unfortunately, as with elite sport, it is difficult to establish reliable figures in terms of prevalence of AAS use. Data from harm reduction programmes, such as needle exchange clinics, offer some indication to the extent of use. In addition to examining AAS use in gymnasia, Korkia (1994) also surveyed syringe exchange clinics. Of the 88 clinics that responded 59 per cent declared that AAS users had contact with the clinic. Later, McVeigh and colleagues (2003) revealed an increase in individuals attending syringe exchange clinics in the northwest of England (Cheshire and Merseyside) for AAS injecting equipment between the years 1991 and 2001. Such increases cannot necessarily be attributed to increased AAS use but clearly illustrate the success of harm reduction programmes in attracting different types of recreational drug users.

9.9 Designer steroids

The term 'designer steroids' first became widely recognised in response to the BALCO affair during the early part of this century. The term refers to the use and development of AAS, specifically to evade detection by anti-doping authorities. Tetrahydrogestrinone (THG), otherwise known as 'the clear', was supplied as a sublingual AAS preparation by BALCO, a US-based company, to athletes for the purpose of enhancing performance. Since THG was never marketed, its existence from an anti-doping perspective was unknown and it was therefore undetectable during routine doping control analysis. Indeed, its existence as a performance-enhancing agent was only possible as a consequence of a 'whistle-blower' who alerted the anti-doping authorities, who were then able to determine its molecular structure and subsequently establish a method for its detection (Catlin et al., 2004). Several high profile athletes tested positive for THG (including the British sprinter Dwain Chambers) and many others were implicated in the affair (including US sprinters Marion Jones and Kelli White) and consequently received sanctions including suspension from competition. In addition to track and field athletes, American football players tested positive for THG and baseball players were implicated in the affair. In addition several athletes were convicted of perjury under state law, in the US. Victor Conte and several coaches were convicted for their part in the distribution of AAS to athletes and received sanctions under state law, including imprisonment.

In addition to DHT, other designer steroids were identified at around the same time, including norbolethone (Catlin et al., 2002) and desoxymethyltestosterone (DMT; Sekera et al., 2005). Desoxymethyltestosterone was also known as Madol and was patented in 1961 but never approved for clinical use in human patients. Probably the first designer steroid, however, was dehydrochloromethyltestosterone (otherwise known as Turinabol), which was used by former-GDR athletes as part of their state-run doping programme (Parr and Schanzer, 2010).

The recent cases involving designer steroids have led to heightened vigilance by anti-doping organisations and WADA-accredited laboratories clearly improving the prospect of early detection. Nevertheless, the most important issue relates to the fact that as un-marketed steroids there is limited, if any, toxicology data and thus safety information. Their use by athletes therefore poses a significant, yet unknown threat to health.

9.10 Prohormones

Prohormones refer to a group of substances that are precursors to steroid hormones and are now accepted as hormones and indeed AAS in their own right. The prohormones, andros-tenedione (Andro) and dehydroepiandrostenedione (DHEA) are endogenous hormones produced by the gonads and adrenal gland and form an important circulating pool of steroid hormone precursors.

Administration of exogenous prohormones is thought to enhance the circulating pool of steroid precursors and thus increase the subsequent biotransformation into testosterone. Increased circulating testosterone is then thought to impact positively on skeletal muscle hypertrophy and function. Unfortunately, the scientific literature does not confirm these hypotheses. Whilst there is evidence to show that the ingestion of prohormones can increase the circulating levels of DHEA and Andro, resultant significant elevations in the circulat-ing pool of testosterone has only been demonstrated in females (Morales et al., 1998).

This could be explained by the fact that in females a significant proportion (up to 100 per cent) of circulating testosterone is as a consequence of peripheral conversion of weaker androgens, namely DHEA (Labrie et al., 2005). However, in males, circulating testosterone is almost entirely based upon its production in the gonads (and to a lesser extent by the adrenal cortex) (Kicman, 2008).

Despite the positive outcomes, in terms of increased circulating testosterone in females, there has been no indication that this might manifest itself in gains in muscle size and strength (King et al., 1999). The efficacy of prohormones as PIEDs is further weakened by the evidence by some scientists that they may induce a number of negative side effects. King et al. (1999) revealed an adverse effect on blood lipid profiles and increased levels of circulating oestrogens following the administration of 300mg.d[-1] administration of Andro over an eight-week period.

Prohormones are commonly included as ingredients in, and marketed as, nutritional sports supplements in order to avoid the necessary controls required in the manufacture and sale of pharmaceutical products. As sports supplements they are available from sports supplements shops and via the internet and used amongst the sports and fitness community. Clearly, such widespread availability poses problems in terms of both the intentional and unintentional use of AAS in elite athletes and potential failed drug tests as a consequence.

9.11 Detection of anabolic androgenic steroids

Detection of exogenous AAS is generally based upon direct quantification of a particular AAS and its metabolites in urine. However, in the case of endogenous AAS it is reliant on the investigation of various steroid profiles in order to establish possible androgen misuse. The concentration of testosterone and its stereoisomer, epitestosterone, is determined together with additional endogenous androgens, including androsterone, etiocholanolone, 5α-androstane-3α,17β-diol (5αAdiol) and 5β-androstane-3α,17β-diol (5βAdiol). In addition to reporting endogenous AAS, ratios of several endogenous androgens are also determined, including the ratio of testosterone to epitestosterone (T:E), androsterone to testosterone (A:T), 5αAdiol to 5βdiol and 5αAdiol to epitestosterone. An individual steroid profile is established as part of the steroidal module of the Athlete Biological Passport (see Chapter 5). Alteration of the endogenous androgens or ratios may constitute doping and further confirmatory analysis maybe warranted (WADA, 2015).

The endogenous AAS, 19-norandrosterone also poses its own unique problem in that it may also be present in urine as a metabolite of the exogenous AAS 19-nortestosterone. A urinary threshold for 19-norandrosterone is therefore set a 2ng.ml[-1].

Micro-dosing using topical application of testosterone via dermal patches and gels is a particular concern to anti-doping personnel not least because of the short half-life of the drug and thus the potential to evade a positive drugs test.

Clearly the introduction of out-of-competition drug testing was in some way effective in catching those administering exogenous AAS (or in acting as a deterrent to potential users) since the use of AAS as PIED is most effective during training and in the lead-up to competition. Before the advent of out-of-competition testing many athletes would therefore simply abstain from use leading up to a competition in order to avoid detection during an in competition test. However, the arrival of designer steroids would prove particularly difficult since their existence as a PIED was unknown and therefore would not appear on a urine drug screen. A proactive approach involving research and intelligence will no doubt help to limit the effects of such events in the future.

9.12 Selective Androgen Receptor Modulators

Selective Androgen Receptor Modulators (SARMs) remain under development and do not have full clinical approval. Nevertheless, as with many doping agents their lack of availability as therapeutic agents are typically no barrier to their potential use as PIED. Consequently their chemical characterisation and methods for their detection have been developed (Thevis et al., 2013a; 2014; Thevis and Schanzer, 2017). Indeed, recent anti-doping testing figures confirm that SARMs have been detected in doping control samples thus providing clear evidence of their misuse in sport (Table 9.3; WADA, 2016b).

Selective androgen receptor modulators may offer a possible advantage over AAS both clinically and as PIED due to their potential for tissue selectivity and in promoting anabolic rather than androgenic effects. They are also designed to be administered orally with reduced hepatotoxicity.

9.13 Beta-2 agonists

Several drugs classified as β_2-agonists are also included on the WADA Prohibited List as anabolic agents, namely clenbuterol and zilpaterol (Table 9.1; WADA, 2016a). Beta-2 agonists are typically used to combat respiratory conditions due to the stimulation of the β_2-adrenergic receptors of the bronchioles and their bronchodilatory effects (see Chapter 11). However, when administered orally, clenbuterol has been shown to possess anabolic effects in animals (Choo et al., 1992). Indeed, both clenbuterol and zilpaterol are used as growth promoters in livestock (Davis et al., 2008). Despite the evidence to support their use as anabolic agents in animals there is limited evidence for this use in humans. Nevertheless, within the bodybuilding fraternity there use is relatively widespread as both an anabolic and repartitioning agent.

The consumption of meat infected with prohibited growth promoters and the impact on doping control

Given the inclusion of a number of livestock growth promoters on the WADA Prohibited List what is the likelihood for the consumption of meat containing such agents culminating in a positive drugs test? This is an obvious concern to athletes subject to doping control tests. Indeed, Parr et al. (2009) demonstrate that there is a real possibility that consuming meat from cattle that have been given clenbuterol may lead to a positive drugs test. In light of this, they suggest the need to introduce a threshold for clenbuterol in an attempt to limit the possibility of an inadvertent doping offence. An alternative approach to limit inadvertent doping requiring further research might be to differentiate between clenbuterol from direct pharmaceutical origin and that from ingested food (Thevis et al., 2014).

It is ironic that there is now concern regarding the possibility of false positives from a doping perspective as a direct consequence of improved analytical methods. The potential to detect minute traces of prohibited substances brings in to question the anti-doping movement's guiding principle of strict liability, particularly as the possibility of prohibited substances entering the body unintentionally, in such small quantities, is considered significant.

During the 2011 FIFA U17 World Cup clenbuterol was detected in over half of the doping control samples. This was attributed to the ingestion of food contaminated with the drug as indicated by food analysis (Thevis et al., 2013b). Risk of inadvertent clenbuterol doping is deemed to be a particular risk in countries where the use of the drug in livestock is not regulated. The European Union prohibits the use of hormonal active growth promoters in livestock (Stephany, 2010). However, in China, where clenbuterol use in livestock is prohibited, it still remains a real risk to athletes (Guddat et al., 2012).

Zeranol is a synthetic compound used in some countries as a growth promoter in livestock. Whilst there have been cases of its presence in doping control samples there is suggestion that this might be as a consequence of food contamination with a mycotoxin, zearalone (Thevis et al., 2011).

9.14 Tibolone

Tibolone is a synthetic steroid hormone with an affinity for oestrogen receptors and is used in the symptomatic relief of the menopause and in the prevention of osteoporosis in women. However, whilst tibolone is indicated for its oestrogenic properties it also has weak androgenic properties hence its inclusion in class S1 of the WADA Prohibited List (Table 9.1; WADA, 2016a).

9.15 Summary

Whilst the WADA classification of Anabolic Agents consist of some new and emerging drugs of abuse, AAS remain the major class of drugs misused by many who seek improvements in terms of muscle size and strength. Despite improvements in terms of drug detection and the unfolding evidence in relation to health concerns surrounding the use of AAS there are no signs to suggest that their use is abating. Indeed, their use amongst those engaged in recreational sport or exercise, particularly gym goers, for purposes largely related to image enhancement appears to be burgeoning.

The scientific literature clearly supports the use of AAS as PIEDs; however, there remains some way to go before there is clear evidence to categorically link the use of AAS with serious, long-term and even life-threatening health effects. Potentially the most disturbing issues in relation to the non-therapeutic use of anabolic agents is the availability of 'black market' products where there is no evidence of their legitimacy and thus their safety. Indeed, the use of new and emerging drugs not yet trialled, such as SARMs, offer no assurances in relation to safety.

9.16 References

ACMD (2010) Consideration of the anabolic steroids report. Available at: https://www.gov.uk/government/publications/advisory-council-on-the-misuse-of-drugs-consideration-of-the-anabolic-steroids--2 (Accessed on 25 July 2017).

Alesci, S., Koch, C.A., Bornstein, S.R. and Pacak, K. (2001) Adrenal androgens regulation and adrenopause. *Endocrine Regulations* 35: 95–100.

Angell, P., Chester, N., Green, D. et al. (2012a) Anabolic steroids and cardiovascular risk. *Sports Medicine* 42: 119–134.

Angell, P., Chester, N., Sculthorpe, N. et al. (2012b) Performance enhancing drug abuse and cardiovascular risk in athletes: Implications for the clinician. *British Journal of Sports Medicine* 46: i78–i84.

Angell, P.J., Chester, N., Green, D.J. et al. (2012c) Anabolic steroid use and longitudinal, radial and circumferential cardiac motion. *Medicine Science Sports and Exercise* 44(4): 583–590.

Basaria, S., Wahlstrom, J.T. and Dobs, A.S. (2001) Anabolic-androgenic steroid therapy in the treatment of chronic diseases. *Journal of Clinical Endocrinology and Metabolism* 86(11): 5,108–5,117.

Berning, J.M., Adams, K.J. and Stamford, B.A. (2004) Anabolic steroid usage in athletics: Facts, fiction and public relations. *Journal of Strength and Conditioning Research* 18(4): 908–917.

Bhasin, S., Storer, T.W., Berman, N. et al. (1996) The effects of supraphysiologic doses of testosterone on muscle size and strength in normal men. *The New England Journal of Medicine* 335: 1–7.

Buckley, W.E., Yesalis, C.E., Friedl, K.E. et al. (1988) Estimated prevalence of anabolic steroid use among male high school seniors. *JAMA* 260: 3,441–3,445.

Cabasso, A. (1994) Peliosis hepatis in a young adult bodybuilder. *Medicine Science Sports and Exercise* 26(1): 2–4.

Calfee, R. and Fadale, P. (2006) Popular ergogenic drugs and supplements in young athletes. *Pediatrics* 117(3): e577–e589.

Catlin, D.H., Ahrens, B.D. and Kucherova, Y. (2002) Detection of norbolethone, an anabolic steroid never marketed, in athletes' urine. *Rapid Communications in Mass Spectrometry* 16(13): 1,273–1,275.

Catlin, D.H., Sekera, M.H., Ahrens, B.D. et al. (2004) Tetrahydrogestrinone: Discovery, synthesis, and detection in urine. *Rapid Communications in Mass Spectrometry* 18: 1,245–1,249.

Choo, J.J., Horan, M.A., Little, R.A. et al. (1992) Anabolic effects of clenbuterol on skeletal muscle are mediated by β_2-adrenoceptor activation. *American Journal of Physiology* 263: E50–E56.

Clark, R.V. (2009) Anabolic-androgenic steroids: Historical background, physiology, typical use and side effects. In: J.L. Fourcroy (ed.) *Pharmacology, Doping and Sports: A Scientific Guide for Athletes, Coaches, Physicians, Scientists and Administrators*. London, Routledge, 23–35.

Davis, E., Loiacono, R. and Summers, R.J. (2008) The rush to adrenaline: Drugs in sport acting on the β-adrenergic system. *British Journal of Pharmacology* 154: 584–597.

Dimeo, P. (2007) *A History of Drug Use in Sport 1876–1976: Beyond Good and Evil*. Oxford, Routledge.

Egner, I.M., Bruusgaard, J.C., Eftestol, E. and Gunderson, K. (2013) A cellular memory mechanism aids overload hypertrophy in muscle long after an episodic exposure to anabolic steroids. *Journal of Physiology* 591(24): 6,221–6,230.

Elsharkawy, A.M., McPherson, S., Masson, S. et al. (2012) Cholestasis secondary to anabolic steroid use in young men. *British Medical Journal* 344: e463.

Evans-Brown, M., Kimergard, A. and McVeigh, J. (2009) Elephant in the room? The methodological implications for public health research of performance-enhancing drugs derived from the illicit market. *Drug Testing and Analysis* 1(7): 323–326.

Evans-Brown, M., McVeigh, J., Perkins, C. and Bellis, M.A. (2012) Human enhancement drugs: The emerging challenges to public health. Available at: http://www.cph.org.uk/wp-content/uploads/2012/08/human-enhancement-drugs---the-emerging-challenges-to-public-health---4.pdf (Accessed on 25 July 2017).

Faigenbaum, A.D., Zaichkowsky, L.D., Gardner, D.E. and Micheli, L.J. (1998) Anabolic steroid use by male and female middle school students. *Pediatrics* 101(5): 1–6.

Franke, W.W. and Berendonk, B. (1997) Hormonal doping and androgenization of athletes: A secret program of the German Democratic Republic government. *Clinical Chemistry* 43: 1,262–1,279.

Freed, D.L., Banks, A.J., Longson, D. et al. (1975) Anabolic steroids in athletics: Crossover double-blind trial on weightlifters. *British Medical Journal* 2(5969): 471–473.

George, A. and Mottram, D.R. (2011) Anabolic agents. In: D. Mottram (ed.) *Drugs in Sport*, 5th edition. London, Routledge, 49–81.

Giannotti, S., Ghilardi, M., Dell'Osso, G. et al. (2014) Left ventricular hypertrophy and spontaneous rupture of the Achilles tendon after anabolic steroids in bodybuilder. *European Orthopaedics and Traumatology* 5(4): 363–365.

Graham, M.R., Ryan, P., Baker, J.S. et al. (2009) Counterfeiting in performance and image-enhancing drugs. *Drug Testing and Analysis* 1(3): 135–142.

Guddat, S., Fussholler, G., Geyer, H. et al. (2012) Clenbuterol: Regional food contamination a possible source for inadvertent doping in sports. *Drug Testing and Analysis* 4(6): 534–538.

Hickson, R.C., Czerwinski, S.M, Falduto, M.T. and Young, A.P. (1990) Glucocorticoid antagonism by exercise and androgenic-anabolic steroids. *Medicine Science Sports and Exercise* 22(3): 331–340.

Hoffman, J.R. and Ratamess, N.A. (2006) Medical issues associated with anabolic steroid use: Are they exaggerated? *Journal of Sport Science and Medicine* 5: 182–193.

Hope, V.D., McVeigh, J., Marongiu, A. et al. (2013) Prevalence of and risk factors for HIV, hepatitis B and C infections among men who inject image and performance enhancing drugs: A cross-sectional study. *BMJ Open* 3: e003207.

Johnson, M.D. (1990) Anabolic steroid use in adolescent athletes. *Pediatric Clinics of North America* 37(5): 1,111–1,123.

Kadi, F. (2008) Cellular and molecular mechanisms responsible for the action of testosterone on human skeletal muscle: A basis for illegal performance enhancement. *British Journal of Pharmacology* 154(3): 522–528.

Kanayama, G., Brower, K.J., Wood, R.I. et al. (2009) Anabolic-androgenic steroid dependence: An emerging disorder. *Addiction* 104(12): 1,966–1,978.

Kanayama, G., Barry, S., Hudson, J.I. and Pope, H.G. (2006) Body image and attitudes towards male roles in anabolic-androgenic steroid users. *American Journal of Psychiatry* 163: 697–703.

Kicman, A.T. (2008) Pharmacology of anabolic steroids. *British Journal of Pharmacology* 154: 502–521.

King, D.S., Sharp, R.I., Vukovich, M.D. et al. (1999) Effect of oral androstenedione on serum testosterone and adaptations to resistance training in young men: A randomized controlled trial. *JAMA* 281(21): 2,020–2,028.

Korkia, P. (1994) Anabolic steroid use in Britain. *International Journal of Drug Policy* 5(1): 6–10.

Kuipers, H., Wijnen, J.A.G., Hartgens, F. et al. (1991) Influence of anabolic steroids on body composition, blood pressure, lipid profile and liver functions in bodybuilders. *International Journal of Sports Medicine* 12(4): 413–418.

Labrie, F., Luu-The, V., Belanger, A. et al. (2005) Is dehydroepiandrosterone a hormone? *Journal of Endocrinology* 187: 169–196.

Lane, H.A., Grace, F., Smith, J.C. et al. (2006) Impaired vasoreactivity in bodybuilders using androgenic anabolic steroids. *European Journal of Clinical Investigation* 36(7): 483–488.

Laseter, J.T. and Russell, J.A. (1991) Anabolic steroid-induced tendon pathology: A review of the literature. *Medicine Science Sports and Exercise* 23(1): 1–3.

Lenders, J.W.M., Demacker, P.N.M., Vos, J.A. et al. (1988) Deleterious effects of anabolic steroids on serum lipoproteins, blood pressure and liver function in amateur body builders. *International Journal of Sports Medicine* 9(1): 19–23.

McCabe, S.E., Brower, K.J., West, B.T. et al. (2007) Trends in non-medical use of anabolic steroids by U.S. college students: Results from four national surveys. *Drug and Alcohol Dependence* 90(2-3): 243–251.

McCreary, D.R. and Sasse, D.K. (2000) An exploration of the drive for muscularity in adolescent boys and girls. *Journal of American of American College Health* 48(6): 297–304.

McVeigh, J., Beynon, C. and Bellis, M.A. (2003) New challenges for agency based syringe exchange schemes: Analysis of 11 years of data (1991-2001) in Merseyside and Cheshire, United Kingdom. *International Journal of Drug Policy* 14(5): 399–405.

Maior, A.S., Carvalho, A.R., Marques-Neto, S.R. et al. (2013) Cardiac autonomic dysfunction in anabolic steroid users. *Scandinavian Journal of Medicine and Science in Sports* 23: 548–555.

Montisci, M., El Mazloum, R., Cecchetto, G. et al. (2012) Anabolic androgenic steroids abuse and cardiac death in athletes: Morphological and toxicological findings in four fatal cases. *Forensic Science International* 217: e13–e18.

Morales, A.J., Haubrich, R.H., Hwang, J.Y. et al. (1998) The effect of six months treatment with a 100 mg daily dose of dehydroepiandrosterone (DHEA) on circulating sex steroids, body composition and muscle strength in age-advanced men and women. *Clinical Endocrinology* 49: 421–432.

Moriarty, D., Fairall, D. and Galasso, P.J. (1992) The Canadian Commission of Inquiry into the use of drugs and banned practices intended to increase athletic performance. *Journal of Legal Aspects of Sport* 2(1): 23–31.

Nasr, J. and Ahmad, J. (2009) Severe cholestasis and renal failure associated with the use of the designer steroid Superdrol (Methasteron): A case report and literature review. *Digestive Diseases and Sciences* 54(5): 1,144–1,146.

Omole, T. (2011) Drug use. In E. Fuller (ed.) *Smoking, Drinking and Drug Use among Young people in England in 2010.* London, NHS Information Centre for Health and Social Care, 141–179. Available at: http://www.esds.ac.uk/doc/6883/mrdoc/pdf/6883report_of_findings.pdf (Accessed on 25 July 2017).

Parr, M.K. and Schanzer, W. (2010) Detection of the misuse of steroids in doping control. *Journal of Steroid Biochemistry and Molecular Biology* 121: 528–537.

Parr, M.K, Opfermann, G. and Schanzer, W. (2009) Analytical methods for the detection of clenbuterol. *Bioanalysis* 1(2): 437–450.

Pope, H.G., Gruber, A.J., Choi, P.Y. et al. (1997) Muscle dysmorphia: An unrecognised form of body dysmorphic disorder. *Psychosomatics* 38: 548–557.

Pope, H.G. and Katz, D.L. (1988) Affective and psychotic symptoms associated with anabolic steroid use. *American Journal of Psychiatry* 145(4): 487–490.

Riebe, D., Fernhall, B. and Thompson, P.D. (1992) The blood pressure response to exercise in anabolic steroid users. *Medicine Science Sports and Exercise* 24(6): 633–637.

Sachtleben, T.R., Berg, K.E., Elias, B.A. et al. (1993) The effects of anabolic steroids on myocardial structure and cardiovascular fitness. *Medicine Science Sports and Exercise* 25(11): 1,240–1,245.

Sanchez-Osorio, M., Duarte-Rojo, A., Martinez-Benitez, B. et al. (2008) Anabolic-androgenic steroids and liver injury. *Liver International* 28(2): 278–282.

Salameh, W.A., Redor-Goodman, M.M., Clarke, N.J. et al. (2010) Validation of a total testosterone assay using high-turbulence liquid chromatography tandem mass-spectrometry: Total and free testosterone reference ranges. *Steroids* 75: 169–175.

Sekera, M.H., Ahrens, B.D., Chang, Y.C. et al. (2005) Another designer steroid: Discovery, synthesis and detection of 'madol' in urine. *Rapid Communications in Mass Spectrometry* 19(6): 781–784.

Shahidi, N.T. (2001) A review of the chemistry, biological action and clinical applications of anabolic-androgenic steroids. *Clinical Therapeutics* 23(9): 1,355–1,390.

Stephany, R.W. (2010) Hormonal growth promoting agents in food producing animals. *Handbook of Experimental Pharmacology* 195: 355–367.

Striegel, H., Simon, P., Frisch, S. et al. (2006) Anabolic ergogenic substance use in fitness-sports: A distinct group supported by health care system. *Drug and Alcohol Dependence* 81: 11–19.

Thevis, M., Fussholler, G. and Schanzer, W. (2011) Zeranol: Doping offence or mycotoxin? A case-related study. *Drug Testing and Analysis* 3: 777–783.

Thevis, M., Piper, T., Beuk, S. et al. (2013a) Expanding sports drug testing assays: Mass spectrometric characterization of the selective androgen receptor modulator drug candidates RAD140 and ACP-105. *Rapid Communications in Mass Spectrometry* 27(11): 1,173–1,182.

Thevis, M., Geyer, L., Geyer, H. et al. (2013b) Adverse analytical findings with clenbuterol among U-17 soccer players attributed to food contamination issues. *Drug Testing and Analysis* 5: 372–376.

Thevis, M., Kuuranne, T., Geyer, H. and Schanzer, W. (2014) Annual banned-substance review: analytical approaches in human sports drug testing. *Drug Testing and Analysis* 6: 164–184.

Thevis, M. and Schanzer, W. (2017) Detection of SARMs in doping control analysis. *Molecular and Cellular Endocrinology.* Available at https://www.ncbi.nlm.nih.gov/pubmed/28137616 (Accessed on 20 October 2017).

Thigpen, A.E., Silver, R.I., Guileyardo, J.M. et al. (1993) Tissue distribution and ontogeny of steroid 5α-reductase isoenzyme expression. *Journal of Clinical Investigation* 92: 903–910.

Toth, M. and Zakar, T. (1982) Relative binding affinities of testosterone, 19-nortestosterone and their 5 alpha-reduced derivatives to the androgen receptor and to other androgen-binding proteins: A suggested role of 5 alpha-reductive steroid metabolism in the dissociation of 'myotropic' and 'androgenic' activities of 19-nortestosterone. *Journal of Steroid Biochemistry* 17(6): 653–660.

van Amsterdam, J., Opperhuizen, A. and Hartgens, F. (2010) Adverse health effects of anabolic-androgenic steroids. *Regulatory Toxicology and Pharmacology* 57: 117–123.

WADA (2015) WADA Technical Document: TD2016EAAS. Available at: https://www.wada-ama.org/sites/default/files/resources/files/wada-td2016eaas-eaas-measurement-and-reporting-en.pdf (Accessed on 25 July 2017).

WADA (2016a) The 2017 Prohibited List International Standard. Available at: https://www.wada-ama.org/sites/default/files/resources/files/2016-09-29_-_wada_prohibited_list_2017_eng_final.pdf (Accessed on 25 July 2017).

WADA (2016b) 2015 Anti-Doping Testing Figures: Laboratory Report. Available at: https://www.wada-ama.org/sites/default/files/resources/files/2015_wada_anti-doping_testing_figures_report_0.pdf (Accessed on 25 July 2017).

Wilson, J.D. (1988) Androgen abuse by athletes. *Endocrine Reviews* 9(2): 181–199.

Woerdeman, J. and de Ronde, W. (2011) Therapeutic effects of anabolic androgenic steroids on chronic disease associated with muscle wasting. *Expert Opinion on Investigational Drugs* 20(1): 87–97.

Wood, T.O., Cooke, P.H. and Goodship A.E. (1988) The effect of exercise and anabolic steroids on the mechanical properties and crimp morphology of the rat tendon. *American Journal of Sports Medicine* 16: 153–158.

Yates, W.R., Perry, P. and Murray, S. (1992) Aggression and hostility in anabolic steroid users. *Biological Psychiatry* 31: 1,232–1,234.

Chapter 10

Peptide hormones, growth factors and related substances

David R. Mottram and Neil Chester

10.1 Introduction

The World Anti-Doping Agency prohibits the use of a number of peptide hormones and related substances (Table 10.1), most of which occur naturally in the body.

Table 10.1 The list of peptide hormones, growth factors, related substances and mimetics on the WADA Prohibited List (January 2017)

The following substances, and other substances with similar chemical structure or similar biological effect(s), are prohibited:

1. Erythropoietin-receptor agonists:

    1.1 Erythropoiesis-stimulating agents (ESAs) including e.g.

    Darbepoetin (dEPO);
    Erythropoietins (EPO);
    EPO-Fc;
    EPO-mimetic peptides (EMP), e.g. CNTO 530 and peginesatide;
    GATA inhibitors, e.g. K-11706;
    Methoxy polyethylene glycol-epoetin beta (CERA);
    Transforming Growth Factor-β (TGF-β) inhibitors, e.g. sotatercept, luspatercept;

    1.2 Non-erythropoietic EPO-receptor agonists, e.g.

    ARA-290;
    Asialo EPO;
    Carbamylated EPO.
2. Hypoxia-inducible factor (HIF) stabilisers, e.g. cobalt, molidustat and roxadustat FG-4592); and HIF activators, e.g. argon and xenon.
3. Chorionic gonadotrophin (CG) and luteinizing hormone (LH) and their releasing factors, e.g. buserelin, gonadorelin and leuprorelin, in males.
4. Corticotrophins and their releasing factors, e.g. corticorelin.
5. Growth hormone (GH) and its releasing factors including:

    • Growth hormone releasing hormone (GHRH) and its analogues, e.g. CJC-1295, sermorelin and tesamorelin;
    • Growth hormone secretagogues (GHS), e.g. ghrelin and ghrelin mimetics, e.g. anamorelin and ipamorelin;
    • GH-releasing peptides (GHRPs), e.g. alexamorelin, GHRP-6, hexarelin and pralmorelin (GHRP-2).

Additional prohibited growth factors:

    Fibroblast growth factors (FGFs);
    Hepatocyte growth factor (HGF);
    Insulin-like growth factor-1 (IGF-1) and its analogues;
    Mechano growth factors (MGFs);
    Platelet-derived growth factor (PDGF);
    Vascular-endothelial growth factor (VEGF) and any other growth factor affecting muscle, tendon or ligament protein synthesis/degradation, vascularisation, energy utilization, regenerative capacity or fibre type switching.

This class of substances includes hormones with significant effects on the body, particularly in the early stages of bodily development. The primary medical uses for these substances include treatment of chronic kidney disease, acute anaemia, short stature and aiding those born prematurely. Inappropriate use of these potent agents by athletes carries severe potential side effects and health risks.

10.2 Erythropoiesis-stimulating agents

Erythropoiesis-stimulating agents (ESA) include the endogenous peptide erythropoietin (EPO), which is commercially available as recombinant-EPO and the synthetically produced darbepoetin (dEPO) and methoxy polyethylene glycol-epoetin beta (CERA).

Mode of action of erythropoietin (EPO)

EPO increases oxygen supply to muscles, thereby increasing an athlete's endurance and performance (Elliott, 2008). EPO works synergistically with other growth factors to cause maturation and proliferation of red blood cell precursors. The net effect is an increase in the number of red blood cells (erythrocytes) that are produced and in the rate at which they are released into the circulation. Consequently, EPO increases the oxygen supply for muscle tissue, allowing muscles to work longer before they build up lactic acid (Tsitsimpikou, 2011).

Recombinant erythropoietin

The gene responsible for the synthesis of erythropoietin was cloned in 1985. Recombinant human erythropoietin (rHuEPO) was first patented by Amgen in 1989. There are currently three generations of rHuEPO in production, the prototype (erythropoietin), novel erythropoiesis stimulating protein (NESP) and continuous erythropoietin receptor activator (CERA). Second generation NESP (darbepoetin, Aranesp™) differs from EPO in having an additional 8-sialic acid residue. Third generation CERA differs in having a long polymer chain (methoxy polyethylene glycol) incorporated into the molecule. These genetically engineered modifications have increased the elimination half-lives from 8.5 to 25.3 to 142 hours, respectively. This has decreased the frequency of initial intravenous dosing from three times weekly to once weekly to once every two weeks, respectively.

Adverse effects of ESAs

EPO poses significant short- and long-term health problems to the abuser. Adverse effects of recombinant human EPO include injection site reactions, nausea, headache, dizziness, arthralgia, allergic and anaphylactic reactions (Birzniece, 2015). Since ESAs stimulate erythropoiesis, the resulting increase in red blood cells increases the viscosity of the blood and therefore raises the risk of microcirculation blockage (thromboembolism), heart failure and strokes (Wells, 2008).

EPO-stimulated erythropoiesis vastly augments the demands of the sportsperson for ferrous iron for the synthesis of haemoglobin. To meet such demands, iron must be injected, leading to potential iron overload. There is evidence from both France (Dine, 2001) and Italy (Cazzola, 2001) that elite cyclists have exhibited ferritin levels indicative of severe iron overload.

Detection of EPO

The first tests for EPO at the Olympic Games were introduced in Sydney in 2000. To be deemed culpable, the athlete had to test positive in both blood (Parisotto et al., 2001) and urine tests (Lasne and de Ceaurriz, 2000). In 2003, WADA's Executive Committee accepted the results from an independent report that urine testing alone could be used to detect the presence of recombinant EPO. In 2009, WADA published a Technical Document entitled "Harmonization of the method for the identification of recombinant erythropoietins (i.e. epoetins) and analogues (e.g. darbepoetin and methoxypolyethylene glycol-epoetin beta)" in which the methodology for detection was specified as were the results for the major commercially available epoetins (rEPO, Aranesp™ and Mircera™). Demonstration of the presence of an epoetin is based upon isoelectric focusing and chemiluminescence (Figure 10.1).

These techniques may be complemented with a further technique known as SDS-PAGE (sodium dodecyl sulfate polyacrylamide gel electrophoresis) (Fig. 10.2).

Note that the technique can identify not only r-HuEPO, NESP and CERA but also biosimilars (e.g. Hemax™ and Dynepo™).

More recently, the use of Athlete Biological Passports (ABPs) to detect EPO and other hormones, using an "endocrine module" is described by Pitsiladis et al. (2014); Saugy et al. (2014) and Vernec (2014). New methods for the direct detection of ESAs are reviewed by Reichel (2014).

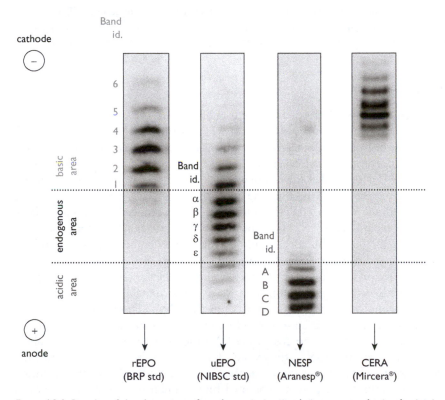

Figure 10.1 Results of the detection of erythropoiesis stimulating agents obtained using isoelectric focusing and chemiluminescence

Source: TD2014EPO - WADA Technical Document on harmonization of analysis and reporting of recombinant erythropoietins (i.e. epoetins) and analogues (e.g. Darbepoetin, Pegserpoetin, Peginesatide, EPO-Fc) by electrophoretic techniques

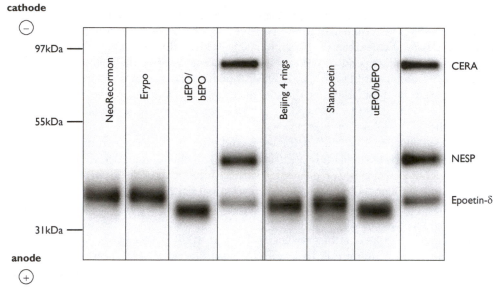

Figure 10.2 Results of the detection of erythropoiesis stimulating agents obtained using SDS-PAGE

Source: TD2014EPO - WADA Technical Document on harmonization of analysis and reporting of recombinant erythropoietins (i.e. epoetins) and analogues (e.g. Darbepoetin, Pegserpoetin, Peginesatide, EPO-Fc) by electrophoretic techniques

Abuse of EPO in sport

The first reports on the clinical use of EPO were published in 1987. The drug company Amagen received a licence for the production of r-HuEPO in 1989. In 1990, the IOC added EPO to the list of banned substances. Around this time, there were several newspaper articles which linked the deaths of 18 Belgian and Dutch cyclists with rumours of EPO abuse in the peloton (Leith, 1992). It is unlikely that the magnitude of the increase in red blood cell production was accurately controlled at this time and the haematocrit (Hct) may have been raised to dangerously high levels. Values of 60 per cent were rumoured. Indeed, one cyclist, Marco Pantani, was found to have an Hct of 60.1 per cent when admitted to hospital after an accident in a 1995 race (Rendell, 2006). This concentration would cause significant increases in both systolic blood pressure and blood viscosity. In the short-term there would be an increased risk of thrombosis and stroke. In the long-term, chronically elevated Hct and blood viscosity could lead to left ventricular hypertrophy and, ultimately, to left ventricular failure and death.

There was much conjecture about abuse of EPO in the 1990s. The former professional cyclist Paul Kimmage referred in his book, *Rough Ride* (1998), to such suspicions within the peloton. He also referred to the Donati dossier (1994), which was an account of EPO abuse involving elite Italian cyclists. Proof of the extent of abuse of EPO did not exist until the 1998 Tour de France in what became known as the "Festina affair". Subsequent detention of the Festina team *soigneur* Willy Voet, prompted him to publish a personal account of drug abuse within the peloton (Voet, 2001). He stated that provision and administration of EPO were formalized within the team and provided evidence of drugs, doses and deductions from salaries according to drugs administered. It is difficult to imagine that other teams could compete with Festina without recourse to EPO, since there was evidence of the ergogenic benefit derived from EPO (e.g. Ekblom and Berglund, 1991; Birkeland et al., 2000).

The ergogenic effects of recombinant human EPO (r-HuEPO) were compared to those of transfusional polycythaemia by Ekblom and Berglund (1991) who reported that r-HuEPO increased Hb concentration equivalent to those evoked by re-infusion of 1350 ml of autologous blood. In a later study, time to exhaustion was increased from 493 ± 74 s to 567 ± 82 s following doses of r-HuEPO (Ekblom, 1997).

There have been many examples of positive tests (adverse analytical findings) for ESAs from athletes in a number of different sports including cross-country skiers, biathletes, swimmers, rowers and athletics including marathon runners, 5000m runners, 400m runners and 400m hurdlers. Confirmation that abuse of EPO is not restricted to participants in endurance events was demonstrated by USA sprinters Marion Jones and Kelli White who tested positive for EPO.

Given that there are well defined methods for the detection of erythropoiesis stimulating agents, why do athletes continue to abuse these drugs and risk sanctions? A possible explanation is that the athletes believe that they can avoid detection by means of diluting red cell concentration using plasma volume expanders. A more subtle strategy is to a microdosing regime which renders EPO undetectable within a short period of administration, as demonstrated in the Lance Armstrong case (Mottram, 2013). Studies by Ashenden et al. (2006 and 2011) have demonstrated that a microdose regime could be utilised to avoid detection of EPO use even when monitored by Athlete Biological Passport (ABP) software. An approach such as this, whilst relatively simple to conduct within a laboratory setting, requires a degree of sophistication and support well beyond the compass of the athlete alone. In the past, this has been thought to involve the coaching and medical support staff.

New techniques for the detection of the use of recombinant human erythropoietin, using biomarkers, is being developed (Durussel et al., 2016).

Cases of EPO abuse in sport

Since the first reports of EPO use in cycling, associated with the "Festina affair" (Voet, 2001), there have been a number of high profile cases.

Box 10.1   Lance Armstrong (2012)

On 24 August 2012 the United States Anti-Doping Agency (USADA) announced that it had imposed on Lance Armstrong a sanction of lifetime ineligibility and disqualification of competition results achieved since August 1998. Despite having never tested positive for a prohibited drug, USADA cited all anti-doping rule violations except those directly relating to the presence of a drug in a sample or evasion of doping tests. One of the drugs most extensively used by Armstrong and the US Postal Services Cycling Team was EPO, which Armstrong subsequently admitted to using. The evidence behind the headlines concerning the Lance Armstrong case is described by Mottram (2013).

Box 10.2   Johannes Duerr (2014)

The Austrian cross-country skier tested positive for recombinant EPO at the 2014 Sochi Winter Olympic Games. Duerr was disqualified by the IOC from the events in which he competed and was excluded from the Games. Subsequently, the International Ski Federation imposed a two-year ban.

10.3 Hypoxia-inducible factor (HIF) stabilizers

Erythropoietin production is regulated by oxygen availability within the body. Oxygen availability is recognised by a gene product called hypoxia-inducible factor (HIF), which is found in the cells that make erythropoietin. Erythropoietin levels in the body can therefore be elevated by HIFs which increase erythropoietin gene expression and therefore increase red blood cell levels (Jelkmann, 2016). Pharmaceutical companies are developing these "HIF-stabilizers" as potential medicinal agents for the treatment of anaemias. Such potential performance enhancing agents have become the target for athletes who cheat, indeed, one such HIF-stabilizer, roxadustat (FG-4592) was detected in four cases arising from WADA laboratory statistics for 2015 (see Table 10.2).

Experimental research has also suggested that the elements argon and xenon can activate HIF, although their effect is considered a minor issue (Jelkmann, 2014). However, a more recent study on the effects of xenon on healthy volunteers showed significant increase in erythropoietin levels (Stoppe et al., 2016). WADA has included these elements on their Prohibited List (see Table 10.1). Other elements, including cobalt and nickel are potential inducers of HIF and are the target for some athletes seeking performance enhancement (Jelkmann and Thevis, 2016). A study by Thevis et al. (2016), in which analysis was made of 19 products obtained online, showed widespread inclusion within these products of prohibited substances such as EPO, HIF stabilizers and metals such as cobalt and nickel.

10.4 Chorionic gonadotrophin (CG)

Chorionic gonadotrophin (CG) is produced by placental trophoblast cells during pregnancy and also by a number of different types of tumour cell. Its major physiological role is stimulation of the corpus luteum in pregnant females, to maintain synthesis and secretion of the hormone progesterone during pregnancy. However, when injected into males, CG also stimulates the Leydig cells of the testes to produce testosterone and epitestosterone, and so it can mimic the natural stimulation of testicular hormone produced by luteinizing hormone (LH). This increase in synthesis is rapid, a 50 per cent increase in plasma testosterone concentration has been measured two hours after intramuscular injection of 6,000 IU of CG (Kicman et al., 1991). Injection of CG also stimulates production of nandrolone (19 nortestosterone) metabolites and this may indicate that it can stimulate production of endogenous nandrolone itself (Reznik et al., 2001). An excellent review of CG has been published by Stenman et al. (2008).

Therapeutic use

CG is used to stimulate ovulation in conjunction with FSH in infertile women. Occasionally, CG is used to stimulate testicular hormone production when puberty is delayed.

CG abuse in sport

CG has been used because it stimulates the secretion from the testes of both testosterone and epitestosterone. This led to the banning of CG by the IOC in 1987. A standard doping regime for CG has been described (Brooks et al., 1989) in which the abuser firstly injects testosterone. Apart from any gains in strength or competitiveness the testosterone causes inhibition of LH secretion from the pituitary. When testosterone is withdrawn before competition (to avoid detection) the athlete would be at a disadvantage with lower than normal plasma testosterone levels. However, administration of CG stimulates testicular testosterone secretion. In a small, elegant experiment, Kicman et al. (1991) reproduced this situation in three normal men and showed that CG can stimulate the testosterone substitution claimed by abusers and retain the testosterone/epitestosterone ratio within WADA limits. In all three cases, the CG could be detected in the urine by radioimmunoassay as long as plasma testosterone levels were raised. Brower (2000) described three separate regimes to restore endogenous testosterone secretion to normal following its suppression due to administration of testosterone or anabolic steroids. He has recorded descriptions of CG 50 IU/Kg producing a doubling of endogenous testosterone secretion within three to four days of administration.

A review by Handelsman (2006) concluded that whilst CG produces marked increases in blood testosterone levels in men, the effects are negligible in women and therefore prohibition and testing for CG should be restricted to men.

Handelsman et al. (2009) showed a prominent dose-dependent and sustained effect on blood and urine CG, LH and testosterone levels after administration of recombinant CG. They further concluded that testosterone:LH ratio measurements may be a sensitive test to detect CG administration for at least one week after injection.

Side effects of CG in sport

The side effects of CG will be similar to those for anabolic steroids. However, the incidence of gynaecomastia may be greater as CG also stimulates oestradiol production by the Leydig cells. The increase of oestradiol may be linked to nandrolone metabolite production in the process of aromatization (Reznik et al., 2001).

10.5 Luteinizing hormone (LH) and its use in sport

Luteinizing hormone (LH) is produced by the gonadotroph cells of the anterior pituitary in both males and females. In males LH stimulates testicular sperm production and the synthesis and secretion of testosterone, while in females it stimulates ovulation and the production of progesterone. There are structural similarities between LH and CG and a detailed comparison is made by Kicman and Cowan (1992). LH secretion is subject to negative feedback control by testosterone, therefore as plasma testosterone levels rise, so LH secretion is reduced. A recent study on the effects of single doses of recombinant LH, up to 750 IU, had no influence on serum or urine LH or testosterone (Handelsman et al., 2009)

LH abuse is limited by its scarcity and its high costs and because its plasma half-life is 50 per cent less than CG (Kicman and Cowan, 1992). "Designer" synthesis of LH, a dual chain peptide, is difficult owing to the complexity of its structure. Problems associated with the detection of LH are reviewed at length by Stenman et al. (2008).

It is much more likely that LH releasing hormone, the substance regulating LH release, will become a drug of abuse. It could be used to stimulate endogenous LH release which will in turn stimulate the testes to secrete testosterone in males withdrawing from anabolic steroid abuse. Brower (2000) has described several LH treatment regimes, which could be used to restore testosterone secretion in males suffering anabolic steroid withdrawal syndromes or in those who need to restore normal testosterone before an event or test.

10.6 Corticotrophins

The peptide hormone Adrenocorticotrophic Hormone (ACTH) is produced and secreted by the corticotroph cells of the anterior pituitary. It is a polypeptide consisting of 39 amino acids, of which only the 24 N-terminal amino acids are necessary for its biological activity. ACTH stimulates the reticularis and fasciculata cells of the adrenal cortex to synthesize and secrete corticosteroids such as cortisol and corticosterone.

Administration of ACTH

ACTH itself is never used for treatment or abuse, instead a synthetic derivative, the peptide tetracosactrin consisting of the first 24 N-terminal amino acids of ACTH, is administered by injection. Tetracosactrin administration stimulates a rise in blood cortisol and corticosterone concentration within two hours.

Abuse of ACTH

ACTH abuse is limited to short term boosting of plasma cortisol and corticosterone in an attempt to reduce lethargy and produce "positive" effects on mood during training and competition. It is for this reason that it is banned by WADA along with corticosteroids. ACTH and corticosteroids are unsuitable for chronic use because they decrease muscle protein synthesis, leading to skeletal muscle wasting.

10.7 Growth hormone (GH)

Introduction

Growth hormone (GH) is one of the major hormones influencing growth and development in humans. The period of human growth extends from birth to the age of 20 years. A large number of hormones influence this period producing many complex interactions. Besides GH, testosterone, oestradiol, cortisol, thyroxine and insulin have important roles at different stages of growth and development. The exact role of GH is difficult to evaluate, because of the many different developmental and metabolic processes which GH can influence. A review of GH and its abuse in sport has been published by Holt and Sonksen (2008). The regulation of muscle mass by GH and growth factors has been reviewed by Velloso (2008).

Release of growth hormone

The anterior pituitary, a small endocrine gland at the base of, but not part of, the brain, contains somatotroph cells which secrete growth hormone. Release of GH is under the control of two hypothalamic hormones: somatostatin, which inhibits secretion, and somatocrinin, which stimulates its secretion. Oestradiol also stimulates GH secretion while testosterone has very little effect. Various brain neurotransmitter systems influence GH secretion. This is thought to occur via a controlling influence on the hypothalamic production of somatostatin and somatocrinin, but direct effects on the somatotroph cells cannot be ruled out. The factors influencing GH secretion have been reviewed in detail by Macintyre (1987) and Muller (1987).

Daily GH secretion is episodic, the highest levels occurring 60-90 mins after the onset of sleep. GH is metabolized in the liver; the plasma half-life is only 12-45 minutes.

The physiological regulation of GH release is complex. Systemic factors stimulating GH secretion include hypoglycaemia, a rise in blood amino acid concentration, stress and exercise, while conversely GH secretion is inhibited by hyperglycaemia. Both endurance exercise and resistance training have been shown to cause an increase in GH secretion in female athletes (Consitt et al., 2002).

Growth hormone action

The most obvious action of GH is that it stimulates somatic growth in pre-adolescents but it also has metabolic effects. The importance of these metabolic actions in homeostatic regulation of fuel usage and storage is unclear as is the overall role of GH in the adult, this is discussed in detail by Macintyre (1987). Receptors for GH are present on the surface of every cell in the body (Holt, 2004). GH stimulates the release, mainly from the liver, of two hormonal polypeptides, somatomedin C (or insulin-like growth factor I (IGF-1)) and somatomedin A (insulin-like growth factor II (IGF-2)) and a full account of this is provided by Kicman and Cowan (1992). Growth hormone exerts its anabolic actions through the generation of IGF-I (Le Roith et al., 2001), although Sonksen (2001) expressed doubt as to whether many, if any, of the important metabolic effects of GH are mediated via IGFs. IGFs are carried in the plasma in two different forms: as ternary complexes and simpler low molecular weight complexes (Boisclair et al., 2001).

Effects on muscle

GH and IGF-1 have an effect on muscle growth that appears similar to that of insulin in that it promotes amino acid uptake and stimulates protein synthesis resulting, in children, in an increase in the length and diameter of muscle fibres, while only the latter growth occurs in adults. The action of insulin is more likely to be an anti-catabolic effect on muscle protein rather than a direct stimulatory effect on muscle protein synthesis (Sonksen, 2001).

Effects on bone

GH stimulates the elongation of bone in pre-adolescents both directly and via the IGFs. This is achieved by a stimulation of cartilage proliferation in the epiphyseal plates situated at each end of each long bone. Cartilage cells possess receptors for GH and IGFs.

Effects on metabolism

The actions of GH on metabolism at both the cellular and organ level are complex and appear to be biphasic. In the first or acute phase, which seems to involve the action of GH alone, amino acid uptake into muscle and liver is stimulated, and there is increased glucose uptake into muscle and adipose tissue together with reduced fat metabolism (Smith and Perry, 1992). During the second, chronic phase, mediated by the IGFs, there is increased lipolysis (triglyceride breakdown) in adipose tissue resulting in a rise in the plasma concentration of fatty acids and increased fatty acid utilization, thus sparing glucose.

Effects on adipose tissue

Treatment of GH deficient adults has shown that GH can increase lean body mass by several kilograms and decrease fat mass, especially visceral fat, by an equivalent amount

(Marcus and Hoffman, 1998). Treatment with GH causes a rise in blood free fatty acid levels or a rise in the blood glucose level and a reduction in the triglyceride content of adipose tissue which contributes to a decrease in adipose tissue mass and an increase in fat-free weight (Kicman & Cowan, 1992).

Effects of exercise on growth hormone

GH levels rise within 20 minutes of beginning exercise to 75-90 per cent VO_2max. The intensity of the response depends on age, level of fitness and body composition. The type of exercise undertaken also produces varying GH responses. Intermittent intense exercise is claimed to result in the highest GH levels (Macintyre, 1987).

Growth hormone disorders

Inadequate secretion of GH is one of the causes of the conditions known as dwarfism. This disorder is usually recognized in childhood when the rate of growth is below the 90th percentile for that child's age, race and sex. The treatment is regular administration of synthetic GH until the end of puberty. Treatment after adolescence is ineffective in stimulating growth in stature because by this time the epiphyseal plates in the long bones have fused, terminating any further bone growth.

Overproduction of GH as a result of a tumour may occur in puberty and adolescence when it gives rise to gigantism; the individual is well above average adult height for their age, sex and race, and the limbs and internal organs are also enlarged.

In late adulthood, a tumour of the anterior pituitary causing increased GH secretion results in the condition known as acromegaly. The affected individual does not grow any taller because the epiphyses have fused but their internal organs enlarge (especially the heart), the fingers grow and the skin thickens. Metabolic disorders occur which often precipitate Type II diabetes mellitus.

A deficiency in GH secretion in adulthood has been recognized in elderly people, some of whom have responded favourably to GH therapy (Marcus and Hoffman, 1998; Gotherstrom et al., 2005). The investigations of this syndrome while providing interesting data on the effects of GH have not indicated a universal benefit for the elderly of GH treatment.

Administration and supply of Growth Hormone

GH is a peptide and must be injected. Therapeutically, GH administration is usually recommended as either three single injections, intramuscularly (i.m.) or subcutaneously (s.c.) or daily s.c. injections in the evening.

Human GH is produced synthetically. In sport, many GH supplies are known to be illicitly obtained by theft from pharmaceutical company production lines and from retail pharmacies (Sonksen, 2001). The prevalence of GH use by athletes is difficult to determine as much of the evidence arises through anecdotal reports (McHugh et al., 2005).

10.8 The abuse of growth hormone in sport

There appear to be four major abuses of GH in sport: (1) to increase muscle mass and strength, (2) to increase lean body mass, (3) to improve the "appearance of musculature",

(4) to increase final adult height. However, scientific evidence to support these potential benefits to athletes is sparse and contradictory.

As early as 1988, Cowart reviewed anecdotal reports by bodybuilders of increases in strength following GH administration. Lombardo et al., (1991) describe experiments where GH administration has caused significant reductions in "fat weight", and increases in fat free weight compared to placebo. When Yarasheski et al. (1993) examined resistance training schedules before and during GH administration in elderly men they found GH did not further enhance muscle strength improvements induced by exercise regimes. In younger adult men there is a similar picture. Sixteen healthy men, aged 21–34 years, who had not previously trained were given GH (0.56 IU/kg/12 weeks) or placebo during 12 weeks of heavy resistance training. At the end of the study, lean body mass and total body water increased in the GH group compared to placebo, but there was no difference in muscle strength or limb circumference (Yarasheski et al., 1992). Negative results have also been obtained with male power athletes where no increases in biceps or quadriceps maximal strength occurred in the GH group compared to placebo (Deyssig et al., 1993). Ehrnborg et al. (2000) reviewed previous research on GH use and concluded that the studies were "too short and included too few subjects" to reach meaningful conclusions.

The potential performance enhancing effects of GH may be attributed to other substances used in combination with GH (Schnirring, 2000; Saugy et al., 2006). In 2003, Rennie questioned whether the adverse effect of GH outweighed the potential performance enhancing effects and Liu et al. (2008) concluded, following a systematic review, that scientific literature did not support claims of enhancement of physical performance by GH.

In 2010, Meinhardt et al. demonstrated that GH administration in recreationally trained athletes resulted in statistically significant improvements in sprint capacity. Birzniece et al. (2011) reported that GH administration has positive effects on aerobic exercise capacity and fat metabolism and that a potential benefit for elite athletes could be improved recovery from intensive exercise. On the other hand, a review by Baumann (2012) concluded that scientific evidence had failed to demonstrate an ergogenic effect with supraphysiological doses of GH, although doses studied may have been lower than those used by athletes.

The desire to produce tall offspring either for cosmetic reasons, athletic potential or so they that they can qualify for a vocation where there is a minimum height limit has prompted GH abuse amongst children. An apparent drive for "bigness" and "tallness" in sport and society by selective and drug-induced means is discussed in a review by Norton and Olds (2001) and by Rogol (2014).

In 2015, Momaya et al. concluded that the use of GH in sport continues despite the lack of evidence-based medicine to support its use in athletes and that many of the purported benefits may apply only to those who are greatly hormone deficient and not to athletes.

Side-effects associated with growth hormone abuse in sport

Between 40 and 80 per cent of healthy adults who have received GH in controlled prospective studies report side effects and most of the acute side effects arise from fluid retention (Birzniece, 2015). The long-term risks of GH in athletes are not well known since epidemiological data derived from users in sport are not available (Saugy et al., 2006).

Major side-effects include skeletal changes, enlargement of the fingers and toes, growth of the orbit and lengthening of the jaw. The internal organs enlarge and the cardiomegaly which is produced is often one of the causes of death associated with GH abuse. Although the skeletal muscles increase in size, there are often complaints of muscle weakness. Adverse biochemical changes include impaired glucose regulation (usually hyperglycaemia), hyperlipidaemia and insulin resistance. The changes described above contribute to the prevalence of diabetes in GH abusers. Arthritis and impotence often occur after chronic GH abuse (Kicman and Cowan, 1992).

A consequence of the increased protein synthesis during GH abuse is changes to the skin. This includes thickening and coarsening – the so-called "elephant epidermis" – which has been known to make the skin almost impenetrable by standard gauge syringe needles (Taylor, 1988). Other skin effects include activation of naevocytes and an increase in dermal viscosity (Ehrnborg et al., 2000).

It is believed that many athletes use doses of GH many times higher than those used therapeutically and it is reasonable to expect that serious side effects may develop (Holt and Sonksen, 2008). It is likely that the longer-term effect of GH administration would also occur with IGF-I (Holt and Sonksen, 2008), as described in clinical trials for mecasermin rinfabate, a drug consisting of recombinant IGF-1 and IGF Binding Protein 3 (Kemp, 2007).

Who abuses growth hormone and why?

The reasons for GH abuse appear to be based on some false premises that it is as effective as anabolic steroids, with fewer side-effects and is less easily detected. Abusers believe GH may protect the athlete who has abused anabolic steroids and who wishes to stop "muscle meltdown", when anabolic steroids are withdrawn.

There are few scientific studies available on the prevalence of GH abuse in sport. In 1997, Korkia and Stimson reported that 2.7 per cent of the anabolic steroid abusers in their UK survey were also abusing GH while Evans (1997) found concordant abuse of anabolic steroids and GH in 12.7 per cent of abusers in his gymnasia survey.

Five per cent of adolescents in a survey (Rickert et al., 1992) admitted using GH and 24.5 per cent claimed to know of someone who was abusing it. Fifty per cent of the abusers could not name one side effect of GH. Those who abused GH were most likely to be involved in wrestling or American football and to have obtained their information about GH from another person such as a coach. There was also some evidence of co-abuse of anabolic steroids and GH in the same adolescent sample.

A study by Brennan et al. (2011) reported that among young weightlifters, illicit GH use has become a common form of substance abuse, frequently associated with both anabolic androgenic steroids dependence as well as dependence on other substances of abuse such as opioids, cocaine and ecstasy.

Since a validated test for GH has not been available until recently, reports of GH abuse have been mostly anecdotal or as observations by anti-doping agencies (Stow et al., 2009). On a number of occasions, athletes have confessed to using GH having tested positive for other substances. This was the case with Ben Johnson after the 1988 Seoul Olympics and for a number of high-profile athletes after the BALCO affair in 2003. A review of the use of GH by athletes can be found in Holt et al. (2009).

Abuse by athletes of IGF-1 has been assumed to be lower than for GH because of its lower availability, however research by Ernst and Simon (2013) suggested IGF-1 use amongst professional track and field sprinters.

10.9 Growth hormone releasing factors (GHRFs)

In 2010, Henninge et al. reported that several peptide drugs were being manufactured as releasing factors for GH. The authors identified the peptide marketed under the name CJC-1295, within an unknown pharmaceutical preparation and believed that it was being used within the bodybuilding community. Further examples of GHRFs, such as GHRP-2 were identified in unlabelled pharmaceutical products (Gaudiano et al., 2013). There is evidence that GHRFs are being marketed on the "life-style" drug market (Evans-Brown et al., 2012) a fact that, it is recommended, needs drawing to the attention of athlete support personnel, such as healthcare professionals (Stensballe et al., 2015).

10.10 Detection of growth hormone abuse

Human GH is a peptide which has a very short half-life within the blood and appears in very low concentrations in the urine. Furthermore, secretion of naturally occurring GH from the pituitary gland is pulsatile. Therefore, blood levels fluctuate significantly. Since GH secretion is affected by factors such as emotion, stress, sleep and nutritional status, there is a high variability within individuals and between individuals (Saugy et al., 2006). In addition, exercise can influence GH secretion (Wallace et al., 2001).

Up to the 2004, Athens Olympic Games a validated method to detect GH was not used, despite significant attempts to develop such a method. After the 1996, Atlanta Olympic Games a research project, entitled GH-2000, was set up comprising a consortium of endocrinologists, with expertise in growth hormone research, from four European countries, with collaboration from two leading pharmaceutical companies (Holt et al., 2009). The project team reported their results in 1999, with a proposal for a test based on the measurement of two markers for GH, IGF-1 and type III pro-collagen (P-III-P; Powrie et al., 2007). Despite significant support for the proposed test, it was recommended that further research was required to ensure the test would work in ethnic groups other than Caucasians and that the test was not affected by injury.

Following the establishment of WADA in 1999, a second phase of research into GH testing was set up, entitled GH-2004, with significant financial support from the US Anti-Doping Agency. GH-2004 directed its efforts towards the "biomarker" approach to GH testing. At the same time, WADA supported an "isoform" approach to testing (Barroso et al., 2009).

The direct "isoform" approach to GH doping detection

This approach involves immunoassays to quantify different types of GH isoforms that differentiate between naturally secreted GH and recombinant GH that has been injected by the athlete.

This test was used, experimentally, at the Athens Olympic Games in 2004 and at the Turin Winter Olympic Games in 2006 (Saugy et al., 2006). To fulfil WADA requirements, two double tests were applied to serum samples. The first test quantified the 22kDa isoform that is derived from recombinant GH. The second test measured the other isoforms derived from naturally occurring GH. When recombinant GH is administered, endogenous growth hormone secretion is inhibited, therefore, the ratio of 22kDa to total GH increases. The ratio between these isoforms is calculated. A second double sample test was used for confirmatory purposes (Bidlingmaier and Strasburger, 2000).

The direct test was also used at the 2008, Beijing Olympic Games. However, as in Athens and Turin, no positive test results were detected. It has been suggested that this was unsurprising as this method has a relatively short (less than 24 hr) window of opportunity. Therefore, any athlete who discontinues their use of GH on the day before the test would not be detected (Holt et al., 2009).

The indirect "biomarker" approach to GH doping detection

The indirect approach does not aim to detect GH itself but to build up a database of the normal range of a number of markers for GH. It has been suggested that this approach would not stand up in a court as an absolute proof of doping (Saugy et al., 2006). However, the results of the GH-2000 and GH-2004 studies supported the choice of IGF-I and P-III-P as markers to detect recombinant GH administration (Erotokritou-Mulligan et al., 2007).

The GH Biomarker test was introduced for the first time at the London 2012 Olympic and Paralympic Games. This test detects increases in the biomarkers for GH which are IGF-1 and procollagen-3 n-terminal peptide (P3NP) (Powrie et al., 2007; Erotokiritou-Mulligan et al., 2007). Unlike previous tests for GH, which could only detect the use of the hormone for a very short period of time, the Biomarker Test detects GH use for at least one week after it has been taken.

Two athletes at the London 2012 Paralympic Games tested positive for GH and were excluded from the Games (see Box 10.4), marking a successful introduction at a major event for the new GH Biomarker Test. In 2014, WADA announced that advances had been made to the GH Biomarker Test based on liquid chromatography – tandem mass spectrometry (WADA, 2014) (Cox et al., 2014).

Another approach being adopted by International Federations is longitudinal studies on athletes' biological profiles. By regularly monitoring haematological and steroidal profiles, any abnormalities would reveal potential doping activity. This technique of Athlete Biological Passports (ABPs) is described in Chapter 5. The use of ABPs to detect GH and other hormones, using an "endocrine module" is described by Pitsiladis et al. (2014); Saugy et al. (2014) and Vernec (2014).

With the development of effective tests for detecting GH, Guha et al. (2013) have highlighted the potential increase in abuse of IGF-1.

Cases of growth hormone abuse in sport

The problems associated with the development of a robust, validated test for GH abuse has meant that few cases have been recorded.

Box 10.3   Terry Newton (2010)

Terry Newton was the first case of GH use resulting in an athlete sanction. This rugby league player was tested out-of-competition in November 2009, when GH was detected in a blood sample. Newton accepted the charge of doping and was banned for two years. Sadly, Newton committed suicide during this period and whilst not directly attributed to his positive drug test, it was clearly a factor in his tragic death.

The UK Anti-Doping Chief Executive stated that "The positive finding was a combination of intelligence, target testing and a strong partnership with anti-doping scientific community and the Rugby Football League" (http://www.ukad.org.uk/news/article/newton-gets-two-years-for-world-first-hgh-finding).

A validated test for GH, robust enough to withstand legal challenge, was introduced in 2012.

Box 10.4   Nikolay Marfin and Vadim Rakitin (2012)

These Russian powerlifters tested positive for GH a week before the start of the London 2012 Paralympic Games. Before the test results were announced, Rakitin had competed in the men's under-90kg class, finishing seventh but Marfin was prevented from competing in the 100-plus kg class. Both athletes were subsequently given two-year bans.

These cases were the first successes for the newly developed "Biomarker Test" for GH, as described earlier in this chapter.

10.11 Growth factors

In addition to IGF-1 there are a wide range of growth factors that are prohibited in sport (Table 10.1). Their prohibition is due to their role in muscle-specific signal transduction pathways involved in the growth and development of skeletal muscle. The mammalian target of rapamycin (mTOR) and myostatin pathways are the most important in terms of muscle growth.

The mTOR pathway integrates signals in response to exercise and energy levels, namely IGF-1, insulin, mechano growth factor (MGF; which is expressed in response to the stimulus of muscle stretch during exercise), dietary protein and energy levels. The overall effect is an increase in muscle protein synthesis. The myostatin pathway unsurprisingly has a negative effect on protein synthesis and thus muscle growth. Potential pharmacological and gene therapy to inhibit myostatin would be of great interest to the unscrupulous athlete and are therefore discussed further in Chapters 12 and 16.

Whilst early research showed that hypertrophy in response to resistance exercise was associated with increased IGF-1 expression, it was unable to distinguish between the different types of growth factors. In fact the increased IGF-1 reflected an increase in MGF, a local signalling molecule (i.e. an autocrine) derived from the IGF-1 gene. Mechano growth factor promotes hypertrophy and repair associated with exercise-induced muscle damage by activating muscle stem cells and anabolic processes (Goldspink, 2005). Although MGF has not been approved for therapeutic use it is commercially available on the black market (Esposito et al., 2012). As yet no test has been developed for its detection.

Insulin-like growth factor-1 has a central role in promoting muscle anabolism as well as glycogen synthesis and mediates the actions of GH. In addition, IGF-1 is involved in the proliferation and differentiation of myocytes (Engert et al., 1996). Nevertheless, evidence to support its efficacy as a performance- and image-enhancing drug (PIED) in humans is limited, although enhanced muscle growth has been demonstrated in an animal model (Adams and McCue, 1998). Its use as a PIED has been reported amongst gym users in the UK and USA (Brennan et al. 2011; Bates and McVeigh, 2014) although to a lesser extent than GH. In an interesting paper by Ernst and Simon (2013) it was claimed that recent improvements in sprinting performance in track and field athletics were indicative of the arrival of IGF-1 to the marketplace as an approved pharmaceutical in 2005.

Deer antler velvet, used in traditional Chinese medicine, is reported to contain IGF-1. However, in a study by Cox and Eichner (2013) it was discovered that deer antler velvet products had been adulterated with pharmaceutical IGF-1. Over recent years there have been reports of the use of supplements containing deer antler velvet by athletes in an attempt to benefit from IGF-1. However, few studies have examined its performance-enhancing effects and those that have are limited in terms of scientific rigour (Gilbey and Perezgonzalez, 2012). The potential for IGF-1 bioavailability via sublingual absorption suggests that athletes should exercise caution when considering its use.

Other growth factors that have been identified which play their part in enhancing muscle size and function include: transforming growth factor-β (TGF-β), platelet-derived growth factor (PDGF), fibroblast growth factor (FGF), epidermal growth factor (EGF), vascular endothelial growth factor (VEGF) and endothelial cell growth factor. Such growth factors are particularly important in the regenerative process following trauma as a consequence of exercise-induced muscle damage and injury.

Fibroblast growth factor 1 (FGF-1) is one such growth factor which has local effects in terms of promoting muscle repair angiogenesis. Whist FGF-1 is not an approved pharmacological agent, recent analysis of black market products has isolated FGF-1 and found it to be slightly different from recombinant FGF-1, thus highlighting the real risk that individuals take when using unlicensed products from the black market (Walpurgis et al., 2011).

The practice of blood spinning has been the topic of much discussion within anti-doping circles in recent years. Blood spinning is the controversial practice of creating platelet-rich plasma (PRP) from an individual's blood by centrifugation and injecting it at a site of injury. Platelet-rich plasma is known to contain high concentrations of growth factors which are believed to enhance the healing process. Whilst this practice in the treatment of injury is currently not prohibited, the use of growth factors *per se* is. For this reason there are concerns as to whether the practice of intramuscular application of PRP influence systemic circulating growth factors (Schippinger et al., 2012). Indeed recent work by Wasterlain et al. (2013) has found that serum IGF-1, VEGF and FGF-2 were significantly elevated after PRP administration, thus demonstrating potential ergogenic effects. Further research in this area will enable WADA to make an informed decision regarding the status of PRP administration in athletes.

Other than their potential as doping agents, the possible down-side of the use of growth factors, particularly in targeting the mTOR pathway, is that by increasing protein synthesis, widespread growth, not solely on skeletal muscle is promoted. Clearly stimulation of growth may have negative effects in tissues and since the mTOR pathway is the focus for anti-cancer drugs (Lui et al., 2009) it is conceivable that growth factors may have carcinogenic effects.

10.12 Prevalence of peptide hormone use in sport

Statistics on the number of adverse analytical findings (AAFs) relating to peptide hormones, as recorded by WADA accredited laboratories, between 2006 and 2012, are shown in Table 10.2.

Table 10.2 WADA statistics for the number of positive results for substances classed as peptide hormones, growth factors and related substances (2009–2015)

	2009	2010	2011	2012	2013	2014	2015
Erythropoietin (EPO)	56	36	43	45	56	57	41
Erythropoietin (active transcription factor)	–	–	1	–	–	–	–
Darbepoetin (dEPO)	4	8	5	4	5	7	5
Micera (CERA)	8	1	–	–	2	3	–
Chorionic gonadotrophin (CG)	25	33	47	93	124	17	12
Leutinising hormone (LH)	6	5	23	29	15	–	17
Insulins*	–	–	–	2	–	–	–
Growth hormone (GH)	1	3	6	8	–	1	4
GH-releasing peptides (GHRPs)	–	–	–	–	6	10	–
FG-4592	–	–	–	–	–	–	4
Ipamorelin	–	–	–	–	–	–	3
Ibutamoren	–	–	–	–	–	–	2
Total	100	86	125	181	202	91	98

*Insulins were re-classified as hormone and metabolic modulators by WADA in 2013

In general, there is an increasing trend towards the detection of peptide hormones, in part due to improved methods of analysis. The extension of the use of Athlete Biological Passports will further improve rates of detection, particularly for EPO, although Ashenden et al. (2011) suggested that improvements are needed to identify doping with EPO through microdosing.

10.13 Peptide hormones as potential targets for gene doping

A review by van der Gronde et al. (2013) highlights peptide hormones as potential targets for gene doping since many of these hormones are being investigated for their beneficial use in gene therapy. A detailed explanation of gene doping is presented in Chapter 16 of this book.

10.14 Summary

- A number of peptide hormones that occur naturally in the body are included on the WADA prohibited list.
- Erythropoietin (EPO) increases red blood cell counts, thereby enhancing oxygen supply to muscles and other tissues.
- Illicit use of EPO can be detected in the laboratory either directly or through recording of Athlete Biological Passport markers.
- Chorionic gonadotrophin (CG) and luteinizing hormone (LH) have the potential to increase endogenous testosterone levels.
- Growth hormone (GH) has a number of significant biological effects, including increase in muscle mass and strength. It also possesses serious potential side effects.
- The effects of GH are mediated through Insulin-like Growth Factor-1 (IGF-1), which is used to detect GH use through the Biomarker Test.

- Localized growth factors that are central to increased muscle size and function would appear to be infiltrating the muscle-building supplements market. The need for a validated test for their detection is therefore necessary.
- The practice of injecting platelet-rich plasma in the treatment of injury would appear to be widespread yet the effects on the systemic circulation of growth factors would suggest that this may offer a potential performance-enhancing effect.

10.15 References

Adams, G.R. and McCue, S.A. (1998) Localised infusion of IGF-1 results in skeletal muscle hypertrophy in rats. *Journal of Applied Physiology* 84(5): 1,716–1,722.

Ashenden, M., Gough, C.E., Garnham, A. et al. (2011) Current markers of Athlete Blood Passport do not flag microdose EPO doping. *European Journal of Applied Physiology* 111: 2,307–2,314.

Ashenden, M., Varlet-Marie, E., Lasne, F. & Audran, M. (2006). The effects of microdose recombinant human erythropoietin regimens in athletes. *Haematologica* 91(8): 1,143–1,144.

Barroso, O., Schamasch, P. and Rabin, O. (2009) Detection of GH abuse in sport: Past, present and future. *Growth Hormone and IGF Research* 19: 369–374.

Bates, G. and McVeigh, J. (2016) Image and performance enhancing drugs 2015 survey results. Available at: http://www.cph.org.uk/wp-content/uploads/2016/07/IPEDs-2015-survey_final1.pdf (Accessed on 28 July 2017).

Baumann, G.P. (2012) Growth hormone doping in sports: A critical review of use and detection strategies. *Endocrine Review* 33: 155–186.

Bidlingmaier, M., Wu, Z. and Strasburger, C.J. (2000) Test method: GH. *Best Clinical Endocrinology and Metabolism* 14: 99–109.

Birkeland, K.I., Stray-Gundersen, J., Hemmersbach, P. et al. (2000). Effect of r-HuEPO administration on serum levels of sTfR and cycling performance. *Medicine and Science in Sports and Exercise* 32(7): 1,238–1,243.

Birzniece, V., Nelson, A.E. and Ho, K.K. (2011) Growth hormone and physical performance. *Trends in Endocrinological Metabolism* 22: 171.

Birzniece, V. (2015) Doping in sport: Effects, harm and misconceptions. *Internal Medicine Journal* 45: 239–248.

Boisclair, Y.R., Rhoads, R.P., Ueki, I., et al. (2001) The acid labile subunits (ALS) of the 150 KDq IGF-binding protein complex: An important but forgotten component of the circulating IGF system. *Journal of Endocrinology* 170: 3–70.

Brennan, B.P., Kanayama, G., Hudson, J.I. and Pope, H.G. (2010) Human growth hormone abuse in male weightlifters. *The American Journal on Addiction* 20: 9–13.

Brooks, R.V., Collyer, S.P., Kicman, A.T. et al. (1989) CG doping in sport and methods for its detection. In P. Bellot, G. Benzi and A. Ljungqvist (eds) *Official Proceedings of Second IAF World Symposium on Doping in Sport*, London, 37–45.

Brower, K.J. (2000) Assessment and treatment of anabolic steroid abuse, dependence and withdrawal. In C. Yesalis (ed.) *Anabolic Steroids in Sport and Exercise*, 2nd edition. Champaign, Illinois, Human Kinetics, 305–332.

Cazzola, M. (2001). Erythropoietin pathophysiology, clinical uses of recombinant human erythropoietin, and medical risks of its abuse in sport. *International Society for Laboratory Hematology (ISLH) XIVth International Symposium*, 21.

Consitt, L.A., Copeland, J.L. and Tremblay, M.S. (2002) Hormonal responses to exercise in women. *Sports Medicine* 32: 1–22.

Cowart, V. (1988) Human growth hormone: The latest ergogenic aid? *Physician and Sport Medicine* 16: 175–185.

Cox, H.D. and Eichner, D. (2013) Detection of human insulin like growth factor-1 in deer antler velvet supplements. *Rapid Communications in Mass Spectrometry* 27(19): 2,170–2,178.

Cox, H.D., Lopes, F. and Woldermariam, G.A. (2014) Interlaboratory agreement of insulin-like growth factor 1 concentrations measured by mass spectrometry. *Clinical Chemistry* 60(3): 541–548.

Deyssig, R., Firsch, H., Blum, W.F. et al. (1993) Effect of growth hormone treatment and hormonal parameters, body composition and strength in athletes. *Acta Endocrinologica (Copenhagen)* 128: 313–318.

Dine, G. (2001). Biochemical and haematological parameters in athletes. *International Society for Laboratory Hematology (ISLH) XIVth International Symposium*, 24.

Durussel, J., Haile, D.W., Mooses, K. et al. (2016) Blood transcriptional signature of recombinant human erythropoietin administration and implications for antidoping strategies. *Physiological Genomics* 48(3): 202–209.

Ehrnborg, C., Bengtsson, B.A. and Rosen, T. (2000) Growth hormone abuse. *Best Clinical Endocrinology and Metabolism* 14: 71–77.

Ekblom, B. and Berglund, B. (1991). Effect of erythropoietin administration on maximal aerobic power. *Scandanavian Journal of Medicine and Science in Sports* 1: 88–93.

Ekblom, B. (1997) Blood doping, erythropoetin and altitude. In T. Reilly and M. Orme (eds) *The Clinical Pharmacology of Sport and Exercise*. Elsevier, Amsterdam, 199–212.

Elliott, S. (2008). Erythropoiesis-stimulating agents and other methods to enhance oxygen transport. *British Journal of Pharmacology* 154: 529–541.

Engert, J.C., Berglund, E.B. and Rosenthal, N. (1996) Proliferation precedes differentiation in IGF-1-stimulated myogenesis. *Journal of Cell Biology* 135(2): 431–440.

Ernst, S. and Simon, P. (2013) A quantitative approach for assessing significant improvements in elite sport performance. Has IGF-1 entered the arena? *Drug Testing Analysis* 5: 384–389.

Erotokritou-Mulligan, I., Bassett, E.E. and Kniess, A. (2007) Validation of the growth hormone (GH)-dependent marker method of detecting GH abuse in sport through the use of independent data sets. *Growth Hormone and IGF Research* 17: 416–423.

Esposito, S., Deventer, K. and Van Eenoo, P. (2012) Characterization and identification of a C-terminal amidated mechano growth factor (MGF) analogue in black market products. *Rapid Communications in Mass Spectrometry* 26(6): 686–692.

Evans, N.A. (1997) Gym and tonic: A profile of 100 anabolic steroid users. *British Journal of Sports Medicine* 31: 54–58.

Evans-Brown, M., McVeigh, J., Perkins, C. and Bellis, M.A. (2012) *Human enhancement drugs: The emerging challenges to public health*. Liverpool, North West Public Health Observatory.

Gaudiano, M.C., Valvo, L. and Borioni, A. (2013) Identification and quantification of the doping agent GHRP-2 in seized unlabelled vials by NMR and MS: A case-report. *Drug testing Analysis* 6: 295–300.

Gilbey, A. and Perezgonzalez, J.D. (2012) Health benefits of deer and elk velvet antler supplements: A systematic review of randomised control studies. *New Zealand Medical Journal* 125(1367): 80–86.

Goldspink, G. (2005) Research on mechano growth factor: Its potential for optimising physical training as well as misuse in doping. *British Journal of Sports Medicine* 39: 787–788.

Gotherstrom, G., Bengtsson, B.-A., Sunnerhagen, K.S. et al. (2005) The effect of five-year growth hormone replacement theray on muscle strength in elderly hypopituitary patients. *Clinical Endocrinology* 62: 105–113.

Guha, N., Cowan, D.A., Sonksen, P.H. et al. (2013) Insulin-like growth factor-1 (IGF-1) misuse in athletes and potential methods for detection. *Analytical and Bioanalytical Chemistry* 405(30): 9,669–9,683.

Handelsman, D.J. (2006) The rationale for banning human chorionic gonadotrophin and estrogen blockers in sport. *Journal of Clinical Endocrinology and Metabolism* 91: 1,646–1,653.

Handelsman, D.J., Goebel, C., Idan, A. et al. (2009) Effects of recombinant human LH and CG on serum and urine LH and androgens in man. *Clinical Endocrinology* 71: 417–428.

Henninge, J., Pepaj, M., Hullstein, I. and Hemmersbach, P. (2010) Identification of CJC-1295, a growth-hormone-releasing peptide, in an unknown pharmaceutical preparation. *Drug Testing Analysis* 2: 647–650.

Holt, R.I.G. (2004) The metabolic effects of growth hormone. *CME Bulletin of Endocrinological Diabetes* 5: 11–17.

Holt, R.I.G. and Sonksen, P.H. (2008) Growth hormone, IGF-1 and insulin and their abuse in sport. *British Journal of Pharmacology* 154: 542–556.

Holt, R.I.G., Erotokritou-Mulligan, I. and Sonksen, P.H. (2009) The history of doping and growth hormone abuse in sport. *Growth Hormone and IGF Research* 19: 320–326.

Jelkmann, W. (2014) Xenon misuse in sports: Increase of hypoxia-inducible factors and erythropoietin, or nothing but "hot air"? *Deutsche Zeitschrift Für Sportmedizin* 65: 267–271.

Jelkmann, W. (2016) Features of blood doping. *Deutsche Zeitschrift Für Sportmedizin* 67: 255–262.

Jelkmann, W. and Thevis, M. (2016) Could nickel become a novel erythropoiesis-stimulating compound for cheating athletes? *Deutsche Zeitschrift Für Sportmedizin* 67: 253–254.

Kemp, S.F. (2007) Mecasermin rinfabate. *Drugs Today* 43:149–155.

Kicman, A.T., Brooks, R.V. and Cowan, D.A. (1991) Human chorionic gonadotrophin and sport. *British Journal of Sports Medicine* 25:73–80.

Kicman, A.T. and Cowan, D.A. (1992) Peptide hormones and sport: Misuse and detection. *British Medical Bulletin* 48: 496–517.

Kimmage. P. (1998) *Rough Ride*. London, Yellow Jersey Press.

Korkia, P. and Stimson, G.V. (1997) Indications and prevalence, practice and effects of anabolic steroid use in Great Britain. *International Journal of Sports Medicine* 18: 557–562.

Lasne, F. and de Ceaurriz, J. (2000). Recombinant erythropoietin in urine. *Nature* 405: 635.

Leith, W. (1992). EPO and cycling. *Athletics* July. 24-26.

Le Roith, D., Bondy, C., Yakar, S. et al. (2001) The somatomedin hypothesis. *Endocrinological Review* 22: 53–74.

Liu, H., Bravata, D.M., Olkin, I. et al. (2008) Systemic review: The effects of growth hormone on athletic performance. *Annals of Internal Medicine* 148: 747–758.

Lombardo, J.A., Hickson, P.C. and Lamb, D.R. (1991) Anabolic/Androgenic steroids and growth hormone. In D.R. Lamb, and M.H. Williams (eds) *Perspectives in Exercise Science and Sports Medicine, Vol.4, Ergogenics: Enhancement of Performance in Exercise and Sport*. New York, Brown & Benchmark, 249–278.

Lui, Q., Thoreen, C, Wang, J. et al., (2009) mTOR mediated anti-cancer drug discovery. *Drug Discovery Today: Therapeutic Strategies* 6(2): 47–55.

Macintyre, J.G. (1987) Growth hormone and athletes. *Sports Medicine* 4: 129–142.

Marcus, R. and Hoffman, A.R. (1998) Growth hormone as therapy for older men and women. *Annual Review of Pharmacology and Toxicology* 38: 45–61.

McHugh, C.M., Park, R.T., Sonksen, P.H. et al. (2005) Challenges in detecting the abuse of growth hormone in sport. *Clinical Chemistry* 51: 1,587–1,593.

Meinhardt, U., Nelson, A.E., Hansen, J.L. et al. (2010) The effects of growth hormone on body composition and physical performance in recreational athletes: A randomised trial. *Annals of Internal Medicine* 152: 568.

Momaya, A., Fawal, M. and Estes, R. (2015) Performance enhancing substances in sports: A review of the literature. *Sports Medicine* 45: 517–531.

Mottram, D.R. (2013) The Lance Armstrong case: The evidence behind the headlines. *Aspetar Sports Medicine Journal* 2(1): 60–65.

Muller, E.E. (1987) Neural control of somatotropic function. *Physiological Review* 3: 962–1,053.

Norton, K. and Olds, T. (2001) Morphological evolution of athletes over the 20th century. *Sports Medicine* 31: 763–783.

Parisotto, R., Wu, M., Ashenden, M.J. et al. (2001). Detection of recombinant human erythropoietin abuse in athletes utilizing markers of altered erythropoiesis. *Haematologica* 86: 128–137.

Pitsiladis, Y., Durussel, J. and Rabin, O. (2014) An integrative "omics" solution to the detection of recombinant human erythropoietin and blood doping. *British Journal of Sports Medicine* 48: 856–861.

Powrie, J.K., Bassett, E.E., Rosen, T. et al. (2007) Detection of growth hormone abuse in sport. *Growth Hormone and IGF Research* 17: 220–226.

Reichel, C. (2014) Detection of peptide erythropoiesis-stimulating agents in sport. *British Journal of Sports Medicine* 48: 842–847.

Rendell, M. (2006). *The Death of Marco Pantani: A Biography*. London, Weidenfeld & Nicolson.

Rennie, M.J. (2003) Claims for the anabolic effects of growth hormone: A case of the emperor's new clothes? *British Journal of Sports Medicine* 37: 100–105.

Reznik, Y., Dehennin, L., Coffin, C., et al. (2001) Urinary nandrolone metabolites of endogenous origin in man: A confirmation by output regulation under human chronic Gonadotrophin stimulation. *Journal of Clinical Endocrinology and Metabolism* 86:146–150.

Rickert, V.I., Pawlak-Morello, C., Sheppard, V., et al. (1992) Human growth hormone: A new substance of abuse among adolescents? *Clinical Paediatrics* 31: 723–726.

Rogol, A.D. (2014) Can anabolic steroids or human growth hormone affect growth and maturation of adolescent athletes? *Paediatric Exercise Science* 26: 423–427.

Saugy, M., Lundby, C. and Robinson, N. (2014) Monitoring of biological markers indicative of doping: the athlete biological passport. *British Journal of Sports Medicine* 48: 827–832.

Saugy, M., Robinson, M., Saudan, C. et al. (2006) Human growth hormone doping in sport. *British Journal of Sports Medicine* 40: i35–i39.

Schippinger, G., Fankhauser, F., Oettl, K. et al. (2012) Does single intramuscular application of autologous conditioned plasma influence systemic circulating growth factors? *Journal of Sports Science and Medicine* 11: 551–556.

Schnirring, L. (2000) Growth hormone doping: the search for a test. *Physician and Sportsmedicine* 28: 1–6.

Smith, D.A. and Perry, P.J. (1992) The efficacy of ergogenic agents in athletic competition. Part II. Other performance enhancing agents. *Annals of Pharmacotherapy* 26: 653–659.

Sonksen, P. (2001) Insulin growth hormone and sport. *Journal of Endocrinology* 170: 13–15.

Stenman, U.-H., Hotakainen, K. and Alfthan, H. (2008) Gonadotrophins in doping: Pharmacological basis and detection of illicit use. *British Journal of Pharmacology* 154: 569–583.

Stensballe, A., McVeigh, J., Breindahl, T. and Kimergard, A. (2015) Synthetic growth hormone releasers detected in seized drugs: New trends in the use of drugs for performance enhancement. *Addiction* 110: 368–370.

Stoppe, C., Ney, J., Brenke, M. et al. (2016) Sub-anesthetic xenon increases erythropoietin levels in humans: A randomised control trial. *Sports Medicine* 46(11): 1,753–1,766.

Stow, M.R., Wojek, N. and Marshall, J. (2009) The UK Sport perspective on detecting growth hormone abuse. *Growth Hormone and IGF Research* 19: 375–377.

Taylor, W.N. (1988) Synthetic human growth hormone: A call for federal control. *Physician and Sports Medicine* 16: 189–192.

Thevis, M., Krug, O., Piper, T. et al (2016) Solutions advertised as erythropoiesis-stimulating products were found to contain undeclared cobalt and nickel species. *International Journal of Sports Medicine* 37(01): 82–84.

Tsitisimpikou, C., Kouretas, D., Tsarouhas, K. *et al.* (2011) Applications and biomonitoring issues of recombinant erythropoietins for doping control. *Therapeutic Drug Monitoring* 33: 3–13.

van der Gronde, T., de Hon, O., Haisma, H.J. et al. (2013) Gene doping: An overview and current implications for athletes. *British Journal of Sports Medicine* 47: 670–678.

Velloso, C.P. (2008) Regulation of muscle mass by growth hormone and IGF-1. *British Journal of Pharmacology* 154: 557–568.

Vernec, A.R. (2014) The athlete biological passport: An integral element of innovative strategies in antidoping. *British Journal of Sports Medicine* 48: 817–819.

Voet, W. (2001) *Breaking the Chain*. London, Yellow Jersey Press.

WADA (2009). Technical Document – TD 2009: EPO harmonization of the method for the identification of recombinant erythropoietins (i.e. epoetins) and analogues (e.g. darbepoetin and methoxypolyethylene glycol-epoetin beta).

WADA (2014) WADA Director General statement on advanced method to hGH Biomarkers Test. Available at: https://www.wada-ama.org/en/media/news/2014-03/wada-director-general-statement-on-advanced-method-to-hgh-biomarkers-test (Accessed February 2017).

Wallace, J.D., Cuneo, R.C., Baxter, R. et al. (1999) Responses of the growth hormone (GH) and insulin-like growth facts axis to exercise, GH administration, and GH withdrawal in trained adult males: A potential test for GH abuse in sport. *Journal of Clinical Endocinology and Metabolism* 84: 3,591–3,601.

Wallace, J.D., Cuneo, R.C., Bidlingmaier, M. et al. (2001) The response of molecular isoforms of growth hormone to acute exercise in trained adult males. *Journal of Clinical Endocinology and Metabolism* 86: 200–206.

Walpurgis, K., Thomas, A., Laussmann, T. et al. (2011) Identification of fibroblast growth factor 1 (FGF-1) in a black market product. *Drug Testing and Analysis* 3(11-12): 791–797.

Wasterlain, A.S., Braun, H.J., Harris, A.H.S. et al. (2013) The systemic effects of platelet-rich plasma injection. *American Journal of Sports Medicine* 41(1): 186–193.

Wells, D.J. (2008) Gene doping: The hype and the reality. *British Journal of Pharmacology* 154: 573–574.

Yarasheski, K.E., Campbell, J.A., Smith, K. et al. (1992) Effect of growth hormone and resistance exercise on muscle growth in young men. *American Journal of Physiology* 262: 261–267.

Yarasheski, K.E., Zachweija, J.J., Angelopoulis, T.J. et al. (1993) Short-term grown hormone treatment does not increase muscle protein synthesis in experienced weightlifters. *Journal of Applied Physiology* 74: 3,073–3,076.

Chapter 11

Beta-2 agonists

Neil Chester and David R. Mottram

11.1 Introduction

Maximum performance in aerobic events, at whatever level of competition, is only achievable if respiratory function is optimal. Competitors will always be concerned about conditions that adversely affect the respiratory system be they major disease, for example, asthma or minor ailment, such as the common cold. Beta-2 agonists are a first line class of drugs used to treat asthma. These drugs produce their therapeutic effect through bronchodilation. Clearly, such an effect has the potential to enhance athletic performance by improving oxygen uptake. Therefore, Beta-2 agonists are included as a category on the World Anti-Doping Agency (WADA) Prohibited List, subject to a complex set of regulations. Since beta-2 agonists are a necessary component in the treatment regimes for asthmatic patients, Therapeutic Use Exemption (TUE) may be required for asthmatic athletes in order to allow them to compete on equal terms with fellow competitors.

Some beta-2 agonists, such as clenbuterol, possess anabolic properties, although through a mechanism that is different from that produced by anabolic steroids. Consequently, they are included under the category of anabolic agents on the WADA Prohibited List.

This chapter will review the condition of asthma and other bronchoconstriction-related conditions and the use of beta-2 agonists in their treatment. The misuse of these drugs in sport will be reviewed and the systems in place for controlling beta-2 agonists as performance-enhancing agents whilst permitting therapeutic use, where appropriate.

11.2 What are beta-2 agonists?

In Chapter 1 of this book, we described how drugs interact through specific targets within the body, known as receptors. In the case of adrenoreceptors, through which the hormone adrenaline (epinephrine) produces its effects in the body, we reviewed the five subclasses of these receptors. This included the sub-class referred to as beta-2 receptors.

Drugs that have been developed to interact selectively on these receptors are known as beta-2 agonists. Table 11.1 lists some of the more commonly prescribed beta-2 agonists.

The table categorises the drugs as short-acting and long-acting, which has a significance regarding their clinical use in the treatment of conditions such as asthma and chronic obstructive pulmonary disease.

Table 11.1 Selective beta-2 agonists

Short-acting
   Salbutamol (Albuterol)
   Terbutaline
   Fenoterol
   Reproterol
   Bitolterol
   Pirbuterol
Long-acting
   Formoterol (Eformoterol)
   Salmeterol
   Bambuterol
   Indacaterol
   Olodaterol
   Tulobuterol
   Procaterol
   Vilanterol

Pharmacology of beta-2 agonists

All selective beta-2 agonists are potent bronchodilators. They differ in their time to onset and duration of action. Salbutamol (Albuterol) and terbutaline are short-acting and the most frequently used beta-2 agonists in many countries. There are many formulations of salbutamol and terbutaline including tablets, slow-release tablets, elixirs, aerosols and dry powder inhalers, solutions for injection and specialised inhalation from a nebuliser. Inhalation is the route of choice because it is the most rapidly effective (1-2 minutes) and is associated with the fewest side-effects. Tremor is the most common side effect after inhalation. However, other side effects of beta-2 agonists are common (Cockcroft, 2006). This led Backer et al. (2007) to conclude that anti-asthmatic treatment should not be used by non-asthmatic elite athletes. Side effects after oral administration include: fine tremor (usually of the hands), nervous tension and headache. Tachycardia, peripheral vasodilation and hypokalaemia may also occur after oral dosing.

The duration of action of salbutamol and terbutaline after aerosol administration is approximately 4 hours. Formoterol (Eformoterol) and salmeterol are the most frequently prescribed long-acting beta-2 agonists with a duration of action of approximately 12 hours.

11.3 Clinical uses of beta-2 agonists

Asthma and its treatment

Definition

Asthma is a chronic inflammatory disorder of the airways. In susceptible individuals, this inflammation causes recurrent episodes of coughing, wheezing, chest tightness and difficulty in breathing. Inflammation makes the airways sensitive to stimuli such as allergens, chemical irritants, tobacco smoke, cold air or exercise. When exposed to these stimuli, the airways may become swollen, constricted, filled with mucus and hyper-responsive to stimuli. The resulting airflow limitation is reversible in most patients, either spontaneously or with treatment. An individualised approach to asthma therapy including regular use of inhaled corticosteroids can ensure that over the long term, symptoms can be reduced in both severity and frequency (Global Initiative for Asthma, 2017).

Pathophysiology

An asthma attack always consists of an early phase and frequently contains a late phase. The early phase, consisting of bronchoconstriction, occurs within minutes of exposure to the trigger factor, reaches a maximum in 15 to 20 minutes and normally resolves within an hour. The late phase, characterised by inflammation of the airways, occurs 2 to 4 hours after exposure to the trigger factor and reaches a maximum after 6 to 8 hours. Appreciation of the change of emphasis from bronchoconstriction to inflammation as the cause of airway obstruction has underpinned the change in approach to the management of asthma.

Trigger factors

There are numerous factors which can trigger an asthma attack. The most common are allergens, which can be either inhaled (e.g. pollens and animal dander such as hairs and feathers) or ingested (e.g. dairy produce or strawberries). Viral, but not bacterial, infection of the upper respiratory tract can trigger asthma. Indeed, the initial presenting feature of asthma may be a persistent wheeze after a self-limiting, upper respiratory tract, viral infection. Occupational pollution can also cause asthma. Asthma attacks can be precipitated by emotional factors. This should not be misinterpreted as an indication that asthma is psychosomatic. Rather it is a reflection of neuroendocrine changes which, as yet, are poorly understood. Certain drugs may precipitate an asthma attack such as beta-blockers and non-steroidal anti-inflammatory drugs (NSAIDs), particularly aspirin. Beta-blockers cause bronchoconstriction by blocking the bronchodilating beta-2 receptors on airway smooth muscle and should not be administered to asthmatics. The mechanism by which NSAIDs evoke bronchospasm is hypothetical but may involve a shift in balance between bronchodilating and bronchoconstricting metabolites of arachidonic acid. Approximately 10 per cent of asthmatics are aspirin-sensitive and will bronchoconstrict if given the drug. For this reason, aspirin and other NSAIDs should be used with caution in asthmatics. An asthmatic may be sensitive to a variety of trigger factors or to just one.

Management of asthma

Non-drug treatment of asthma involves avoidance of known trigger factors. Drug treatment of asthma is primarily directed at arresting and reversing the inflammatory process with the emphasis shifting from the excessive and inappropriate use of beta-2 agonist bronchodilator therapy towards the earlier use of anti-inflammatory drugs. Beta-2 agonists merely relieve the symptoms of asthma without addressing the underlying inflammation. Guidelines for treatment of chronic asthma have been prepared in several countries. They constitute a systematic approach to the treatment of increasing severity of symptoms.

Essentially, the first step involves the occasional use of short-acting inhaled beta-2 agonists to relieve the symptoms of bronchoconstriction. Thereafter, depending on the severity of symptoms, more regular use of short-acting beta-2 agonists is recommended, with the addition of inhaled corticosteroids. If the symptoms are more severe, long-acting beta-2 agonists or other bronchodilators are used with inhaled corticosteroids. Corticosteroids are subject to WADA regulations, as described in Chapter 20 of this book.

It must be remembered that the treatment of asthma can also be stepped down if the severity of the symptoms declines.

Exercise-induced asthma (EIA) and exercise-induced bronchoconstriction (EIB)

Exercise-induced asthma (EIA) can be defined as a lower airway obstruction and symptoms of cough, wheezing or dyspnoea induced by exercise in patients with underlying asthma (Schwartz et al., 2008). The same presentation of symptoms in individuals without asthma can be defined as exercise-induced bronchoconstriction (EIB). EIB probably includes an interplay between environmental training factors, such as allergens, temperature, humidity and air pollutants and an athlete's personal risk factors such as genetic and neuroimmunoendocrine determinants (Moreira et al., 2011).

In 2014, a systematic review by Price et al. (2014) investigated the impact of EIB on athletic performance. The authors concluded that, whilst it was reasonable to suspect that EIB does impact on athletic performance, there was insufficient evidence to provide a definitive answer.

Diagnosis of asthma and EIB

A major issue with respect to ensuring the effective healthcare of individuals with respiratory conditions such as asthma relates to accurate diagnosis. There is, however, no standardised diagnosis of asthma as a consequence of the fact that no consistent definition of the symptoms exists (British Thoracic Society, 2012). As well as a clinical history, individuals who present themselves with asthma symptoms to their clinician will typically undertake a simple peak flow assessment. Unfortunately a normal peak flow recorded whilst an individual is asymptomatic does not preclude them from a positive diagnosis of asthma. There are, however, a number of tests that include the assessment of lung function pre and post a bronchoprovocation challenge. A marked reduction in lung function from baseline (typically >10% drop in FEV_1) is required in order for an individual to test positive to a specific bronchoprovocation challenge and thus form the basis of a diagnosis of asthma or EIB. Broncoprovocation challenges may include the administration of Histamine, Mannitol, Metacholine and saline or a bout of exercise. Whilst an exercise challenge is the most ecologically valid test it is difficult to control factors such as ventilation and environmental conditions. The Eucapnic Voluntary Hyponea (EVH) challenge has been established to mimic exercise in a controlled manner and involves an individual attaining a minute ventilation equivalent to 85 per cent of their predicted maximal voluntary ventilation rate for six minutes during which dry, CO_2-rich air (<2% relative humidity; 5% CO_2) is inhaled. The EVH challenge has been shown to be particularly sensitive in the assessment of EIB in athletes and has subsequently been adopted as the method of choice by the IOC Medical Commission in the diagnosis of EIB and support of subsequent prescription of inhaled beta-2 agonists (Whyte, 2013).

Implementation of such tests have not only unearthed previously undiagnosed asthma, but also misdiagnosis (Dickinson et al., 2011). In a significant number of individuals previously diagnosed with asthma, there was no confirmation following detailed assessment.

In such cases it is likely that individuals may suffer from dysfunctional breathing brought on by stressful situations during exercise.

Dysfunctional breathing is a loose term also known as overt episodic hyperventilation, chronic hyperventilation syndrome and disproportionate breathlessness (Morgan, 2002). It includes several breathing abnormalities associated with the following symptoms: breathlessness, chest tightness, chest pain, unsteady and irregular breathing and non-diaphragmatic respiratory effort (Thomas et al., 2005). Whilst dysfunctional breathing commonly accompanies asthma, it may also exist in those without asthma (Thomas et al., 2005). No gold standard method of diagnosis exists, however the Nijmegen questionnaire (van Dixhoorn and Duivenvoorden, 1985) is commonly used to identify those with symptoms. Together with an objective test to diagnose asthma and EIB (involving a provocation challenge), the Nijmegan questionnaire may be used to identify those exhibiting symptoms associated with dysfunctional breathing only. Clearly, the significance of establishing a criterion method of diagnosis lies in the notion that methods of treatment, other than pharmacotherapy, may be prescribed. Further research is needed, not only in its diagnosis, but in the development and application of non-pharmacological treatment including breathing technique training.

Prevalence of EIA and EIB in athletes

A consistent body of evidence has shown that elite athletes have an increased risk of asthma when compared to the general population, especially those taking part in endurance sports or winter sports (Carlsen et al., 2008a). A review of previous studies, by Parsons and Mastronarde (2005), revealed that prevalence rates for brochospasm related to exercise ranged from 11 to 50 per cent. Furthermore, up to 90 per cent of individuals with asthma will have exercise–induced asthma. The highest prevalence of exercise-induced asthma (EIA) has been noted in athletes competing in the winter season, due to exposure to cold, dry air (Weiler and Ryan, 2000). The high prevalence of asthma in swimmers and other athletes training in indoor pools can be explained by exposure to chlorine and its derivatives (Langdeau and Boulet, 2001; Balcerek et al., 2015). Pedersen et al. (2008) believe that elite swimmers do not have particularly susceptible airways when they take up competitive swimming when young but develop respiratory symptoms, airway inflammation and airway hyperresponsiveness during their swimming careers. Similarly, Fitch (2006) reported that of the 193 athletes who met the IOC's criteria for the use of beta-2 agonists at the 2006 Winter Olympics, only 32.1 per cent had childhood asthma and 48.7 per cent of athletes reported onset at age 20 years or older. This led the authors to speculate that years of intense endurance training may be a causative factor in bronchial hyperreactivity.

The higher prevalence of airway hyperresponsiveness measured in athletes coupled with the use of subjective methods to diagnose asthma may mean that the prevalence of respiratory problems in athletes is under-diagnosed (Langdeau and Boulet, 2003). A review by Carlsen et al. (2008a) confirms the view that the prevalence of asthma and bronchial hyperresponsiveness is markedly increased in athletes, especially within endurance sports and that environmental factors often contribute to this increase. These authors also provide recommendations for the diagnosis of asthma in athletes. A review by Fitch (2012) concludes that asthma is the most common chronic medical condition experienced by Olympic athletes, affecting between 7 and 8 per cent of Olympic athletes and that years of endurance training may be a contributory factor. Furthermore, Fitch (2012) concluded that athletes with asthma were not overly disadvantaged by their medical condition and that evidence from recent Games shows that they have outperformed their non-asthmatic rivals.

The increased exposure, through sporting activity, to environmental agents such as cold dry air in skiers and chlorine compounds in swimmers, increases symptoms and signs of asthma and bronchial hyper-responsiveness either worsening existing asthma or leading to a novel disease in a previously healthy athlete (Carlsen et al., 2011).

Management of exercise-induced asthma (EIA) and exercise-induced bronchoconstriction (EIB)

The management of EIB should involve preventative/non-pharmacological measures as well as treatment with drugs, such as beta-2 agonists (Schumacher et al., 2011; Anderson and Kippelen, 2012; Ansley et al., 2013).

Non-drug treatment

Fitness does not prevent EIA. However, aerobic fitness does improve lung function, retards deterioration in lung function with age (in non-asthmatics) and enables asthmatics to exercise with less EIA. There is no evidence to suggest that aerobic training is deleterious to asthmatics provided that their treatment is optimal and that they have a satisfactory management plan which includes access to appropriate bronchodilator therapy, if required.

Minimisation of the cooling and drying of the airways can be achieved by nasal breathing, whenever possible. Susceptible individuals should seek to avoid exercising in a cold, dry environment. If this is unavoidable then a face mask may reduce cooling and drying of the airways.

The inhalation of particulate matter, a key component of air pollution, may have a detrimental effect on exercising athletes. Cutrufello et al. (2012) provide some useful advice for athletes on how to avoid the inhalation of particulate matter during exercise.

Drug treatment for EIA and EIB with beta-2 agonists

A review by Carlsen et al. (2008b) of the treatment of exercise-induced asthma concluded that it should be treated in athletes following the same principles as for non-athletes since there is little evidence for improvement in athletic performance by inhaled beta-2 agonists.

Beta-2 agonists are the most effective prophylactic treatment of EIA preventing asthma symptoms in 90 per cent of patients (Lacroix, 1999). Short-acting beta-2 agonists (Table 11.1) should be administered 15 to 30 minutes before commencing exercise (Rupp, 1996; Lacroix, 1999). They induce bronchodilation within five minutes and afford protection against EIA for approximately three to six hours. They should be available to the athlete for rapid relief of symptoms should they develop despite pre-exercise treatment. Salmeterol, a long-acting beta-2 agonist, should be taken 30 minutes before exercise and is effective for up to nine hours (Nelson et al., 1998). Because of its slower onset of action, salmeterol should not be used as a rescue medication to relieve symptoms of an asthma attack.

Fitch (2016) reviews the restrictions that the WADA Code places on the prescription of drugs to prevent and to treat asthma in athletes and provides useful information for respiratory physicians who manage elite and sub-elite athletes with asthma.

11.4 The illicit use of beta-2 agonists in sport

Prevalence of beta-2 agonists in sport

Beta-2 agonists have been a target for athletes for many years. They have appeared in large numbers on the WADA annual statistics for adverse analytical findings (Table 11.2).

These annual figures for positive test results for beta-2 agonists do include cases where athletes have received permission to use the drugs for therapeutic purposes. However, it has been acknowledged that there has been a marked increase by athletes in the application to use short-acting beta-2 agonists (Fitch et al., 2008). Figures for the percentage of all athletes applying to inhale beta-2 agonists at summer Olympic Games show 3.6 per cent at Atlanta in 1996; 5.7 per cent at Sydney in 2000 and 4.6 per cent at Athens in 2004 (Carlsen et al., 2008a). The equivalent figures for winter Olympic Games were higher, with 5.6 per cent at Nagano in 1998, 6.3 per cent at Salt Lake City in 2002 and 8.3 per cent at Turin in 2006 (Carlsen et al., 2008a), perhaps reflecting the higher incidence of EIA in cold conditions. However, recent changes in WADA legislation means that common beta-2 agonists such as salbutamol, formoterol and salmeterol may be inhaled in therapeutic doses without the need for a TUE (Table 11.3).

Regardless of the specific need for beta-2 agonists for the treatment of asthma under particular conditions, the incidence of adverse analytical findings for beta-2 agonists extends across all sports, with relatively higher incidences in certain sports (Figure 11.1).

Cases involving beta-2 agonists

There are few high profile cases involving those drugs commonly used to combat the symptoms of asthma. However, in response to a case involving the detection of high levels of salbutamol in a rugby league player there has been renewed interest into the possible misuse of such drugs.

Table 11.2 WADA statistics for the number of adverse analytical findings for substances classed as beta-2 agonists (2006–2015)

	2006	2007	2008	2009	2010	2011	2012	2013	2014	2015
Salbutamol	391	60	56	29	9	6	6	11	8	16
Terbutaline	175	182	163	157	111	130	117	103	93	87
Formoterol	42	107	91	84	78	84	–	–	–	–
Salmeterol	16	37	30	23	6	1	3	9	7	1
Fenoterol	5	11	10	5	5	2	5	15	9	10
Reproterol	2	2	–	3	–	1	–	–	–	1
Ritodrine	–	–	–	1	–	–	–	–	–	–
Pirbuterol	–	–	–	1	–	–	–	–	–	–
Bambuterol	–	–	–	–	–	1	–	–	–	–
Tulobuterol	–	–	–	–	–	–	–	–	5	–
Total	631	399	350	303	209	225	131	138	122	115

Results on beta-2 agonists include adverse findings for which the athlete may have been granted Therapeutic Use Exemption under WADA regulations

Table 11.3 WADA Prohibited List (2017) regulations relating to beta-2 agonists

All selective and non-selective beta-2 agonists, including all optical isomers, are prohibited. Including, but not limited to:

Fenoterol
Formoterol
Higenamine
Indacaterol
Olodaterol
Procaterol
Reproterol
Salbutamol
Salmeterol
Terbutaline
Vilanterol.

Except: • Inhaled salbutamol: maximum 1600 micrograms over 24 hours, not to exceed 800 micrograms every 12 hours; • Inhaled formoterol: maximum delivered dose of 54 micrograms over 24 hours; • Inhaled salmeterol: maximum 200 micrograms over 24 hours. The presence in urine of salbutamol in excess of 1,000 ng/mL or formoterol in excess of 40 ng/mL is presumed not to be an intended therapeutic use of the substance and will be considered as an adverse analytical finding (AAF) unless the Athlete proves, through a controlled pharmacokinetic study, that the abnormal result was the consequence of the use of the therapeutic dose (by inhalation) up to the maximum dose indicated above.

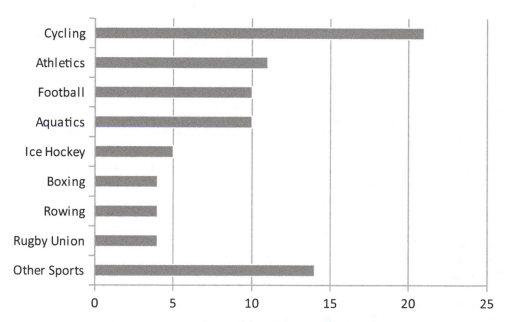

Figure 11.1 Numbers of adverse analytical findings for beta-2 agonists in 2015

Data obtained from WADA 2015 Anti-Doping Testing Figures. Available at: https://www.wada-ama.org/sites/default/files/resources/files/2015_wada_anti-doping_testing_figures_report_0.pdf (Accessed: July 2017)

Box 11.1   Ian Sibbit (2009)

Despite holding a TUE for the use of salbutamol Ian Sibbit, an RFL (Rugby Football League) player, was accused of misusing the drug and not following prescription guidelines. However, confusion exists as it is typically prescribed on an as needed basis or *pro re nata* (PRN). This can be misunderstood and viewed as permission to use the drug as many times as required which may ultimately lead to the administration of doses in excess of the recommended maximal therapeutic doses (400 μg up to four times daily) by individuals with poorly controlled asthma. The player was eventually acquitted following appeal and advised on how to manage his condition more effectively.

Box 11.2   Simon Yates (2016)

The British cyclist, Simon Yates, tested positive for terbutaline during the Paris–Nice race in March 2016. He was prescribed the drug for asthma but the drug was not declared on a TUE form. His team admitted that they were responsible for the error; however, strict liability rules were applied and, although the UCI concluded it was a "non-intentional" violation, Yates was given a 4-month ban.

Most high profile cases involve the use of the beta-2 agonist, clenbuterol, which is misused typically for its anabolic effects, hence its inclusion on the WADA Prohibited List as an anabolic agent (Chapter 9).

Do beta-2 agonists enhance performance?

Several studies have investigated the effects of inhaled beta-2 agonists, both in asthmatic and in healthy athletes. Few studies have reported an increase in exercise performance following inhaled treatment (Signorile et al., 1992; van Baak et al., 2004). The majority of studies failed to show an ergogenic effect (Morton and Fitch, 1992; Norris et al., 1996; Larson et al., 2005; Carlsen et al., 2008b, Kippelen et al., 2012). Inhaled salbutamol, even in high doses, did not have a significant effect on endurance performance in non-asthmatic, highly trained cyclists (Goubault et al., 2001). These authors did note that salbutamol had a slight but significant bronchodilator effect, which may be sufficient to improve respiratory adaptation at the beginning of exercise. However, they further concluded that it is unlikely that such minimal effects were unlikely to be responsible for the widespread use of salbutamol by athletes. A study by Elers et al. (2012a) concluded that no ergogenic effect of a high dose of salbutamol on aerobic capacity was found in healthy trained men. Dickinson and colleagues (2014c) examined the effect of long-term administration (6 weeks) of high dose inhaled salbutamol (4 × 400 μg daily) on measures of endurance, strength and power performance in non-elite, male athletes following a structured training programme and found no improvement. A review in which 20 randomised, placebo controlled studies were evaluated, only three studies reported a performance-enhancing effect of inhaled beta-2 agonists (Kindermann and Meyer, 2006), although methodological shortcomings were cited as being factors in the findings. These authors concluded that there is no ergogenic potential of inhaled beta-2 agonists in non-asthmatic athletes and questioned the inclusion of inhaled beta-2 agonists on the WADA Prohibited List.

In cold environments, where athletes with exercise-induced asthma are more likely to experience symptoms of the condition, inhaled formoterol did not improve endurance performance in healthy, well-trained male athletes (Tjørhom et al., 2007). The authors therefore concluded that formoterol could be used in competitive sports without fear of a possible performance-enhancing effect.

Fitch (2012) reported that Olympic athletes with asthma and airway hyper-responsiveness have consistently out-performed their peers, which research suggests is not due to their treatment enhancing sports performance. Although a review by Collomp et al. (2010) reported that almost all research trials after acute or short-term oral administration at therapeutic dosage levels demonstrated significant improved performance, whatever the exercise intensity, most studies using inhaled beta-2 agonists have generally failed to show improved performance (Dickinson et al., 2014b; Koch et al., 2015). On the other hand, systemic use of beta-2 agonists may have a positive effect on physical performance in healthy subjects (Pluim et al., 2011). Oral administration of salbutamol has been shown to have a significant positive effect on sprint capacity in recreational athletes (Sanchez et al., 2012). Similarly, Hostrup et al. (2016) investigated acute and 2-week administration of oral salbutamol on exercise performance and muscle strength in athletes and concluded that salbutamol taken by that route benefits athletes' sprint ability.

Anabolic effects of beta-2 agonists

Beta-2 agonists possess anabolic activity, although the extent of this varies between drugs. Anabolic effects of oral beta-2 agonists has have been clearly demonstrated in animals (Ryall et al., 2006). Clenbuterol is a long-acting, beta-2 agonist, which is licensed for the treatment of asthma in some countries. It is not licensed for human use in either the UK or the USA. However, it is licensed for veterinary use (Ventopulmin®, Boehringer Ingelheim) in horses for the treatment of bronchoconstriction caused by several equine respiratory diseases.

Clenbuterol, as a beta-2 agonist has side-effects which are typical of this group of drugs i.e. tremor, restlessness, agitation, headache, increased blood pressure and palpitations. These side-effects are dose-related and purported to decrease after 8 to 10 days. This is due to a decrease i.e. down-regulation of beta-2 receptors, a consequence of which is also a decrease in the anabolic effect of the drug. Other potential adverse, dose-dependent effects include tissue desensitization and cell necrosis in heart and slow-twitch soleus muscle as demonstrated in an animal model (Burniston et al., 2005).

Zilpaterol, like clenbuterol, was introduced as a growth promoter in cattle. It has a similar pharmacological profile to clenbuterol (Davies et al., 2008). It has a reputation as an anabolic agent with bodybuilders, despite little published work on its efficacy in this respect.

With respect to the anabolic effects of beta-2 agonists, it is dependent on the receptor density of muscles (Beerman, 2002). Since chronic administration of beta-2 agonists produces downregulation of receptors (Johnson, 2006), this may limit the effectiveness and therefore the value of beta-2 agonists as anabolic agents (Davies, et al., 2008).

Box 11.3   The "Festina affair" (1998)

Clenbuterol was one of the frequently used drugs cited by Willy Voet in his account of the notorious "Festina affair" in the 1998 Tour de France cycle race (Voet, 2001).

Box 11.4   Jessica Hardy (2008)

Jessica Hardy was dropped from the US Olympic team one month before the 2008 Beijing Olympic Games having tested positive for clenbuterol. She claimed that she had accidentally ingested the banned substance when taking a nutritional supplement. The Arbitration Panel for Sport accepted her claim and reduced her suspension from two years to one year.

Box 11.5   Alberto Contador (2010)

The Spanish professional cyclist, Albert Contador tested positive for Clenbuterol during the 2010 Tour de France, the event that he won. His victory was subsequently annulled and he received a two-year suspension from competition. Contador's defence included the claim that his positive test was as a consequence of the contaminated meat in his diet.

11.5 Beta-2 agonists and the WADA Prohibited List

From an anti-doping perspective the status of inhaled beta-2 agonists has changed over recent years. Whilst terbutaline remains prohibited at all times several other common beta-2 agonists, such as salbutamol, salmeterol and formoterol are permitted by inhalation for therapeutic use. The WADA Prohibited List (2017) regulations relating to beta-2 agonists are shown in Table 11.3.

Clearly, athletes who require treatment with beta-2 agonists have recourse, under WADA regulations, to use salbutamol, formoterol or salmeterol. However, the WADA regulations are designed to ensure that athletes who require bronchodilation with these drugs limit their use to recommended therapeutic dose regimes. Other beta-2 agonists, such as terbulatine, are subject to Therapeutic Use Exemption (TUE) regulations. Similarly, the administration of salbutamol, formoterol or salmeterol by routes other than inhalation is also subject to TUE regulation.

In an attempt to differentiate between misuse and recommended therapeutic use urinary thresholds have been introduced for salbutamol and formoterol. Any athlete exceeding the threshold or indeed the decision limit (a concentration set above the recognised WADA threshold) will be asked to perform a controlled pharmacokinetic study in an attempt to establish whether the positive test was as a consequence of administering the drug up to a maximal therapeutic dose by inhalation.

Unfortunately there is evidence to suggest a high inter-individual variation exists in terms of urinary drug levels following the inhalation of therapeutic doses of beta-2 agonists to the extent that exceeding the thresholds in such circumstances is likely (Elers et al., 2012b; Dickinson et al., 2014a; Fitch, 2017). This likelihood is increased further through poor management of respiratory conditions and the prescribing of many short-acting beta-2 agonists *pro re nata*. As a prophylactic and when used by those with poorly controlled asthma, doses may exceed recommended maximal daily doses and thus risk an anti-doping rule violation. Whilst this may be deemed misuse, it does not necessarily constitute intentional doping.

The issue of dehydration and prohibited substances that are subject to threshold limits is an important one raised by Fitch (2017). Dickinson and colleagues et al. (2014a) clearly demonstrated the impact of dehydration on the urinary salbutamol concentrations. Salbutamol levels surpassed the urinary threshold following therapeutic dosing under conditions of dehydration and high urinary specific gravity. This supports the need to correct urinary drug levels for specific gravity.

McKenzie and Fitch (2011) have proposed that there is no pharmacological difference between permitted and prohibited beta-2 agonists, therefore asthmatic athletes are being managed differently, based on a WADA directive that has no foundation in pharmacological science or in clinical practice.

The WADA Prohibited List states that all optical isomers of beta-2 agonists are prohibited. It has been reported (Jacobson and Fawcett, 2016) that the permitted beta-2 agonists, salbutamol, formoterol and salmeterol are chiral compounds containing 50:50 racemic mixtures of active and inactive isomers. If athletes use single active enantiomers of these drugs they can double the effect of the drug whilst remaining within allowable urinary threshold limits.

Kalsen et al. (2014) drew attention to the potential performance-enhancing effects of using combinations of salbutamol, formoterol and salmeterol, each within their respective permitted dose regimes, which should be considered when making future anti-doping regulations.

Beta-2 agonists such as clenbuterol, zeranol and zilpaterol appear on the WADA Prohibited List under class S1 Anabolic Agents, reflecting their potential anabolic properties.

11.6 Summary

- Beta-2 agonists are first line drugs in the treatment of asthma and other obstructive airways diseases because of their bronchodilatory activity.
- Exercise-induced asthma and bronchoconstriction are conditions prevalent in elite athletes, involved in high volumes of training. It is particularly prevalent in those engaged in winter sports and swimming.
- The performance-enhancing potential for beta-2 agonists is dependent on the dose and route of administration of the drugs. This is reflected in WADA's regulations concerning the prohibition of this class of drugs, including the criteria for Therapeutic Use Exemption.

11.7 References

Anderson, S.D. and Kippelen, P. (2012) Assesment and prevention of exercise-induced bronchoconstriction. *British Journal of Sports Medicine* 46: 391–396.

Ansley, L., Rea, G. and Hull, J.H. (2013) Practical approach to exercise-induced bronchoconstriction in athletes. *Primary Care Respiratory Journal* 22(1): 122–125.

Backer, V., Lund, T. and Pedersen, L. (2007) Pharmaceutical treatment of asthma symptoms in elite athletes: Doping or therapy? *Scandanavian Journal of Medicine and Science in Sports* 17: 615–622.

Balcerek, T., Lutomski, P. and Grzesiak, M. (2015) Asthma in athletes and the use of asthma treatment. *Trends in Sport Sciences* 1(22): 13–18.

Beerman, D.H. (2002) β-Adrenergic receptor agonist modulation of skeletal muscle growth. *Journal of Animal Science* 80E (Suppl 1): e18–e23.

British Thoracic Society (2012) British Guideline on the Management of Asthma. https://www.brit-thoracic.org.uk/document-library/clinical-information/asthma/btssign-asthma-guideline-2012/ (Accessed on 1st December 2017).

Burniston, J.G., Chester, N., Clark, W.A. et al. (2005) Dose-dependent apoptotic and necrotic myocyte death iduced by the β_2-adrenergic receptor agonist, clenbuterol. *Muscle Nerve* 32: 767–774.

Carlsen, K.H., Anderson, S.D., Bjermer, L. et al. (2008a) Exercise induced asthma, respiratory and allergic disorders in elite athletes: Part I of the report from the Joint Task Force of European Respiratory Society (ERS) and European Academy of Allergy and Clinical Immunology (EAACI) in cooperation with GA²LEN. *Allergy* 63: 387–403.

Carlsen, K.H., Anderson, S.D., Bjermer, L. et al. (2008b) Treatment of exercise induced asthma, respiratory and allergic disorders in sports and the relationship to doping: Part II of the report from the Joint Task Force of European Respiratory Society (ERS) and European Academy of Allergy and Clinical Immunology (EAACI) in cooperation with GA²LEN. *Allergy* 63: 492–505.

Carlsen, K.H., Hem, E. and, Stensrud, T. (2011) Asthma in adolescent athletes. *British Journal of Sports Medicine* 45: 1,266–1,271.

Cockcroft, D.W. (2006) Clinical concerns with β_2-agonists: Adult asthma. *Clinical Reviews in Allergy and Immunology* 31(2-3): 197–207.

Collomp, K., Le Panse, B., Candau, R. et al. (2010) Beta-2 agonists and exercise performance in humans. *Science and Sports* 25: 281–290.

Cutrufello, P.T., Smoliga, J.M. and Rundell, K.W. (2012) Small things make a big difference: Particulate matter and exercise. *Sports Medicine* 42(12): 1,041–1,058.

Davies, E., Loiacono, R. and Summers, R.J. (2008) The rush to adrenaline: Drugs in sport acting on the β-adrenergic system. *British Journal of Pharmacology* 154: 584–597.

Dickinson, J., McConnell, A. and Whyte, G. (2011) Diagnosis of exercise-induced bronchoconstriction: eucapnic voluntary hyperpnoea challenges identify previously undiagnosed elite athletes with exercise-induced bronchoconstriction. *British Journal of sports Medicine* 45: 1,126–1,131.

Dickinson, J., Chester, N., Hu, J. et al. (2014a) Impact of ethnicity, gender and dehydration on the urinary excretion of inhaled salbutamol with respect to doping control. *Clinical Journal of Sports Medicine* 24(6): 482–489.

Dickinson, J., Hu, J., Chester, N. et al. (2014b) Acute impact of inhaled short acting β_2-agonists on 5Km running performance. *Journal of Sports Science and Medicine* 13: 271–279.

Dickinson, J., Molphy, J., Chester, N. et al. (2014c) The ergogenic effect of long-term use of high dose salbutamol. *Clinical Journal of Sports Medicine* 24(6): 474–481.

Elers, J., Morkeberg, J., Jansen, T. et al. (2012a) High-dose inhaled salbutamol has no acute effects in aerobic capacity or oxygen uptake kinetics in healthy trained men. *Journal of Medical Science in Sports* 22: 232–239.

Elers, J., Pedersen, L., Henninge, J. et al. (2012b) The pharmacokinetic profile of inhaled and oral salbutamol in elite athletes with asthma and non-asthmatic subjects. *Clinical Journal of Sports Medicine* 22: 140–145.

Fitch, K. (2006) β_2-agonists at the Olympic Games. *Clinical Reviews in Allergy and Immunology* 31(2-3): 259–268.

Fitch, K., (2012) An overview of asthma and airway hyper-responsiveness in Olympic athletes. *British Journal of Sports Medicine* 46: 413–416.

Fitch, K. (2016) The World Anti-Doping Code: Can you have asthma and still be an elite athlete? *Breathe* 12: 148–158.

Fitch, K. (2017) The enigma of inhaled salbutamol and sport: Unresolved after 45 years. *Drug Testing and Analysis* 9(7): 977–982.

Fitch, K., Sue-Chu, M., Anderson, S. et al. (2008) Asthma and the elite athlete: Summary of the International Olympic Committee's Consensus Conference, Lausanne, Switzerland, January 22-24, 2008. *Journal of Allergy and Clinical Immunology* 122: 254–260.

Global Initiative for Asthma. (2017) 2017 Pocket Guide for Asthma Management and Prevention. Available at: http://www.ginasthma.org/gina-reports/ (Accessed on 1 December 2017).

Goubault, C., Perault, M-C., Leleu, E. et al. (2001) Effects of inhaled salbutamol in exercising non-asthmatic athletes. *Thorax* 56: 675–679.

Hostrup, M., Kalsen, A., Auchenberg, M. et al. (2016) Effects of acute and 2-week administration of oral salbutamol on exercise performance and muscle strength in athletes. *Scandanavian Journal of Medicine and Science in Sports* 26: 8–16.

Jacobson, G.A. and Fawcett, J.P. (2016) Beta2-agonist doping control and optical isomer challenges. *Sports Medicine* 46: 1,787–1,795.

Johnson, M. (2006) Molecular mechanisms of β_2-adrenergic receptor function, response and regulation. *Journal of Allergy and Clinical Immunology* 117: 18–24.

Kalsen, A., Holstrup, M., Bangsbo, J. and Backer, V. (2014) Combined inhalation of beta$_2$-agonists improve swim ergometer sprint performance but not high-intensity swim performance. *Scandanavian Journal of Medicine and Science in Sports* 24: 814–822.

Kindermann, W. and Meyer, T. (2006) Inhaled β_2 agonists and performance in competitive athletes. *British Journal of Sports Medicine* 40(Suppl 1): i43–i47.

Kippelen, P., Fitch, K.D., Anderson, S.D. et al (2012) Respiratory health of elite athletes: Preventing airway injury – a critical review. *British Journal of Sports Medicine* 46: 471–476.

Koch, S., MacInnis, M.J., Sporer, B.C. et al. (2015) Inhaled salbutamol does not affect athletic performance in asthmatic and non-asthmatic cyclists. *British Journal of Sports Medicine* 49: 51–55.

Lacroix, V.J. (1999). Exercise-induced asthma. *The Physician and Sportsmedicine* 27 (12): 75–92.

Langdeau, J.-B. and Boulet, L.-P. (2001) Prevalence and mechanisms of development of asthma and airway hyperresponsiveness in athletes. *Sports Medicine* 31(8): 601–616.

Langdeau, J.-B. and Boulet, L.-P. (2003) Is asthma over- or under-diagnosed in athletes? *Respiratory Medicine* 97: 109–114.

Larsson, K., Carlsen, K.H. and Bonini, S. (2005) Anti-asthmatic drugs: Treatment of athletes and exercise-induced bronchoconstriction. *European Respiratory Monthly* 33: 73–88.

McKenzie, D.C. and Fitch, K.D. (2011) The asthmatic athlete: Inhaled beta-2 agonists and doping. *Clinical Journal of Sports Medicine* 21(1): 46–50.

Moreira, A., Delgardo, L. and Carlsen, K.H. (2011) Exercise-induced asthma: Why is it so frequent in Olympic athletes? *Expert Review of Respiratory Medicine* 5(1): 1–3.

Morgan, M.D.L. (2002) Dysfunctional breathing in asthma: Is it common, identifiable and correctable? *Thorax* 57(Suppl II): ii31–ii35.

Morton, A.R. and Fitch, K.D. (1992) Asthmatic drugs and competitive sport: An update. *Sports Medicine* 14: 228–242.

Nelson, J.A., Strauss, L., Skowronski, M., et al. (1998). Effect of long-term salmeterol treatment on exercise-induced asthma. *New England Journal of Medicine* 339: 141–146.

Norris, S.R., Petersen, S.R. and Jones, R.L. (1996) The effects of salbutamol on performance in endurance cyclists. *European Journal of Applied Physiology and Occupational Physiology* 73: 364–368.

Parsons, J.P. and Mastronarde, J.G. (2005) Exercise-induced bronchoconstriction in athletes. *Chest* 128: 3,966–3,974.

Pedersen, L., Lund, T.K., Barnes, P.J. et al. (2008) Airway responsiveness and inflammation in adolescent elite swimmers. *Journal of Allergy and Clinical Immunology* 122: 322–327.

Pluim, B.M., de Hon, O., Stael, J.B. et al. (2011) Beta(2)-agonists and physical performance: A systematic review and meta analysis of randomised control trials. *Sports Medicine* 41: 39–57.

Price, O.J., Hull, J.H., Backer, V. et al. (2014) The impact of exercise-induced bronchocontriction on athletic performance: A systematic review. *Sports Medicine* 44: 1,749–1,761.

Rupp, N.T. (1996). Diagnosis and management of exercise-induced asthma. *The Physician and Sportsmedicine* 24 (1): 77–87.

Ryall, J.G., Sillence, M.N. and Lynch, G.S. (2006) Systemic administration of β_2-adrenoceptor agonists, formoterol and salmeterol, elicit skeletal muscle hypertrophy in rats at micromolar doses. *British Journal of Pharmacology* 147: 587–595.

Sanchez, A.M., Collomp, K., Carra, J. et al. (2012) Effect of acute and short term oral salbutamol treatments on maximal power output in non-asthmatic athletes. *European Journal of Applied Physiology* 112(9): 3,251–3,258.

Schumacher, Y.O., Pottgeisser, T. and Dickhuth, H. (2011) Exercise-induced bronchoconstriction: Asthma in athletes. *International Sports Medicine Journal* 12(4): 145–149.

Schwartz, L.B., Delgardo, L., Craig, T. et al. (2008) Exercise-induced hypersensitivity syndromes in recreational and competitive athletes: A PRACTALL consensus report. *Allergy* 63(8): 953–961.

Signorile, J.F., Kaplan, T.A., Applegate, B. et al. (1992) Effects of acute inhalation of the bronchodilator, albuterol, on power output. *Medicine and Science in Sports and Exercise* 24: 638–642.

Thomas, M., McKinley, R.K., Freeman, E., Foy, C. and, Price, D. (2005) The prevalence of dysfunctional breathing in adults in the community with and without asthma. *Primary Care Respiratory Journal* 14: 78–82.

Tjørhom, A., Riiser, A. and Carlsen, K.H. (2007) Effects of formoterol on endurance performance in athletes at an ambient temperature of -20°C. *Scandanavian Journal of Medicine and Science in Sports* 17: 628–635.

Van Baak, M.A., de Hon, O.M., Hartgens, F. et al. (2004) Inhaled salbutamol and endurance cycling performance in non-asthmatic athletes. *International Journal of Sports Medicine* 25: 533–538.

Van Dixhoorn, J. and Duivenvoorden, H.J. (1985) Efficacy of Nijmegan questionnaire in recognition of the hyperventilation syndrome. *Journal of Psychosomatic Research* 29: 199–206

Voet, W. (2001). *Breaking the Chain*. London, Yellow Jersey Press, London.

Weiler, J.M. and Ryan, E.J., III (2000) Asthma in United States Olympic athletes who participated in the 1998 Olympic winter games. *Journal of Allergy and Clinical Immunology* 106: 267–271.

Whyte, G. (2013) Asthma, EIB and the athlete: Diagnosis, prevalence, treatment and anti-doping. *Aspertar Sports Medicine Journal* 2(3): 334–338.

Chapter 12

Hormone and metabolic modulators

Neil Chester

12.1 Introduction

According to the WADA Prohibited List both S1 and S2 classes of doping agents are comprised of by and large naturally occurring hormones and their synthetic derivatives. The S4 class entitled, 'Hormone and Metabolic Modulators' (Table 12.1) contains several groups of synthetic compounds, or otherwise, which act by modulating various endogenous hormonal pathways and local muscle-specific transduction pathways. The aim of such modulators is in most cases to enhance exercise performance, however in the case of aromatase inhibitors, selective oestrogen receptor modulators (SERMs) or other anti-oestrogenic substances, it may be to counteract the unwanted side effects of anabolic androgenic steroid (AAS) administration.

12.2 Hormone and metabolic modulators and the WADA Prohibited List

The class of doping agents categorised as Hormone and Metabolic Modulators (S4) are prohibited at all times, both within competition and out-of-competition. Previously, all doping agents in this class, except for the metabolic modulators including insulins, were classified as Hormone Antagonists and Modulators and introduced to the WADA Prohibited List in

Table 12.1 Class S4 of the 2017 WADA List of prohibited substances and methods (WADA, 2016a)

S4. Hormone and metabolic modulators

1 Aromatase inhibitors including but not limited to: 4-androstene-3,6,17 trione (6-oxo); aminoglutethimide; anastrozole; androsta-1,4,6-triene-3,17-dione (androstatrienedione); androsta-3,5-diene-7,17-dione (arimistane); exemestane; formestane; letrozole; testolactone
2 Selective estrogen receptor modulators (SERMS) including, but not limited to: raloxifene; tamoxifen; toremifene
3 Other anti-estrogenic substances including, but not limited to: clomiphene; cyclofenil; fulvestrant
4 Agents modifying myostatin function(s) including, but not limited, to: myostatin inhibitors
5 Metabolic modulators:

   1 Activators of the AMP-activated protein kinase (AMPK), e.g. AICAR; and Peroxisome Proliferator Activated Receptor δ (PPARδ) agonists, e.g. GW 1516;
   2 Insulins and insulin mimetics;
   3 Meldonium;
   4 Trimetazidine

2008. Prior to this many of these substances were classed as Agents with Anti-oestrogenic Activity. These substances were combined as a class in 2012 and included metabolic modulators, namely peroxisome proliferator activated receptor δ (PPARδ) agonists and activators of AMP-activated protein kinase (AMPK), which were formerly classified under the prohibited method of gene doping since their introduction to the Prohibited List in 2009. Insulin was added as a metabolic modulator in 2013 after formerly being included as Peptide Hormones, Growth Factors and Related Substances. The most notable recent additions to this classification of prohibited substances were Trimetazidine in 2015, having previously been classified within the Stimulants category in 2014 and Meldonium added in 2016.

As regards to the positive drug tests attributed to the use of substances within this class, the most common is that of the SERM, tamoxifen, which accounted for almost 40 per cent of the total number of adverse analytical findings (AAFs) reported by WADA-accredited laboratories in 2015. There was however, significant representation, in terms of AAFs, from anti-oestrogenic substances (e.g. clomiphene) and aromastase inhibitors (e.g. anastrozole, letrozole and androstatrienedione) (WADA, 2016b; Table 12.2). Although not represented in the latest WADA-accredited laboratory testing figures (WADA, 2016b) there has been a spate of positive cases for meldonium since its introduction to the Prohibited List in 2016 (Thevis et al., 2017).

12.3 Aromatase inhibitors

Androgens are readily converted to oestrogens by the enzyme aromatase. Aromatase inhibitors are therefore a class of drugs that limit this conversion by binding to aromatase and rendering it inactive. As a doping agent, they are only of potential benefit to males and are typically used in an attempt to elevate testosterone levels and to combat some of the unwanted side-effects attributed to the use of anabolic androgenic steroids (AAS).

Table 12.2 Prohibited hormone and metabolic modulators identified by WADA-accredited laboratories in 2015 (WADA, 2016b)

Hormone and metabolic modulator	Occurrences	Per cent within class
1 **Aromatase inhibitors**		
Anastrozole	16	10.5%
Letrozole	10	6.6%
Androstatrienedione	6	4.0%
Androstene-3,6,17 trione (6-oxo)	2	1.3%
5a-androst-2-en-17-one metabolites	1	0.7%
Arimistane	1	0.7%
Exemestane	1	0.7%
Testolactone	1	0.7%
2 **SERMs**		
Tamoxifen	59	38.8%
3 **Other anti-oestrogenic substances**		
Clomiphene	37	24.3%
4 **Agents modifying myostatin function**		
5 **Metabolic modulators**		
Trimetazidine	11	7.2%
GW1516	6	4.0%
Insulin (aspart)	1	0.7%

Clinical use of aromatase inhibitors

Aromatase inhibitors have been used in the treatment of breast tumours, particularly in post-menopausal women. Since oestrogens have been implicated in the development and progression of such tumours, the objective of treatment is to deprive the tumour of oestrogens. This can be accomplished by inhibiting aromatase, the enzyme that catalyses the final step in the biosynthesis of oestrogen (Njar and Brodie, 1999). Post-menopausal women tend to have tumours that are positive for oestrogen receptors and are therefore more responsive to treatment involving hormone antagonism.

Aromatase inhibitors include both steroidal and non-steroidal mechanism-based inhibitors. The steroidal agents are mostly analogs of androstenedione and include testolactone, formestane, exemestane and atamestane, whilst the non-steroidal analogues include fadrozole, letrozole, anastrozole, vorozole and finrazole (Handelsman, 2006).

Use of aromatase inhibitors in sport

Natural androgens, such as testosterone and androstenedione, are the precursors of the principal oestrogen, estradiol, and this conversion is achieved by the enzyme aromatase. Clearly, the inhibition of aromatase will lead to elevated levels of the endogenous androgens, testosterone and androstenedione, thereby increasing potential anabolic effects. The most potent natural androgen, dihydrotestosterone, cannot be aromatised and therefore cannot be converted to an oestrogen (Handelsman, 2008).

Aromatase inhibitors may also be used by AAS users in an attempt to treat the development of breast tissue (gynaecomastia), a common side effect associated with androgen use in men, although the clinical efficacy for this is debatable (Handelsman, 2008).

12.4 Selective Oestrogen Receptor Modulators

Selective Oestrogen Receptor Modulators (SERMs) are particularly attractive anti-oestrogen drugs since they target specific tissues without affecting other organs. Tamoxifen is by far the most common SERM, misused by elite athletes subject to doping control measures (Table 12.2) and gym users alike.

Clinical use of Selective Oestrogen Receptor Modulators

The first drugs to be used clinically as blockers of oestrogen receptors were non-steroidal drugs such as clomiphene and tamoxifen. Newer anti-oestrogens such as raloxifene, toremifene, droloxifene and lasoxifene have been developed. These drugs also possess partial agonist activity and therefore became collectively described by the term selective oestrogen receptor modulators. Most SERMs act as an oestrogen receptor antagonist in breast tissue whilst acting as an oestrogen receptor agonist in bone, resulting in increases in bone mineral density. As such, they are widely used in the management of breast cancer and osteoporosis in postmenopausal women (Pickar et al., 2010). There are however safety concerns with the use of SERMs, for example, long-term use of tamoxifen has been associated with an increased risk of endometrial cancer (Bundred and Howell, 2002). The partial agonist effect of tamoxifen has also been associated with the development of 'tamoxifen resistence', where the drug ceases to inhibit tumour growth and appears to promote it (Bundred and Howell, 2002).

Use of Selective Oestrogen Receptor Modulators in sport

As anti-oestrogens, SERMs have the potential to elevate testosterone levels through competitive binding of oestrogen hypothalamic and pituitary receptors, thus blocking the negative feedback loop and stimulating follicle-stimulating hormone (FSH) and luteinising hormone (LH) release (Mazzarino et al., 2011). Nevertheless, this is only evident in males since in females circulating testosterone is derived largely from the adrenal cortex and peripheral conversion of circulating androgens and is not controlled by homeostatic feedback (Handelsman, 2006).

Despite the potential effects on testosterone, use of SERMs as performance and image-enhancing drugs has tended to centre on the treatment of adverse side effects attributed to AAS use. Indeed, tamoxifen is widely used in the treatment of gynecomastia and was attributed to widespread use in a survey of recreational gym users in South Wales (Baker et al., 2006). Indeed, 22 per cent of respondents who reported AAS use also reported using tamoxifen. In a survey conducted by Bates and McVeigh (2017) it was reported that a high proportion of performance- and image-enhancing drug users in the UK were also administering tamoxifen.

12.5 Other anti-oestrogenic substances

As already mentioned anti-oestrogens are drugs that act as oestrogen receptor antagonists to block the action of oestrogen. Whilst SERMs are selective in terms of their target tissue, traditional anti-oestrogens are non-selective and include clomiphene, cyclofenil and fulvestrant.

Clinical use of anti-oestrogenic substances

This sub-class of drugs is also used primarily for the treatment of breast cancer in post-menopausal women. Fulverstrant is an oestrogen receptor antagonist that competitively binds to the receptors with an affinity similar to that of oestradiol but higher than that of tamoxifen (McKeage et al., 2004). The binding of fulvestrant to the oestrogen receptor sets off a series of changes to down regulate receptor function. Unlike tamoxifen, fulvestrant has no partial oestrogen receptor agonist activity and therefore has fewer side effects. Clomiphene is an approved drug in the treatment of ovulatory dysfunction in females.

Use of anti-oestrogenic substances in sport

Synthetic anabolic steroids are used by athletes, primarily for their anabolic effects. However, most have some androgenic effects that inhibit the release of gonadotropin-releasing hormone from the hypothalamus and follicle-stimulating hormone and leutinising hormone from the anterior pituitary gland. With prolonged use, the resulting hypogonadotropic state results in testicular atrophy. This decreases serum testosterone levels, causing impotence and decreased libido. Clomiphene has been reported to be used to treat these conditions by an anti-oestrogen effect on the hypothalamus resulting in increased gonadotropin-releasing hormone release and oestrogen-like effects on the pituitary increasing the sensitivity to gonadotropin-releasing hormone (Bickelman et al., 1995). The relatively high numbers of samples testing positive for clomiphene at WADA-accredited laboratories suggest widespread use by athletes (Table 12.2).

In women, it has been argued that there is no convincing evidence that oestrogen blockers cause any consistent, biologically significant increase in blood testosterone concentrations (Handelsman, 2008). Furthermore, Handelsman suggests that oestrogen blockade poses no unusual medical risks to female athletes and there is therefore no basis on which to ban oestrogen blockade in female athletes.

12.6 Agents modifying myostatin function(s)

As introduced in Chapter 10, the myostatin signalling pathway is important in the regulation of skeletal muscle growth. As its name suggests, myostatin is involved in the inhibition of muscle growth, opposing the mTOR pathway. In a healthy individual there is a balance between both pathways to ensure that normal muscle growth is maintained. As a local signalling molecule, myostatin initiates protein breakdown through its binding with a membrane-bound receptor on skeletal muscle. As demonstrated in animals such as thoroughbred horses, myostatin deficiency manifests itself in muscle hypertrophy and heightened physical performance (Hill et al., 2010). Therefore the myostatin gene is the focus of much attention with regards to gene therapy and doping, however the focus in this chapter relates to agents with the potential to inhibit myostatin function.

Clinical uses of agents modifying myostatin function

Myostatin is a member of the transforming growth factor-β group of proteins that regulates muscle growth during embryogenesis (Matsakas et al., 2005). Myostatin contributes both to muscle development during growth and regulation of muscle growth in adulthood and protects against uncontrolled cellular proliferation.

Myostatin is upregulated in disease states and during prolonged bed rest where muscle wasting is symptomatic (Han and Mitch, 2011). It is also present in relatively high levels, in the muscle of aging individuals (Yarasheski et al., 2002). It therefore follows that inhibition of myostatin would have a huge potential in promoting health.

The clinical applications for the development of myostatin-based medicines include muscular dystrophy, cachexia (muscular atrophy associated with AIDS and other chronic diseases), myopathies resulting from inflammation and sarcopenia, the loss of muscle associated with increasing age (Wagner, 2005). However, drugs that manipulate myostatin signalling are also being considered as lifestyle drugs in anti-aging therapies and for their potential to enhance physical performance in athletes (Matsakas and Diel, 2005). Therapies for inhibiting myostatin function are under clinical investigation however as yet there are no reliable treatments available (Han and Mitch, 2011). Follistatin appears to be an attractive therapeutic agent for the future that works by blocking the activation of the myostatin pathway (Rodino-Klapac et al., 2009).

Use of agents modifying myostatin in sport

In humans, resistance or endurance training has been shown to suppress myostatin expression (Raue et al., 2006). This allows muscle to grow in size. It is not surprising, therefore, that suppression of myostatin function is deemed to be a potential method for increasing the growth response to training or even to stimulate muscle growth independently of training. It is for this reason that WADA introduced agents modifying myostatin function(s) to the Prohibited List in January 2008 despite there being no therapeutic agents at present. Nevertheless, the sale of potential counterfeit myostatin inhibitor (Follistatin 344) has been identified via the internet (Graham et al., 2012).

12.7 Metabolic modulators

As the name suggests this class of substances are concerned with controlling metabolic processes and pathways. Until recently the metabolic modulators comprised of two distinct groups, namely insulins and peroxisome proliferator activated receptor delta (PPARδ) agonists and activators of AMP-activated protein kinase (AMPK). In 2015, Trimetazidine was included as a metabolic modulator, followed by Meldonium in 2016. Although pharmacologically different, both of these drugs are used therapeutically for their anti-ischemic effects.

Clinical use of metabolic modulators

Insulin is a commonly used therapy in the millions of individuals worldwide who suffer from diabetes mellitus. Insulin therapy can take several forms and is typically based upon the type of diabetes that an individual suffers from. Type I diabetes, often termed insulin-dependent diabetes, requires regular daily insulin injections to combat the body's inability to produce insulin. Type II diabetes may vary in the therapeutic approach to reflect the condition of the patient. In mild cases alternative strategies to drug therapy might be considered, such as lifestyle changes including exercise and weight loss. However, drug therapy including insulin is usually prescribed. Insulin is administered subcutaneously via injection or an infusion pump.

Whilst insulin was exclusively derived from animals (i.e. bovine and porcine pancreases) it now tends to be human insulin produced by recombinant DNA technology. Analogues of insulin are also manufactured in order to modify the action of insulin in terms of its onset and duration of action. Insulin may also be categorised according to its onset and duration of action. There are generally considered to be three general types:

1   Rapid-acting (onset of action: 12 to 30min; duration of action: 3 to 5h);
2   Intermediate-acting (onset of action: 30min to 2h; duration of action: 12 to 16h); and
3   Long-acting (onset of action: 1 to 2h; duration of action: up to 36h).

Regular human insulin has a time for onset of action of 30 to 60 minutes with a duration of action of between five and eight hours. An ultra-long acting treatment (Degludec) is a new generation insulin with a time for onset of action of 30 to 90 minutes and a duration of action of greater than 42 hours (Cahn et al., 2015).

Both PPARδ and activators of AMPK are relatively new drugs whose capabilities as therapeutic agents (and otherwise) are currently being developed. PPARδ agonists are a class of drugs that have the potential to treat both cardiovascular and metabolic diseases. By and large these drugs show great promise, although they are not without their problems. Indeed, clinical trials of the PPARδ agonist, GW501516, which was developed by GlaxoSmithKline, were stopped due to concerns over potential carcinogenic effects (Geiger et al., 2009). Nevertheless, this has not prevented its availability and illicit use as a performance and image-enhancing drug.

The activator of AMPK, Aminomidazole carboxamide ribonucleotide (AICAR), has undergone clinical trials for the treatment of ischemia-reperfusion injury during heart surgery (Alkhulaifi and Pugsley, 1995). It has also been considered as a possible treatment for a wide range of diseases including diabetes mellitus (Pold et al., 2005) and cancer (Jose et al., 2011).

Both meldonium and trimetazidine are recent additions to the WADA Prohibited List and both are anti-ischemic drugs designed as a cardioprotective drug in the treatment of problems associated with cardiovascular disease such as angina (Dambrova et al., 2016; Jarek et al., 2014). Trimetazidine works by reducing oxygen demand by shifting energy provision from lipid to carbohydrate metabolism (Jarek et al., 2014). Meldonium inhibits L-carnitine biosynthesis, thus supressing lipid metabolism and enhancing glycolysis and, as such, also reduces the oxygen demand of energy provision (Gorgens et al., 2015).

Use of metabolic modulators in sport

Although insulins are essential in the pharmacotherapy of diabetes mellitus, they are thought to have huge potential as performance-enhancing agents. Indeed, Sonksen (2001) outlined a number of ways in which insulin might enhance exercise performance: 1) increased glucose uptake by skeletal muscle as a consequence of elevated insulin levels would lead to augmented glycogen storage which would be advantageous in prolonged exercise and the recovery between training or competition; 2) the inhibition of protein breakdown by insulin would limit the catabolic effects associated with heavy training and further enhance the effectiveness of resistance training in increasing muscle bulk. Insulin would therefore appear to work in synergy with other anabolic agents such as anabolic androgenic steroids (AAS), growth hormone and insulin-like growth factor-1 (IGF-1).

The use of insulin as anabolic agents was reported by Dawson and Harrison (1997) amongst patents at a needle exchange and support clinic in the UK. Also, it has been reported by Rich et al. (1998) that 25 per cent of AAS users were using insulin concurrently. A recent investigation reported that of 41 non-diabetic insulin users 95 per cent also administered AAS (Ip et al., 2010). Since bodybuilders are a group particularly prone to using insulin in order to increase muscle mass there are particular risks associated with competitive bodybuilders who may be using insulin with concurrent fasting prior to a competition. Clearly this practice poses a particular risk in terms of hypoglycaemia. Indeed, there are reports whereby individuals have suffered from hypoglycaemic coma (Evans and Lynch, 2003).

Insulin was added to the list of prohibited substances by the IOC after concerns regarding its possible misuse at the Nagano Olympics in 1998 (Sonksen, 2001). Clearly athletes with diabetes may use insulin with a valid therapeutic use exemption. From a drug testing perspective it is difficult to differentiate between the endogenous hormone and that which might be administered exogenously. In addition the pulsatile nature of insulin release coupled with its short half-life makes doping control extremely challenging.

PPARδ agonists are important regulators of substrate utilisation and are involved in the regulation of muscle fibre type (Wang et al., 2004). Whilst research involving an animal model, examining the effect of a PPARδ agonist, namely GW501516, resulted in a shift from carbohydrate to fat utilisation in skeletal muscle, no improvement in endurance performance was found in sedentary mice. Nevertheless, endurance performance was improved when exercise training was combined with GW501516 (Narkar et al., 2008). The same research study also demonstrated the effectiveness of the AMPK-agonist, AICAR on enhanced endurance running in mice (Narkar et al., 2008).

AMPK is often described as the master metabolic regulator due to its effect on lipid and glucose metabolism. It is activated in response to changes in energy levels (i.e. low ATP levels) that occur during stress (e.g. exercise). Drugs that target AMPK (and indeed PPARδ) have been termed exercise mimetics due to their ability to activate numerous signalling pathways and regulate the expression of particular genes in a similar way to exercise. It is for this reason that such drugs have become attractive to individuals looking to enhance sports performance.

From a drug testing perspective the first case of GW501516 use was in cycling and coincided with the development of a test for its detection by Thevis et al. (2013). The cyclist in question was the Russian Valery Kaykov, who won European Track Championship team pursuit gold in 2012. AICAR is a naturally occurring AMPK agonist which is readily detected in urine and therefore quantitative analysis and the implementation of a suitable threshold is likely to determine its misuse (Thevis et al., 2009).

In a study by Jarek et al. (2014) the use of trimetazidine was monitored in Polish athletes over a wide spectrum of sports prior to its inclusion on the Prohibited List. Widespread use was determined by the WADA-accredited laboratory in Warsaw between 2008 and 2013 supporting its prohibition in 2015.

Meldonium was placed on the WADA Monitoring Program in 2015 and analysis of athletes' samples from the 2015 European Games in Baku showed a high prevalence of use. In communicating these findings from Baku, Stuart et al. (2016) highlighted that 8.7 per cent of samples tested positive for meldonium and a significant number did not declare the use of the drug on their doping control form. The study further highlights concern over the widespread prescription of the drug in healthy athletes.

The following year meldonium was added to the Prohibited List. A series of positive tests followed, including the former world number one and multiple grand slam tennis champion, Maria Sharapova. Sharapova immediately pleaded ignorance and stated that she was not familiar with the name meldonium, rather a brand name, Mildronate and that she had been using the drug for ten years for therapeutic reasons. Nevertheless, she had concealed the use of the medication to her support staff and had not declared the use of the medicine on the doping control form when tested (Court of Arbitration for Sport, 2016). Subsequently a two-year period of ineligibility was imposed by the International Tennis Federation, which was subsequently reduced to 15 months following an appeal to the Court of Arbitration for Sport. This case was particularly interesting since it suggested that the athlete was not aware of the substance being added to the Prohibited List, nor were her support staff. As a Ukraine-born athlete currently residing in the United States this drug was a registered prescription drug in East European nations including the Ukraine but not in the USA.

The considerable number of positive tests for meldonium during the early part of 2016 led to questions over the pharmacokinetics of the drug. The suggestion that meldonium might be retained in erythrocytes and other tissues causing release of the drug over an extended period of time has been considered as a plausible explanation for the elevated number of positive tests (Thevis et al., 2017).

Both trimetazidine and meldonium are promoted as performance enhancers in sport, particularly endurance sport, through reduced oxygen cost of exercise. However, there is limited evidence to support their efficacy in healthy athletes (Greenblatt and Greenblatt, 2016). Further research is needed to clarify the reputed benefits of such drugs.

12.8 Summary

Hormone and metabolic modulators are a diverse group of substances with a diverse range of therapeutic uses. As performance and image-enhancing drugs they have the potential to boost skeletal muscle growth and function by increasing the availability of testosterone or limiting protein breakdown and increase endurance capacity via PPARδ- and AMPK-agonists. In addition, by modulating oestrogen and its receptors the side effects attributed to androgen use may be tackled. New additions to this category of prohibited substances include the anti-ischemic drugs trimetazidine and meldonium. Although evidence supporting widespread use led to their inclusion on the Prohibited List there is limited evidence to support their use as performance enhancers.

In many respects this group of substances represents a group of emerging performance- and image-enhancing drugs that in many cases remain under development and therefore may prove attractive to athletes in the future. A high profile case involving the drug meldonium highlights the need for athletes and their entourage to be vigilant with regards to the annual updates of the Prohibited List and Monitoring Program.

12.9 References

Alkhulaifi, A.M. and Pugsley, W.B. (1995) Role of acadesine in clinical myocardial protection. *British Heart Journal* 73: 303–304.

Baker, J.S., Graham, M.R. and Davies, B. (2006) Steroid and prescription medicine abuse in the health and fitness community: A regional study. *European Journal of Internal Medicine* 17(7): 479–484.

Bates, G. and McVeigh, J. (2016) Image and performance enhancing drugs 2015 survey results. Available at: http://www.cph.org.uk/wp-content/uploads/2016/07/IPEDs-2015-survey_final1.pdf (Accessed on 28 July 2017).

Bickelman, C., Ferries, L. and Eaton, R.P. (1995) Impotence related to anabolic steroid use in a body builder: Response to clomiphene citrate. *Western Journal of Medicine* 162: 158–160.

Bundred, N. and Howell, A. (2002) Fulvestrant (Faslodex): Current status in the therapy of breast cancer. *Expert Review in Anticancer Therapy* 2(2): 151–160.

Cahn, A., Miccoli, R., Dardano, A. and Del Prato, S. (2015) New forms of insulin and insulin therapies for the treatment of type 2 diabetes. *The Lancet* 3(8): 638–652.

Court of Arbitration for Sport (2016) Maria Sharapova v International Tennis Federation Available at: http://www.tas-cas.org/fileadmin/user_upload/Award_4643__FINAL__internet.pdf (Accessed on 28 July 2017).

Dambrova, M., Makrecka-Kuka, M., Vilskersts, R. et al. (2016) Pharmacological effects of meldonium: Biochemical mechanisms and biomarkers of cardiometabolic activity. *Pharmacological Research* 113: 771–780.

Dawson, R. T. and Harrison, M.W. (1997) Use of insulin as an anabolic agent. *British Journal of Sports Medicine* 31: 259.

Evans, P.J. and Lynch, R.M. (2003) Insulin as a drug of abuse in body building. *British Journal of Sports Medicine* 37: 356–357.

Geiger, L.E., Dunsford, W.S., Lewis, D.J. et al. (2009) Rat carcinogenicity study with GW501516, a PPAR delta agonist. *The Toxicologist* 108(1) Abstract 895.

Gorgens, C., Guddat, S., Dib, J. et al. (2015) Mildronate (Meldonium) in professional sports-monitoring doping control urine samples using hydrophilic interaction liquid chromatography: High resolution/high accuracy mass spectrometry. *Drug Testing and Analysis* 7: 973–979.

Graham, M.R., Davies, B, Grace, F.M. et al. (2012) Exercise, science and designer doping: Traditional and emerging trends. *Journal of Steroids and Hormonal Science* 3(1): 1–10.

Greenblatt, H.K. and Greenblatt, D.J. (2016) Meldonium (Mildronate): A performance-enhancing drug? *Clinical Pharmacology in Drug Development* 5(3): 167–169.

Han, H.Q. and Mitch, W.E. (2011) Targeting the myostatin signalling pathway to treat muscle wasting diseases. *Current Opinion in Supportive and Palliative Care* 5(4): 334–341.

Handelsman, D.J. (2006) The rationale for banning human chorionic gonadotropin and estrogen blockers in sport. *The Journal of Clinical Endocronology and Metabolism* 91: 1,648–1,653.

Handelsman, D.J. (2008) Indirect androgen doping by oestrogen blockade in sports. *British Journal of Pharmacology* 154: 598–605.

Hill, E.W., Gu, J., Eivers, S.S. et al. (2010) A sequence of polymorphism in MSTN predicts sprinting ability and racing stamina in thoroughbred horses. *PLoS One* 5(1): e8645.

Ip, E.J., Barnett, M.J., Tenerowicz, M.J. and Perry, P.J. (2010) Weightlifting's risky new trend: A case of 41 insulin users. *Handbook of Experimental Pharmacology* 195: 209–226.

Jarek, A., Wojtowicz, M., Kwiatkowska, D. et al. (2014) The prevalence of trimetazidine use in athletes in Poland: Excretion study after oral drug administration. *Drug Testing and Analysis* 6: 1,191–1,196.

Jose, C., Hebert-Chatelain, E., Bellance, N. et al. (2011) AICAR inhibits cancer cell growth and triggers cell-type distinct effects on OXPHOS biogenesis, oxidative stress and Akt activation. *Biochimica et Biophysica Acta* 1807: 707–718.

McKeage, K., Curran, M.P. and Plosker, G.L. (2004) Fulvestrant: A review of its use in hormone receptor-positive metastatic breast cancer in postmenopausal women with disease progression following antiestrogen therapy. *Drugs* 64(6): 633–648.

Matsakas, A. and Diel, P. (2005) The growth factor myostatin, a key regulator in skeletal muscle growth and homeostasis. *International Journal of Sports Medicine* 26(2): 83–89.

Mazzarino, M., Bragano, M.C., de la Torre, X. et al. (2011) Relevance of the selective oestrogen receptor modulators tamoxifen, toremifene and clomiphene in doping field: Endogenous steroids urinary profile after multiple oral doses. *Steroids* 76: 1,400–1,406.

Narkar, V.A., Downes, M., Yu, R.T. et al. (2008) AMPK and PPARδ agonists are exercise mimetics. *Cell* 134: 405–415.

Njar, V.C.O. and Brodie A.M.H. (1999) Comprehensive pharmacology and clinical efficacy of aromatase inhibitors. *Drugs* 58(2): 233–256.

Pickar, J.H., MacNeil, T. and Ohleth, K. (2010) SERMs: Progress and future perspectives. *Maturitas* 67: 129–138.

Pold, R., Jensen, L.S., Buhl, E.S. et al. (2005) Long-term AICAR administration and exercise prevents diabetes in ZDF rats. *Diabetes* 54(4): 928–934.

Raue, U., Slivka, D., Jemiolo, B. et al. (2006) Myogenic gene expression at rest and after a bout of resistance exercise in young (18–30 yr) and old (80–89 yr) women. *Journal of Applied Physiology* 101: 53–59.

Rich, J.D., Dinkinson, B.P. and Merriman, N.A. (1998) Insulin use in bodybuilders. *JAMA* 270(20): 1,613–1,614.

Rodino-Klapac, L.R., Haidet, A.M., Kot, J. et al. (2009) Inhibition of myostatin with emphasis on follistatin as a therapy for muscle disease. *Muscle and Nerve* 39(3): 283–296.

Sonksen, P.H. (2001) Insulin, growth hormone and sport. *Journal of Endocrinology* 170: 13–25.

Stuart, M., Schneider, C. and Steinbach, K. (2016) Meldonium use by athletes at the Baku 2015 European Games. *British Journal of Sports Medicine* 50(11): 694–698.

Thevis, M., Kuuranne, T., Geyer, H. and Schanzer, W. (2017) Annual banned-substance review: Analytical approaches in human sports drug testing. *Drug Testing and Analysis* 9: 6–29.

Thevis, M., Moller, I., Beuck, S. and Schanzer, W. (2013) Synthesis, mass spectrometric characterization and analysis of the PPARδ agonist QW1516 and its major human metabolites: Targets in sports drug testing. *Methods in Molecular Biology* 952: 301–312.

Thevis, M., Thomas, A., Kohler, M. et al. (2009) Emerging drugs: Mechanism of action, mass spectrometry and doping control analysis. *Journal of Mass Spectrometry* 44: 442–460.

WADA (2016a) The 2017 Prohibited List International standard. Available at: http://www.wada-ama.org/en/World-Anti-Doping-Program/Sports-and-Anti-Doping-Organizations/International-Standards/Prohibited-List/ (Accessed on 28 July 2017).

WADA (2016b) 2015 Anti-Doping Testing Figures Report. Available at: http://www.wada-ama.org/en/Resources/Testing-Figures/ (Accessed on 28 July 2017).

Wagner, K.R. (2005) Muscle regeneration through myostatin inhibition. *Current Opinions in Rheumatology* 17: 720–724.

Wang, Y.W., Zhang, C.L., Tu, R.T. et al. (2004) Regulation of muscle fibre type and running endurance by PPARδ. *PLoS Biology* 2(10): e294.

Yarasheski, K.E., Bhasin, S., Sinha-Hikim et al. (2002) Serum myostatin-immunoreactive protein is increased in 60–92 year old women and men with muscle wasting. *Journal of Nutrition, Health and Aging* 6(5): 343–348.

Chapter 13

Diuretics and masking agents

David R. Mottram

13.1 Introduction

Diuretics are drugs that act on the kidneys to increase the rate of urine flow. They have a number of important clinical uses, particularly in the treatment of cardiovascular disorders. However, they are also widely misused in sport, as their pharmacological action has led some athletes to believe that increased urine excretion will mask the use of other prohibited substances. Furthermore, diuretics have been misused to temporarily reduce weight in sports where weight categories apply.

In this chapter, the use of diuretics, and other agents which may be used to mask prohibited drug use, will be reviewed along with the World Anti-Doping Agency's regulations to prohibit their use.

13.2 What are diuretics?

The main function of the kidneys is to maintain a constant interior environment to the body by regulating the volume, electrolyte content and pH of extracellular fluid in response to variations in diet and fluctuations in external environmental conditions. The kidneys are also responsible for eliminating waste and noxious products from the body. Within the kidneys, fluid salts and low-molecular weight constituents of the plasma are extracted from the blood and mostly re-absorbed, leaving excess water, ions and "foreign" chemicals to be excreted within the urine.

Diuretics act on the kidneys to increase the rate of urine flow and the excretion of ions, particularly sodium (Na^+). They therefore adjust the volume and composition of body fluids. The different types of diuretics can be classified according to their chemical structure and their clinical use (Table 13.1) The wide range of structures does not pose a problem with respect to doping analysis (Deventer et al., 2002; Morra et al., 2006).

13.3 Action and use of diuretics in sport

Diuretics as masking agents

One of the principal reasons for athletes' use of diuretics is for their masking effect through the production of copious volumes of urine. This attempt at disguising other drugs being excreted is highly unlikely to succeed considering the levels of sensitivity and accuracy exhibited by modern analytical testing regimes. Some diuretics can alter urinary pH and inhibit the passive excretion of acidic and basic drugs in urine (Cadwallader et al., 2010).

Table 13.1 Classification of diuretics and their major clinical uses

Class of diuretic	Examples	Major clinical uses
Loop diuretics	Furosemide Bumetanide Torasemide Etacrynic acid	Chronic heart failure; renal failure
Thiazide and related diuretics	Bendroflumethazide Hydrochlorothiazide Chlortalidone Indapamide Metolazone Chlorothiazide Cyclopenthiazide Xipamide	Hypertension; oedema
Potassium sparing diuretics	Amiloride Triamterene	In conjunction with loop or thiazide diuretics to maintain potassium balance
Aldosterone antagonists (also potassium sparing)	Spironolactone Eplerenone Canrenone	Primary hyperaldosteronism Cirrhosis of the liver
Carbonic anhydrase inhibitors	Acetazolamide Dorzolamide Brinzolamide	Rarely used except orally (Acetazolamide) or topically to treat glaucoma
Osmotic diuretics	Mannitol	Cerebral oedema
Selective vasopressin V2-receptor antagonists	Tolvaptan	Syndrome of inappropriate antidiuretic hormone secretion

Diuretics in sports requiring weight limitation or categorisation

A number of sports require weight categorisation in order to ensure some degree of equivalence between competitors. Most of these sports involve physical contact, such as combat sports, including boxing, judo and wrestling, or compare the ability to lift weights. Combat sports represent about 25 per cent of Olympic medals (Franchini et al., 2012). Such sports require a weigh-in prior to competition. Clearly, athletes must meet the limits of their respective weight category and often need to resort to rapid weight lowering strategies in order to achieve that objective. These strategies have sometimes included the use of diuretics. In a Brazilian study of methods used to reduce body mass by competitive combat sport athletes, it was found that around one third used diuretics or laxatives (Brito et al., 2012). Regardless of the method used for rapid weight loss, procedures may be harmful to performance and health (Franchini et al., 2012).

Another sport in which weight is of prime importance is professional horse racing, where jockeys are required to maintain very precise weight control. All jockeys routinely adopt practices of restricting food intake and sauna-induced sweating. However, a study in which professional jockeys in Australia were questioned on their weight management revealed that 22 per cent of subjects frequently resorted to diuretics for rapid weight loss (Moore et al., 2002). This practice is widespread and reports date back many years (Price, 1973).

Sports federations within which weight control is a factor reserve the right to administer anti-doping tests at the time of the weigh-in as well as at the time of competing, since the weigh-in may take place some period of time before the competition.

Diuretics have been used for weight loss in sports other than those where weight categories apply. In a study by Martin et al. (1998), the use of diuretics by female basketball, softball and volleyball players was investigated, showing that volleyball players (23.6 per cent), in particular, used diuretics for weight loss purposes although in 79.6 per cent of cases this was for appearance enhancement.

Diuretic use with other prohibited substances

Diuretics have a particular appeal as part of the culture of polydrug use in activities such as body building (Delbeke et al., 1995). In this context, the principal function of diuretics is to counter the fluid retentive properties of anabolic steroids. In the case of body builders this is an essential property in order to attain the required "cut" look. A similar result was found in gym users, where polypharmacy was practised by over 80 per cent of steroid users, with 22 per cent using diuretics as part of their regime (Evans, 1997). A review by Birzniece (2015) reported that concomitant use of diuretics with anabolic androgenic steroids and with growth hormone, where fluid retention is a significant factor, is widespread.

Diuretics and altitude acclimatisation

It is important that athletes and their support staff are aware of the serious health risks that can occur when exercising and competing at altitude greater than 1,500m (Da Rosa and Jotwani, 2012).

Acetazolamide is a weak diuretic but has been used for prophylaxsis against acute mountain sickness (AMS) in skiers and mountain climbers (Cadwallader et al., 2010), an indication for which it is not clinically licensed in many countries. However, it is not suitable for altitude acclimatisation. The mechanisms by which acetazolamide reduces the symptoms of AMS are open to discussion and include the induction of metabolic acidosis from renal carbonic anhydrase (CA) inhibition but also improvements in ventilation from tissue respiratory acidosis, improvements in sleep quality from carotid body CA inhibition and effects of diuresis (Leaf and Goldfarb, 2007; Swenson and Teppema, 2007).

A study into the effect of acetazolamide on exercise performance and muscle mass at high altitude concluded that subjects taking acetazolamide had fewer symptoms of acute mountain sickness than controls, although the difference was not statistically significant (Bradwell et al., 1986). The authors also showed that weight loss, including muscle mass, was greater in controls and this correlated with a fall in exercise performance leading to the conclusion that acetazolamide is useful for climbers and trekkers who are acclimatised to high altitudes and that the drug could be most useful at extreme altitudes. There is no published evidence for benefits of acetazolamide at altitudes where other sports are undertaken.

Inter-relationship between exercise and diuretics

Diuretics can have a variety of effects on exercise physiology, including effects on metabolism (thermoregulation and potassium homeostasis) and on the cardiovascular and respiratory systems, mostly as a consequence of volume reduction and electrolyte imbalance and depletion (Cadwallader et al., 2010). These authors also reviewed the significant variety of ways that exercise can affect the pharmacological actions of diuretics, with associated serious side effects.

13.4 Action and uses of masking agents in sport

Table 13.2 shows the principal substances that have been used as masking agents in sport.

The use of diuretics in this context has been described in Section 13.2 of this chapter, other masking agents are reviewed below.

Desmopressin

Desmopressin (1-desamino-8-D-arginine-vasopressin, DDAVP) is a synthetic analogue of the posterior pituitary hormone, vasopressin (antidiuretic hormone, ADH) and is used clinically in the treatment of pituitary ("cranial") diabetes insipidus (Kim et al., 2004). It has a more potent diuretic effect than vasopressin. It works by limiting the amount of water that is eliminated in urine by binding to V2 receptors in renal collecting ducts, thereby increasing water resorption.

In 2010, a landmark study was conducted by Sanchis-Gomar and co-authors to test whether desmopressin-induced haemodilution would alter the concentration of haematological parameters used to detect blood doping in sports (Sanchis-Gomar et al., 2010). After treatment with desmopressin, they found a significant decrease in the haematocrit, haemoglobin and the OFF Hr-Score (method based on the calculation of erythropoietic response, Gore et al., 2003) values which are recorded in Athlete Biological Passports. The authors concluded that desmopressin has a very significant haemodilution effect and recommended that desmopressin should be included on the WADA Prohibited List. WADA introduced desmopressin to the 2011 List of Prohibited Substances and Methods.

In 2011, Sanchis-Gomar et al. confirmed that desmopressin has a very effective haemodilution effect after the administration of recombinant human erythropoietin (rHuEPO) and significantly modifies the haematological values measured by the anti-doping authorities to detect blood doping as part of the WADA Athlete Biological Passport scheme (Gilbert, 2010).

Probenecid

Probenecid is an inhibitor of renal tubular transport mechanisms. Since it inhibits the resorption of uric acid it increases the elimination of urate through the kidneys. This therefore reduces plasma uric acid leading to the likelihood of this substance crystallising out in joints and soft tissue, the effects of which leads to the painful symptoms of gout.

Probenecid has an opposite effect on the elimination of other drugs, such as penicillins, where it inhibits urinary excretion, leading to increased plasma concentrations. This has

Table 13.2 Substances used as masking agents in sport

Desmopressin
Probenecid
Plasma expanders e.g. glycerol and intravenous administration of albumin, dextran, hydroxyethyl starch and mannitol

been used to therapeutic advantage in the case of penicillins, which are otherwise rapidly excreted, leading to the necessity for frequent dosing in order to maintain therapeutically effective plasma levels of the drug.

Probenecid has also been shown to inhibit the urinary excretion of other drugs, including anabolic steroids and their metabolites, and has therefore been used as a masking agent (Ventura and Segura, 2010). However, the urinary excretion of anabolic steroids and their metabolites is not completely inhibited by probenecid, therefore athletes would still record an adverse analytical finding during drug testing. It is therefore not surprising to find that probenecid has, in recent years, rarely appeared in WADA's laboratory statistics (see Table 13.3).

Plasma volume expanders (PVEs)

Plasma volume expanders contain large molecules that, when administered by intravenous infusion, do not readily leave the blood vessels. Within blood vessels they exert osmotic pressure and hold extra fluid in the blood, thereby elevating plasma volume and total blood volume. This can disguise elevated red blood cell levels. This property of plasma expanders was exploited by athletes using erythropoietin (EPO) prior to the validated test for EPO that was introduced in 2000. Before the introduction of this test, evidence for EPO use relied on blood tests showing elevated haematocrit levels (Ventura and Segura, 2010).

Albumin is an endogenous plasma protein. Its concentration in the plasma can be increased through intravenous infusion of albumin solution, derived by extraction from whole blood which has had most other constituents removed. Albumin also has the potential to bind drugs thereby delaying their excretion via the urine. There are a number of side effects associated with albumin infusion, the most serious of which is the risk of hypersensitivity reactions leading to anaphylaxis.

Other plasma expanders include the plasma substitutes dextran, gelatin and hydroxyethyl starch (HES). They expand and maintain increased blood volume and are only slowly metabolised. They also expose the user to the risk of hypersensitivity reactions. HES was added to the Prohibited List in 2000 after reports of its use by athletes. This led to the search for a validated method to identify this substance in urine (Thevis et al., 2000). Rapid screening techniques for HES and dextran are now available (Guddat et al., 2008; Scalco et al., 2010; Esposito et al., 2014).

Botré et al. (2014) reported on two novel types of potential masking strategies based on (1) the use of drug delivery systems, such as liposomes, to transport prohibited substances and (2) unconventional drug–drug interactions to alter the metabolism of a given prohibited drug, referred to as metabolic modulators.

13.5 History of diuretics and masking agents in sport

Masking agents are drugs that do not posses performance-enhancing properties but are taken in an attempt to disguise the fact that other prohibited substances are being used. Athletes quickly realised the potential for this type of subterfuge therefore these drugs have been used for as long as athletes have been subject to drug testing.

The International Olympic Committee (IOC) and then World Anti-Doping Agency (WADA) have classified and re-classified diuretics and masking agents in a variety of ways. Diuretics were first added to the IOC Prohibited List, as a class of doping substances, in 1985.

From 1985 to 2003 diuretics were listed as a class of drugs alongside other major classes of drugs, such as anabolic agents and stimulants. In 2004 they were re-classified under substances prohibited in certain sports. In 1987, probenecid and other masking agents were added under Doping Methods as part of the class referred to as Pharmacological Chemical and Physical Manipulation.

In 2005, WADA combined diuretics with other masking agents under the section of substances and methods prohibited at all times (in- and out-of-competition), where they have remained to the current time (2017 WADA Prohibited List).

The principal reason for the variation in classification described in the previous paragraphs lies in the fact that diuretics have been used over the years not only as masking agents but also as drugs to produce short-term weight loss in sports where weight categories apply. The extent to which diuretics and other masking agents have been used in sport, in recent years, can be gauged by looking at Table 13.3.

During the period 2009 to 2013 diuretics and other masking agents represented between 5.4 per cent and 7.5 per cent of the adverse analytical findings (AAFs) reported by WADA laboratories. In 2014 and 2015, this figure rose to 13 per cent and 12 per cent respectively. This represents a significant proportion of AAFs considering that anabolic agents account for around 50 per cent of the AAFs in each of those years.

It is clear that the most frequently abused diuretics are furosemide and hydrochlorothiazide, which may relate to the fact that they have a short half-life and will be difficult to detect if urine samples are not collected within 24–48 hours after the last administration (Cadwallader et al., 2010).

There have been a number of high profile cases involving this class of prohibited substances.

Case studies involving diuretics and masking agents

Masking agents can act in a variety of ways but their presence generally indicates that the athlete was taking another prohibited substance. The Pedro Delgado case was therefore of interest.

Table 13.3 WADA statistics for the number of positive results for substances classed as diuretics and other masking agents (2009–2015)

	2009	2010	2011	2012	2013	2014	2015
Diuretics							
Furosemide	92	152	123	127	145	128	153
Hydrochlorothiazide	90	120	123	101	125	120	125
Canrenone	21	27	29	24	23	38	33
Triamterene	10	8	10	7	15	5	9
Amiloride	8	13	12	6	18	14	24
Chlorothiazide	12	25	36	24	23	21	20
Indapamide	14	7	4	8	6	10	9
Acetazolamide	8	12	8	8	14	14	9
Others	10	23	19	13	13	33	39
Probenecid	7	2	3	4	5	2	5
Plasma Expanders							
Hydroxyethyl starch (HES)	1	7	1	–	–	1	1
Dextran	–	–	–	–	1	–	–
Glycerol	–	–	–	–	5	3	1
Total	273	396	368	322	393	389	428

Box 13.1   Pedro Delgardo (1988)

In 1988, the professional road race cyclist, Pedro Delgardo tested positive for the masking agent, probenecid, whilst leading on the 12th stage of the Tour de France cycle race. Probenecid was included on the IOC Prohibited List at that time, however, the governing body for cycling, the Union Cycliste International (UCI), did not prohibit the drug. Delgardo was therefore allowed to continue the race, which he eventually won. Remarkably little comment ensued, despite the fact that probenecid possesses no performance-enhancing properties. This should have raised the question as to what the cyclist was trying to mask. This case illustrated the lack of harmonisation that existed in international doping control at that time.

Some cases involve collusion between team members.

Box 13.2   8th Swimming World Championships, Australia (1998)

These Championships were marred by a number of doping-related events surrounding the Chinese swimming team. In addition to the discovery of vials of human growth hormone by Australian Customs officials prior to the Games, out-of-competition pre-testing at the Games resulted in adverse analytical findings for the diuretic, triamterene, in four members of the Chinese squad.

In addition to the athletes themselves, some cases involving the use of masking agents have involved collaboration with team supporters, including medical practitioners.

Box 13.3   World Nordic Skiing Championships, Finland (2001)

At the time before a validated test for EPO had been widely adopted by laboratories, the International Ski Federation had reduced the acceptable "safe" haemoglobin limit in blood to 17.5mg/dl for men in an attempt to control the use of erythropoietin (EPO). Some athletes realised that by combining EPO with plasma volume expanders they could elevate haemoglobin and total blood volume while holding haemoglobin below the legal limit. At the World Nordic Skiing Championships in 2001, six Finnish skiers tested positive for hydroxyl ethyl starch (HES) having not realised that the WADA laboratories had devised a detection method for HES but had not generally announced this fact (Seiler, 2001). In this case, it was further revealed that the use of EPO along with the intravenous administration of HES had been undertaken systematically with the collusion of the Head Coach and two national team doctors. It served to remind that such athlete support personnel can be implicated as accessories to athlete doping.

At least one case has involved an athlete whose adverse analytical finding resulted from the use of a prohibited substance which was later removed from the Prohibited List.

Box 13.4   Zach Lund (2006)

In February 2006, the skeleton sled racer, Zach Lund, was banned from competition for one year, having tested positive for finasteride (a constituent in his hair growth stimulant) on the eve of the Winter Olympic Games in Torino, Italy. The one-year ban was a reduction from the two year ban recommended by WADA since the Court of Arbitration for Sport had determined that Lund "bears no significant fault or negligence". Finasteride was removed from the WADA Prohibited List in January 2009.

There have been cases in which diuretics appear to have been taken inadvertently

Case studies involving inadvertent use of diuretics

The cyclist Franke Schleck was handed a one-year ban by the Luxembourg Anti-Doping Agency after testing positive for the diuretic, xipamide, during the 2012 Tour de France. It had been noted that the drug was present in extremely low concentrations and that the drug may have been taken inadvertently.

The Jamaican sprinter Veronica Campbell-Brown tested positive for the diuretic, furosemide, in May 2013. She was originally given just a public warning by her national agency. However, the IAAF stepped in and awarded a two-year ban. Campbell-Brown appealed against this ban to CAS, claiming that the diuretic was present in a cream that she had been using to treat a leg injury and that she had declared the use of this medication at the time of the test. CAS ruled that she had not been guilty of any violation and overruled the ban.

In 2014, two cases revealed that the diuretic chlorazanil was detected during anti-doping tests. Both athletes denied intake of the drug, however, both declared the use of the antimalarial drug, proguanil. Subsequent investigations showed that the metabolism of proguanil produces a metabolite which is a chemical precursor in the synthesis of chloazanil. It was concluded that the detection of the diuretic in these cases was not a result of illicit drug use (Thevis et al., 2015).

In another case, an athlete tested positive for the diuretic hydrochlorothiazide, having declared ingestion of a non-steroidal anti-inflammatory drugs (NSAID) prior to competing. Subsequent analysis of the NSAID tablets showed that they were contaminated with the diuretic, presumably during the manufacture by the pharmaceutical company. The athlete's claim for inadvertent use was supported.

13.6 WADA classification of diuretics and masking agents

Classification in the 2017 WADA Prohibited List

The substances that are included under Diuretics and Masking Agents in the 2017 WADA Prohibited List is shown in Table 13.4.

Table 13.4 List of substances included under diuretics and other masking agents in the WADA Prohibited List, 2017

The following diuretics and masking agents are prohibited, as are other substances with a similar chemical structure or similar biological effect(s).

Including, but not limited to:

• Desmopressin; probenecid; plasma expanders, e.g. glycerol and intravenous administration of albumin, dextran, hydroxyethyl starch and mannitol;
• Acetazolamide; amiloride; bumetanide; canrenone; chlortalidone; etacrynic acid; furosemide; indapamide; metolazone; spironolactone; thiazides, e.g. bendroflumethiazide, chlorothiazide and hydrochlorothiazide; triamterene and vaptans, e.g. tolvaptan.

Except:

• Drospirenone; pamabrom; and ophthalmic use of carbonic anhydrase inhibitors (e.g. dorzolamide, brinzolamide);
• Local administration of felypressin in dental anaesthesia.

The detection in an athlete's sample at all times or in-competition, as applicable, of any quantity of the following substances subject to threshold limits: formoterol, salbutamol, cathine, ephedrine, methylephedrine and pseudoephedrine, in conjunction with a diuretic or masking agent, will be considered as an adverse analytical finding (AAF) unless the athlete has an approved Therapeutic Use Exemption (TUE) for that substance in addition to the one granted for the diuretic or masking agent.

A new class of diuretics, Vasopressin V_2 Antagonists (Vaptans) was added to the Prohibited List in 2014. WADA removed the word "other" from the title "Diuretics and Other Masking Agents" in 2015, to reflect that diuretics are not only masking agents but can also be abused for other purposes, such as the induction of weight loss.

Exception to prohibition

In 2013, WADA decided that the potential masking effect of felylpressin, an anaesthetic used in dental practice, did not warrant its inclusion as a prohibited substance when administered locally. The 2017 WADA Prohibited List cites four other diuretics/masking agents that are not prohibited. Drospirenone is an analogue of the aldosterone antagonist diuretic, spironolactone and has weak diuretic effects. However, its principal pharmacological effect lies in the fact that it is a progestin, a synthetic version of the hormone progestogen. As such, it is used clinically in combined oral contraceptive pills. The diuretic effect of drospirenone is therefore deemed insufficient, by WADA, to warrant its prohibition as a masking agent. Pamabrom is a weak diuretic that is largely available as a combined over-the-counter medication for pre-menstrual/menstrual symptoms and therefore is not prohibited by WADA.

WADA does not prohibit the carbonic anhydrase inhibitors, dorzolamide and brinzolamide, when used topically, such as in eye drop preparations for the treatment of glaucoma, as they will not be absorbed into the systemic circulation in sufficient quantities to act as masking agents.

Diuretics and Therapeutic Use Exemption

Diuretics have a number of important clinical uses (see Table 13.1) and therefore athletes may apply for Therapeutic Use Exemption (TUE), where appropriate (WADA, 2016).

The WADA Prohibited List pays particular attention to the use of TUEs with diuretics and other masking agents. An athlete may apply for and be granted a TUE for a diuretic or masking agent alone. However, if that diuretic or other masking agent is used with another drug which is subject to a WADA threshold limit (see Table 13.4) the athlete must apply for a TUE for this other drug, regardless of the quantity that is prescribed or whether the drug is taken in-competition or out-of-competition. A TUE for a diuretic can never be approved for an athlete in a sport with weight categories (Fitch, 2012).

13.7 Summary

- Diuretics act on the kidneys to increase urine flow.
- Diuretics may be misused by athletes to mask the use of other prohibited substances but may also be taken to temporarily reduce weight in sports where weight categories apply.
- A number of non-diuretic drugs, such as probenecid, desmopressin and plasma volume expanders, may also be used to attempt to mask prohibited drug use.
- Diuretics are used extensively by those athletes who use illegal performance enhancing drugs, as gauged by WADA's annual laboratory statistics.
- Specific criteria apply with regard to Therapeutic Use Exemption for diuretics. Exceptions are not permitted in sports where weight categories apply.

13.8 References

Birzniece, V. (2015) Doping in sport: Effects, harm and misconceptions. *Internal Medicine Journal* 45: 239–248.

Botré, F., de la Torre, X., Donati, F. and Mazzarino, M. (2014) Narrowing the gap between the number of athletes who dope and the number of athletes who are caught: Scientific advances that increase the efficacy of anti-doping tests. *British Journal of Sports Medicine* 48: 833–836.

Bradwell, A.R., Coote, J.H., Milles, J.J. et al. (1986) Effect of acetazolamine on exercise performance and muscle mass at high altitude. *Lancet* 327, Issue 8488: 1,001–1,005.

Brito, C.J., Roas, A.F.C.M., Brito, I.S.S. et al. (2012) Methods of bady-mass reduction by combat sport athletes. *International Journal of Sport Nutrition and Exercise Metabolism* 22: 89–97.

Cadwallader, A.B., de la Torre, X., Tieri, A. et al. (2010) The abuse of diuretics as performance enhancing drugs and masking agents in sport doping: Pharmacology, toxicology and analysis. *British Journal of Pharmacology* 161: 1–16.

Da Rosa, M.J. and Jotwani, V. (2012) Travelling to high altitude with athletes. *International Journal of Athletic Therapy and Training* 17(5): 11–17.

Delbeke, F.T., Desmet, N. and Debackere, M. (1995) The abuse of doping agents in competing body builders in Flanders (1988–1993). *International Journal of Sports Medicine* 16(1): 66–70.

Deventer, K., Delbeke, F.T., Roels, K. et al. (2002) Screening for 18 diuretics and probenecid in doping analysis by liquid chromatography-tandem mass spectrometry. *Biomedical Chromatography* 16: 529–535.

Esposito, S., Daventer, K., Giron, A. et al. (2014) Investigation of urinary excretion of hydroxyethyl starch and dextran by UHPLC-HRMS in different acquisition modes. *Biology in Sport* 31: 95–104.

Evans, N.A. (1997) Gym and tonic: A profile of 100 male steroid users. *British Journal of Sports Medicine* 31: 54–58.

Fitch, K. (2012) Proscribed drugs at the Olympic Games: Permitted use and misuse (doping) by athletes. *Clinical Medicine* 12(3): 257–260.

Franchini, E., Brito, C.J. and Artioli, G.G. (2012) Weight loss in combat sports: Physiological, psychological and performance effects. *Journal of International Society of Sports Nutrition* 9: 52–58.

Gilbert, S. (2010) The biological passport. *Hastings Central Report* 40: 18–19.

Gore, C.J., Parisotto, R., Ashenden, M.J. et al. (2003) Second-generation blood tests to detect erythropoietin abuse by athletes. *Haematological* 88: 333–344.

Guddat, S., Thevis, M., Thomas, A. et al. (2008) Rapid screening of polysaccharide-based plasma volume expanders dextran and hydroxyethyl starch in human urine by liquid chromatography-tandem mass spectrometry. *Biomedical Chromatography* 22: 695–701.

Helmlin, H-J., Mürner, A., Steiner, S. et al. (2016) Detection of the diuretic hydrochlorothiazide in a doping control urine sample as a result of a non-steroidal anti-inflammatory drug (NSAID) tablet contamination. *Forensic Science International* 267: 166–172.

Leaf, D.E. and Goldfarb, D.S. (2007) Mechanisms of action of acetazolamide in the prophylaxis and treatment of acute mountain sickness. *Journal of Applied Physiology* 102(4): 1,313–1,322.

Kim, R.J., Malattia, C., Allen, M. et al. (2004) Vasopressin and desmopressin in central diabetes insipidus: Adverse effects and clinical considerations. *Pediatric Endocrinology Review* 2 (Suppl. 1): 115–123.

Martin, M., Schlaback, G. and Shibinski, K. (1998) The use of non-prescription weight loss products among female basketball, softball and volleyball athletes from NCAA Division 1 Institutions: Issues and concerns. *Journal of Athletic Training* 33(1): 41–44.

Moore, J.M., Timperio, A.F., Crawford, D.A. et al. (2002) Weight management and weight loss strategies of professional jockeys. *International Journal of Sports Nutrition* 12(1): 1–13.

Morra, V., Davit, P., Capra, P. et al. (2006) Fast gas chromatographic/mass spectrometric determination of diuretics and masking agents in human urine: Development and validation of a productive screening protocol for antidoping analysis. *Journal of Cheromatography* A 1,135: 219–229.

Price, D. (1973) Abuse of diuretics by jockeys. *British Medical Journal* 1(5,856): 804.

Sanchis-Gomar, F., Martinez-Bello, V.E., Nascimento, A.L. et al. (2010) Desmopressin and hemodilution: Implications in doping. *International Journal of Sports Medicine* 31: 5–9.

Sanchis-Gomar, F., Martinez-Bello, V.E., Debre, F. et al. (2011) Rapid hemodilution induced by desmopressin after erythropoietin administration in humans. *Journal of Human Sport and Exercise* 6(2): 315–322.

Scalco, F.B., Simoni, R.E. and de Oliveira, M.C. (2010) Screening for hydroxyethyl starch (HES) doping in sport. *Journal of Science and Medicine in Sport* 13: 13–15.

Seiler, S. (2001) Doping disaster for Finnish Ski Team: A turning point for drug testing? *Sportscience* 5(1): 1–3.

Swensen, E.R. and Teppema, L.J. (2007) Prevention of acute mountain sickness by acetazolamide: As yet an unfinished story. *Journal of Applied Physiology* 102(4): 1,305–1,307.

Thevis, M., Geyer, H., Thomas, A. et al. (2015) Formation of the diuretic chlorazanil from the antimalarial drug proguanil: Implications for sports drug testing. *Journal of Pharmaceutical and Biomedical Analysis* 115: 208–213.

Thevis, M., Opfermann, G. and Schanzer, W. (2000) Detection of plasma volume expander hydroxyethyl starch in human urine. *Journal of Chromatography B: Analytical Technologies in the Biomedical and Life Sciences* 744(2): 345–350.

Ventura, R. and Segura, J. (2010) Masking and manipulation. *Handbook of Experimental Pharmacology*. Berlin, Springer, 327–354.

WADA (2016) International Standard for Therapeutic Use Exemptions. In: *International Standard for Therapeutic Use Exemptions at* https://www.wada-ama.org/en/resources/therapeutic-use-exemption-tue/international-standard-for-therapeutic-use-exemptions-istue. (Accessed January 2017).

Chapter 14

Manipulation of blood and blood components

Yorck Olaf Schumacher

14.1 Introduction

In endurance sports or any strenuous exercise lasting more than one minute, performance is limited by the ability of the organism to provide oxygen to the active muscles. Several factors contribute to oxygen delivery: The ability of the heart to pump blood through the blood circulatory system (the cardiac output), the oxygen transport capacity of the blood and the ability of the muscle to extract the oxygen from the blood.

It has been demonstrated that in well trained individuals, the limiting factor for the maximal oxygen uptake of the muscle is mainly the oxygen-carrying capacity of the blood (di Prampero and Ferretti, 1990).

This transport capacity is determined by the blood's haemoglobin content. Haemoglobin binds oxygen within the red blood cells. The more haemoglobin the body contains, the more oxygen it can transport. A typical endurance athlete will have about 12-14g of haemoglobin per kilogram of bodyweight (Heinicke et al., 2001). It is this total amount of body haemoglobin rather than its relative concentration commonly measured in conventional blood tests which is correlated to the maximal oxygen uptake. When the total haemoglobin is increased, maximal oxygen uptake and thus endurance performance is proportionally improved.

It has been estimated that adding 1g of haemoglobin increases the maximal oxygen uptake by about 3.5ml (Schmidt and Prommer, 2010). A typical blood bag used for blood transfusions in a hospital contains between 50 and 70g of haemoglobin. Thus, as an example, adding this amount of haemoglobin to the blood of an athlete will increase their maximal oxygen uptake by 175-245ml. In terms of performance, this can be modelled to an improvement of 30sec to 1min in a 10km run.

Given the large impact on performance, manipulations of the blood have always been appealing to athletes and have widely been abused in all endurance sports over the last decades. Only in 1986 was the manipulation of blood included in the list of forbidden substances and methods. Since then, the definition of "blood manipulation" or "blood doping" has constantly evolved as new methods and substances were developed and have entered the world of sports.

Currently (as of 2017), WADA addresses the entity of blood manipulations in two sections of the prohibited list. The main section M1 Manipulation of Blood and Blood Components and section S2 Peptide Hormones, Growth Factors, Related Substances, and Mimetics, where certain blood modulating substances are specified further.

Accordingly, the following are prohibited:

1 The Administration or reintroduction of any quantity of autologous, allogenic (homologous) or heterologous blood, or red blood cell products of any origin into the circulatory system.
2 Artificially enhancing the uptake, transport or delivery of oxygen.
   Including, but not limited to, perfluorochemicals, efaproxiral (RSR13) and modified haemoglobin products, e.g. haemoglobin-based blood substitutes and microencapsulated haemoglobin products, excluding supplemental oxygen by inhalation.
3 Any form of intravascular manipulation of the blood or blood components by physical or chemical means.

In the chapter on peptide hormones, the following substance classes are explicitly mentioned: Erythropoietin-Receptor agonists such as Erythropoiesis-Stimulating Agents (ESAs) (e.g. various forms of erythropoietin (EPO)), EPO-Receptor agonists (e.g. Peginesatide) and Hypoxia-inducible factor (HIF) stabilizers and activators (e.g. molidustat and roxadustat).

14.2 Blood transfusions

The most basic method of increasing the amount of haemoglobin of an athlete is the application of a blood transfusion. Such practices were popular in the 1970s and there are numerous reports which involved athletes from a variety of countries. For example, the 5,000m Gold Medallist of the 1972 Munich and 1976 Montreal Olympic Games, Lasse Viren from Finland, openly admitted using blood transfusions to prepare for his races. It has to be highlighted that the infusion of one's own blood was not officially banned at that time. Blood transfusions were also common in most other endurance sports such as cross country skiing or cycling.

Methods of blood transfusion

There are two forms of blood transfusion: autologous and homologous. Autologous blood transfusion is the transfusion of one's own blood, homologous blood transfusion is the transfusion of blood that has been taken from another person with the same blood type. For both methods, blood can be stored (refrigerated or frozen) until needed. Based on the regulations in place in most countries, refrigerated blood can be stored at 4°C for four to six weeks. Frozen blood can be stored for ten years or longer, however the freezing process is more cumbersome, requires special equipment and is only available in very few transfusion centres world-wide.

The method of autologous blood doping involves withdrawing 500 to 1500ml of blood from an athlete. The blood is then treated further (mainly by adding conserving and anti-coagulation solutions and by removing a certain amount of the blood plasma and the white cells). The then-packed red blood cells (RBCs) are stored at 4°C and reinfused prior to important competitions.

The main challenge for cheating athletes who dope with their own blood is to time the withdrawal and reinfusion phases based on their competition schedule, as after the blood withdrawal they will have a reduced performance for a certain time (due to the decreased amount of blood in their circulation). Under normal conditions, it takes a healthy individual around 36 days to recover a blood loss of about 500ml. To counter these performance impairments and address the restraints imposed by the limited storage times for blood, athletes use complex schemes alternating various amounts of blood withdrawal and reinfusion to maintain their haemoglobin levels while still stocking up extra blood for later reinfusion.

The advent of freezing of red blood cells at -80°C permitted storage of blood for up to ten years. Nevertheless, this method is not applied routinely.

Testing for blood transfusions

Given that in autologous blood transfusions the additional blood cells used by the doping athlete originate from the athlete himself, and are thus identical to the ones in his normal circulation, there is currently no direct test for this type of manipulation. Large research efforts are being deployed by the anti-doping authorities to fill this gap; however, all attempts have been proven unsuccessful so far. Testing hypotheses included approaches to detect changes induced by the prolonged storage ("storage lesion") of the newly infused red blood cells.

The only currently practicable approach to test for autologous blood transfusions is the Athlete Biological Passport (ABP), which is discussed in more detail in Chapter 5.

Homologous transfusions, however, can nowadays easily be detected. The test (operational since 2004) relies on differences in secondary blood group antigens between the donor of the blood and the receiving athlete (Nelson et al., 2003). In fact, for any homologous blood transfusion, a match in the major blood group antigens (ABO and Rhesus) between the donor and the recipient are required. In addition to these well-known blood group antigens, there are a number of other, secondary blood group antigens, which are characteristically present or absent in all cells of a person. The presence or absence of certain of these antigens can be measured with cell sorting methodology after immunofluorescent marking of the blood group antigen in question. The presence of a mixed cell population (presence of cells both with and without the antigen) indicates that the tested subject has received blood from a foreign donor.

The most famous case in this context was American cyclist Tyler Hamilton, who was identified having a mixed cell population in 2004 following the Vuelta a Espana cycling race and was subsequently banned.

14.3 Erythropoiesis stimulating agents

The production of recombinant human erythropoietin (EPO) was one of the major drug discoveries of recent decades and the substance has since been one of the most commercially successful drugs ever marketed. In all endurance sports, the commercial introduction of EPO has radically changed the landscape of performance. Gaining the performance increases provided by an increased amount of red cells without the logistical challenges required by blood transfusions was appealing to many athletes. EPO is believed to have entered the arena of world sports shortly after its commercial introduction in 1989. Several scientific studies show its massive impact on endurance capacity (Ekblom and Berglund, 1991), which is best illustrated by a quote from multiple Tour de France winner and cycling world champion Greg Lemond who recalls the 1991 Tour de France: "I was the fittest I had ever been, my split times in spring training rides were the fastest of my career . . . But something was different in the 1991 Tour. There were riders from previous years who could not stay on my wheel which were now dropping me even on modest climbs". This description is matched by the development in peak performances during that time visible in many sports, such as long distance running or speed skating.

Erythropoietin and derivatives

EPO is the human hormone which regulates the amount of red blood cells in the body. It is regulated and secreted by specific cells in the kidney, which monitor oxygen partial pressure in the blood through the hypoxia inducable factor (HIF) pathway (see p. 214). If the oxygen partial pressure drops (such as in situations of anaemia (blood loss) or hypoxia caused by altitude), the production of EPO is increased. When it is increased, the production is reduced.

Since the end of the 1980s, EPO could be genetically manufactured and many different variants have been developed, mainly to overcome the pharmacological limitations of the original EPO. Original EPO is very short acting (plasma half-life 4–10h) and has to be injected repeatedly over a period of several weeks. The newer developed EPO such as Darbepoetin (Aranesp®) and the continuous EPO receptor activator (Mircera®) were therefore longer acting EPO variants, which only had to be administered once per week (Aranesp, plasma half-life 24–26h) or once per month (Mircera, plasma half-life 120-130h). This was achieved by modifying the original EPO molecule (Aranesp) or binding larger molecules to the active EPO molecule (CERA), thereby delaying its excretion and prolonging its action.

Testing for erythropoietin

The various forms of EPO can be detected directly in different matrices by various methods, mostly relying on differences in the glycosylation of the endogenous EPO and the artificial products (Isoelectric focussing, sodium dodecyl sulfate polyacrylamide gel electrophoresis (SDS-PAGE)) (Lasne and de Ceaurriz, 2000; Reichel et al., 2009). Given the short half-life of many of the commercially available erythropoiesis stimulating agents, test timing in relation to the injection rather than analytical methods is key.

Another tool in the detection of EPO is the haematological module of the biological passport (see Chapter 5), which aims to detect changes in certain blood markers triggered by EPO (Schumacher, 2014). The advantage of this method is that it is independent of the doping substance (i.e. EPO, Aranesp, Mircera), as it unmasks the effect of the abused product and not the product itself. It can also be used for targeting purposes, where athletes with suspicious blood values are targeted with conventional EPO anti-doping tests.

14.4 New developments in erythropoietic drugs

Since the commercial introduction of EPO and its large clinical success, research has consistently tried to develop substances with a similar action (increase of red cells), but easier clinical handling: most preparations of EPO and derivates have to be stored refrigerated until applied and can only be administered through injection. A selection of new developments, which are mostly stable at room temperature and can be administered orally or as a topical spray is briefly introduced below (see Jelkmann, 2015 for a concise summary and more details).

EPO receptor agonists

Several peptides have been developed which stimulate the EPO receptor (and thus trigger the same actions than EPO) but show no sequence homology to EPO.

The clinically most advanced product was Peginesatide (Omontys®), which was commercialised in the United States in 2012, but was withdrawn from the market shortly after due to acute hypersensitivity reactions in a number of patients.

Other erythropoietic agents

Luspatercept and Sotatercept are fusion proteins which interact with ligands playing a role in the inhibition of growth factors involved in the late stage of erythropoiesis and the resorption of iron. The substances thereby increase the differentiation and proliferation of erythroid progenitors. Luspatercept is currently in Phase III clinical trials (as of 2017).

HIF stabilisers

Substances impacting the stability of the Hypoxia-inducible factor (HIF) can influence erythropoiesis in a pathway upstream of EPO. HIF is a transcription factor which under conditions of normoxia is almost immediately degraded after its production. Under hypoxia, however, it stabilises and upregulates the transcription of genes which code for processes adapting the organism to low-oxygen environments, such as the increased production of endogenous EPO or the promotion of blood vessel growth.

Molidustat and Roxadustat are substances which inhibit the natural breakdown of HIF by inhibiting prolyl hydroxylase, the enzyme which normally cleavages HIF in conditions of normoxia. This mimics the situation encountered in hypoxic conditions, triggering the downstream action of HIF on the various organ systems.

The substances can be administered orally and several HIF modulators are currently in Phase III clinical trials.

Although no HIF stabilisers are officially commercialised, several athletes have already been found positive for them. Most of the substances can be purchased on the black market.

Testing for new developments

Despite the fact that only very few products of the drug families mentioned above have reached the market yet, doping tests to detect most of these substances are readily available. This is due to a joint initiative by WADA and the pharmaceutical industry, who aim to develop analytical tests for potential doping agents already before their market introduction.

Given that the new products are distinctively different from any endogenous substance, detection is analytically not difficult using methods like mass spectrometry.

14.5 Blood substitutes

Due to problems with the limited supply and storage times of blood for transfusions and the associated risk of infections (e.g. HIV, Hepatitis, Creutzfeldt-Jakob Disease), there has been much research into blood substitutes which can increase tissue oxygenation without having to use human donor material. Historically, there have been many different approaches to develop blood substitutes. The most advanced developments have involved candidate substances that are able to bind and release oxygen either based on chemical constituents or on haemoglobin which has been obtained from animal sources or genetically engineered. However, none of the substances developed in this context has reached the commercial market for broad human use except for some very specific indications in selected countries.

There is not much research investigating the impact of currently developed blood substitutes on performance in athletes. The only study performed in exercising humans for this purpose has been criticised for major methodological flaws. It can be assumed, however, that any clinically functioning blood substitute will transpose its oxygen transport capacities also to the performance of the athlete.

While there is yet to be the first positive case for blood substitutes in doping control, artificial oxygen carriers have been seized on several occasions during drug raids in the sporting community. It has also been reported that several cyclists required intensive care medical support after having self-administered various types of blood substitutes, some of them being approved only for veterinary use.

Perfluorocarbons (PFCs)

The PFCs are synthetic, highly fluorinated, inert organic compounds related to Teflon that can dissolve oxygen and other respiratory gases. There is no chemical interaction between oxygen and the PFC: oxygen is dissolved in the PFC particles, the amount being directly proportional to the partial pressure of oxygen applied. Thus, the PFC will dissolve oxygen in the lungs and then release it in the peripheral tissue. This process will be repeated for the time that the PFC remains in the body. First generation PFCs (e.g. Perfloran) had a long half-life (65 days) but a low capacity to dissolve oxygen (5ml/dl at a pO_2 of 500mmHg). Second generation PFCs (e.g. Perflubron) have a shorter half-life (4-6 hrs) and a higher capacity to dissolve oxygen (16ml/dl at a pO_2 of 500mmHg). This is comparable to the oxygen carrying capacity of whole blood. From these descriptions, it becomes apparent that given the high partial pressure required, PFCs are not readily suitable as a doping product: the 500mmHg of oxygen partial pressure that are required to dissolve oxygen in the PFCs are never reached in healthy, unventilated humans. In fact the normal partial pressure of oxygen in the ambient air ranges around 160mmHg, thus insufficient to dissolve relevant amounts of oxygen in PFC.

Testing for PFCs

PFCs, as inert organic chemicals, are immiscible in water and must be infused as an emulsion. The droplets are removed from the circulation by phagocytosis by the cells of the reticulo-endothelial system (RES). They are not metabolised but gradually released back into the circulation and excreted in the expired air. Therefore, detection in doping controls is not challenging: they can be detected for extended periods of time in both blood and expired air either by gas chromatography or by a combination of gas chromatography and mass spectrometry.

Haemoglobin-Based Oxygen Carriers (HBOCs)

Haemoglobin, the oxygen transport protein of the body, is rather constant in its structure across species and thus, free haemoglobin is easy to obtain, for example from bovine sources. However, in its free form, it will rapidly degrade and will be excreted by the kidney. Given its ability to bind and release oxygen in a partial-pressure depending manner, haemoglobin is also very reactive with its environment. In the normal circulation, it is protected by the membrane and the effectors inside the red cell, which attenuates any direct interaction with other reagents. Once freed from this protective layer in the blood vessel however, haemoglobin will scavenge nitric oxide (NO) (which usually guarantees a stable vascular tone) and thereby induce heavy vasoconstriction, with increases in arterial blood pressure, and subsequently causes organ failure due to micro ischemia induced by the disproportionate narrowing of the small vessels. Furthermore, it has a high redox potential, which further interacts with many metabolic processes. These facts make the use of free haemoglobin for the transport of oxygen impracticable.

Several strategies have therefore been used to overcome these limitations and to allow the use of modified haemoglobin as an artificial oxygen carrier: haemoglobin molecules have been crosslinked, chemically altered or encapsulated into liposomes or other enveloping material to mimic the qualities of the genuine red blood cell. Newer developments include the use of alternative types of haemoglobin, for example from sea worms (which is less reactive due to its larger size), or the partial modification of the haemoglobin molecule to reduce its reactive characteristics.

Despite the research and development efforts in this area of medicine, only a single haemoglobin-based oxygen carrier has been approved for human use (Hemopure®, approved in South Africa for the treatment of acute anaemia).

Testing for haemoglobin-based oxygen carriers

Haemoglobin-based oxygen carriers can be easily detected for several days in blood through capillary electrophoresis and other related methods.

See Schumacher et al., 2001 and Schumacher and Ashenden, 2004 for an overview on the topic of artificial oxygen carriers in sports.

Haemoglobin modifiers

Another approach to improving oxygen delivery is to facilitate its release in the tissue. This can be achieved by altering the affinity of haemoglobin to oxygen. Physiologically, this is caused by changes in pH, temperature, the CO_2- and 2,3 biphosphoglyeric acid (2,3-DPG) level. Changes in these variables shift the oxygen dissociation curve either towards the left or the right. For easier oxygen offloading in the peripheral tissue, a shift to the right is required, that is, the affinity of haemoglobin will decrease at a given oxygen partial pressure, making more oxygen available to the tissue by releasing it earlier.

Efaproxiral (RSR13) mimics the effects of 2,3-BPG and decreases the oxygen affinity of haemoglobin by binding allosterically to the molecule. One study demonstrated a dose-dependent shift in p50 which is the partial pressure of oxygen at which haemoglobin is 50 per cent saturated. The drug was in phase III clinical trials in Canada and the USA but its development has since been suspended as it failed to meet successful endpoint criteria. While there have been no adverse analytical findings for RSR13, there has been one media report of an elite Italian cyclist being in possession of RSR13 in 2001.

Testing for haemoglobin modifiers

The developer of RSR13, Allos Therapeutics, has reported that sensitive and validated methods of detection exist for both human blood and urine using gas chromatography and mass spectrometry.

Artificial red blood cells

Artificial red blood cells generated from pluripotent stem cells are also under development, but still in an early, "proof of concept" development phase. As of 2017, no related product has entered clinical trials at any level. It can nevertheless be assumed that should such products become available; the potential of abuse will be important. Commendably, WADA monitors the research situation as for other substances and is in contact with the inventors to develop anti-doping test methods prior to any commercial release.

14.6 Summary

- The oxygen transport capacity of the blood is the main performance limiting factor in endurance sport.
- Increasing the amount of blood improves endurance performance in a dose dependant manner.
- Blood transfusions are the simplest way of blood doping.
- The transfusion of autologous (one's own) blood cannot be detected in conventional anti-doping tests.
- Erythropoietin (EPO) increases the body's own production of red blood cells.
- There are numerous EPO derivates and new substances which have the same effect.
- Anti-doping tests already exist for most of these new developments.

14.7 References

di Prampero, P.E. and Ferretti, G. (1990) Factors limiting maximal oxygen consumption in humans. *Respiration Physiology* 80(2–3): 113–128.

Ekblom, B. and Berglund, B. (1991) Effect of erythropoietin administration on maximal aerobic power. *Scandinavian Journal of Medicine and Science in Sports* 1(2): 88–93.

Heinicke, K., Wolfarth, B., Winchenbach, P., Biermann, B. et al. (2001) Blood volume and hemoglobin mass in elite athletes of different disciplines. *International Journal of Sports Medicine* 22(7): 504–512.

Jelkmann, W. (2015). The ESA scenario gets complex: From biosimilar epoetins to activin traps. *Nephrology, Dialysis, Transplantation* 30(4): 553–559.

Lasne, F. and de Ceaurriz, J. (2000). Recombinant erythropoietin in urine. *Nature* 405(6,787), 635.

Nelson, M., Popp, H., Sharpe, K. and Ashenden, M. (2003). Proof of homologous blood transfusion through quantification of blood group antigens. *Haematologica* 88(11): 1,284.

Reichel, C., Kulovics, R., Jordan, V., Watzinger, M. and Geisendorfer, T. (2009). SDS-PAGE of recombinant and endogenous erythropoietins: Benefits and limitations of the method for application in doping control. *Drug Testing and Analysis* 1(1): 43–50.

Schmidt, W. and Prommer, N. (2010). Impact of alterations in total hemoglobin mass on VO_2max. *Exercise and Sport Sciences Reviews* 38(2): 68–75.

Schumacher, Y.O. (2014). The athlete biological passport: Haematology in sports. *The Lancet: Haematology* 1(1): e8–e10.

Schumacher, Y.O. and Ashenden, M. (2004) Doping with artificial oxygen carriers: An update. *Sports Medicine (Auckland)* 34(3): 141–150.

Schumacher, Y.O., Schmid, A., Dinkelmann, S., Berg, A. and Northoff, H. (2001) Artificial oxygen carriers: The new doping threat in endurance sport? *International Journal of Sports Medicine* 22(8): 566–571.

Chapter 15

Chemical and physical manipulation

David R. Mottram

15.1 Introduction

Athletes are liable for both targeted and randomised, no-notice drug testing, both in-competition and out-of-competition. Those athletes who use prohibited substances and methods are, unsurprisingly, keen to avoid detection. Procedures that are used for this subterfuge are classified by the World Anti-Doping Agency (WADA) as chemical and physical manipulation and are themselves subject to anti-doping rule violation regulations.

This chapter describes some of the techniques that have been used by individual athletes in an attempt to avoid detection and the methods by which such abuse is monitored and controlled. Attention is also drawn to institutionalised manipulation of the doping control process.

15.2 Current (2017) WADA regulations with respect to chemical and physical manipulation

The 2017 WADA regulations relating to the prohibited methods involving Chemical and Physical Manipulation are shown in Table 15.1.

Needless to say, tampering with samples collected during the doping control procedures contravenes WADA regulations. In addition, manipulation of samples through prior administration of excess volumes of fluid through infusions or injections is also prohibited. This regulation, in part, accounts for the IOC No-needle Policy which is implemented at Olympic Games (https://stillmed.olympic.org/media/Document%20Library/OlympicOrg/IOC/What-We-Do/Protecting-Clean-Athletes/Fight-against-doping/EN-IOC-Needle-Policy-Rio-2016.pdf). Clearly, there are significant legitimate circumstances where

Table 15.1 WADA Prohibited List (2017) regulations relating to chemical and physical manipulation

The following are prohibited:

1 Tampering or attempting to tamper to alter the integrity and validity of samples collected during doping control. Including but not limited to: urine substitution and/or adulteration e.g. proteases.
2 Intravenous infusions and/or injections of more than 50mL per six-hour period except for those legitimately received in the course of hospital admissions, surgical procedures or clinical investigations.

an athlete may require intravenous infusions and/or injections. WADA therefore provides clarification for physicians with respect to these regulations by which athletes and their medical practitioners can seek Therapeutic Use Exemption for procedures, when appropriate (WADA, 2016a).

It is difficult to anticipate the varied and imaginative ways in which athletes may undertake chemical and physical manipulation in order to avoid detection of prohibited drug use. In 2007, Jaffee et al. reported that adulterants and urine substitutes designed to defeat doping control tests were readily available over the internet, including data on their efficacy. However, they concluded that vigilant precautions would be able to detect most instances of tampering.

This chapter provides illustrative case studies in which various manipulative methods have been used by both individual athletes and by institutions.

15.3 Prevalence of chemical and physical manipulation in sport

WADA statistics relating to chemical and physical manipulation by athletes

Table 15.2 shows the numbers of positive test results from WADA-accredited laboratories, relating to chemical and physical manipulation, since 2003.

It is clear that few instances have been identified over the years. To what extent this reflects athletes' disinclination to use such techniques or an inability on behalf of the laboratories to identify such practices is difficult to establish.

Case studies in which chemical and physical manipulation has been attempted

Athletes have attempted to avoid detection of prohibited substances and methods by a wide variety of methods, either alone or in collaboration with other athletes, as in the case of Katrina Krabbe.

Table 15.2 Adverse analytical findings (AAFs) relating to chemical and physical manipulation from WADA statistics 2003–2015

Year	Number of AAFs
2015	1
2014	3
2013	1
2012	1
2011	3
2010	6
2009	5
2008	–
2007	3
2006	4
2005	–
2004	–
2003	2

Box 15.1　Katrina Krabbe (1992)

Katrina Krabbe won three gold medals at the 1990 European Athletic Championships, the last time East Germany competed in track and field athletics under its own flag. Krabbe then won two gold medals for the unified German team at the 1991 World Championships in Tokyo.

Prior to the 1992 Olympic Games, Krabbe and her team mates Grit Breuer and Silke Moeller provided allegedly identical urine samples during a test at a training camp in South Africa. All three athletes were suspended from racing, although the suspensions were lifted four months later on a technicality associated with the test procedure.

Subsequently, Krabbe and Breuer received suspensions having tested positive for clenbuterol before the 1992 Barcelona Olympic Games.

At the 1996 Atlanta Olympic Games, Michelle de Bruin, somewhat unexpectedly in the minds of many observers, won three gold medals in swimming events. Her trainer had been her husband, Eric de Bruin, a former Dutch discus thrower who had served a four-year suspension for failing a drug test for testosterone.

Box 15.2　Michelle de Bruin (née Smith) (1998)

Following the Atlanta Games, Michelle de Bruin missed at least one out-of-competition drug test and received a warning from her governing body, FINA. In January 1998 she was asked to provide a urine sample at her home in Dublin during an unannounced out-of-competition drug test administered by FINA. The sample was analysed at the IOC Accredited Laboratory in Barcelona and was found to have "unequivocal signs of adulteration" and that the concentration of alcohol present "is in no way compatible with human consumption" and that the sample showed "a very strong whiskey odor". A second test on the urine B sample was performed in May 1998, the results being compatible with the January findings. At a hearing in July 1998, a FINA doping panel found that the sample had been manipulated in an uncertain manner by de Bruin.

Michelle de Bruin was banned from national and international competition for four years. She appealed the decision at the Court of Arbitration for Sport (CAS). The hearing revealed that traces of a metabolic pre-cursor of testosterone had been found in three samples from the swimmer during tests taken between November 1997 and March 1998. CAS upheld the ban.

A number of cases have involved athletes sharing urine samples with other athletes.

Box 15.3　Galabin Boevski (2003)

The Bulgarian weightlifters Galabin Boevski, Zlatan Vanev and Georgi Markov were suspended from competition after it was alleged that they provided identical urine samples derived from one person when tested at the World Championships in Vancouver in 2003. Vanev and Markov, both World Champions, were given eighteen-month suspensions. Boevski, who won gold at the 2000 Olympic Games in Sydney, was given an eight-year suspension as it was his second adverse analytical finding since 1995.

Box 15.4   Rebecca Gusmao (2007)

The Brazilian swimmer Rebecca Gusmao underwent a doping control test at the 2007 Pan American Games in Rio de Janeiro, Brazil. The WADA Laboratory at Rio reported the test to be negative. However, the Games were attended by a WADA Independent Observer (IO) Team, whose role was to randomly monitor and report on all phases of the doping control and results management processes in a neutral and unbiased fashion. The IO Team reported to the international swimming federation, FINA, that Ms Gusmao had been tested on multiple occasions prior to and over the course of the Games and that these tests had yielded some suspicious results suggestive of possible manipulation. Upon review of the steroid profiles for the swimmer it appeared that the samples were from two different people.

Urine samples were re-tested to compare genotypes. It was confirmed that they belonged to different donators. Ms Gusmao denied having tampered with the samples and, furthermore, claimed invalidity of the follow-up tests. The FINA Doping Panel rejected her claims and instituted a lifetime ban, Ms Gusmao having already received a previous suspension from FINA.

Other cases have involved substitution of urine samples at the time of testing.

Box 15.5   Olga Yegorova (2008)

Olga Yegorova and seven other leading Russian track and field athletes were suspended by the IAAF after being charged with manipulating urine samples. They were accused of urine substitution when samples taken at the World Championships in Osaka did not match samples taken in out-of-competition tests in May 2007. Yegorova had previously tested positive for erythropoietin at the 2001 World Championships in Edmonton but her suspension for that offence was lifted because incomplete testing procedures had taken place.

In a paper by Thevis et al. (2012), the authors described a number of selected cases of suspected urine manipulation. In one case, the doping offence constituted the substitution by the athlete of a urine sample with non-alcoholic beer, as identified through the presence in the sample of saccharides accompanied by hordenine and Serpine-Z4, while no endogenous steroids were detected, as would be expected within a normal urine sample. Another case identified four urine specimens that returned similar steroid profiles. The results of an investigation into this, using DNA analysis, revealed that a Doping Control Officer had filled the urine collection containers with her own urine.

In September 2013, Devis Licciardi, a long distance runner, had just competed in a 10km road race at Molfetta in the southern region of Puglia when he was asked to take a urine test. The 27-year-old athlete, a member of the Italian air force team, was caught trying to siphon off "clean" urine from a fake penis, which was concealed in his underpants (Squires, 2013). He was subsequently given a three-year ban.

15.4 Institutionalised manipulation of the doping control process

In December 2014, WADA launched an independent commission to establish if there had been any breaches of anti-doping rules following allegations made through a German television documentary which was broadcast on 3 December 2014. The documentary, *Top Secret Doping: How Russia Makes Winners* alleged the existence of a sophisticated and well-established system of state-sponsored doping within the All-Russia Athletics Federation (ARAF), the governing body for the sport of athletics in Russia. Implicated in the documentary were Russian athletes, coaches, national and international sport federations, the Russian Anti-Doping Agency (RUSADA) and the Moscow WADA-accredited laboratory. The WADA Commission began its work in January 2015 (WADA, 2014).

The Commission investigated allegations of corrupt practices around:

- Sample collection and results management;
- Other ineffective administration of anti-doping processes that implicated Russia, the IAAF, athletes, coaches, trainers, doctors and other members of athletes' entourages; and
- The accredited laboratory based in Moscow and RUSADA.

The role of the Commission was extended by WADA in August 2015 following the release of the documentary titled *Doping – Top Secret: The Shadowy World of Athletics*, which contained new allegations regarding widespread doping in international athletics (WADA, 2015a).

The independent Commission published its report in November 2015 (WADA, 2015b). A significant number of findings and recommendations were reported, resulting in WADA taking the following actions:

- Provisionally suspending the Moscow Laboratory and setting up a disciplinary committee;
- Making a recommendation to the Russian Ministry of Sport that the Moscow Laboratory Director, Dr Grigory Rodchenkov, be permanently removed from his position;
- Requesting the IAAF to declare its member organisation, the All Russian Athletics Federation (ARAF), non-compliant; and
- Initiating the process to assess the compliance of the Russian Anti-Doping Agency (RUSADA) – the result of which would be considered by WADA's Foundation Board on 18 November (2015).

Having suspended the laboratory, in April 2016 WADA revoked the accreditation of the Moscow laboratory, thereby prohibiting any WADA-related anti-doping activities, including all analysis of urine and blood samples (WADA, 2016b).

In May 2016, two further media revelations were published alleging doping misconduct by Russian athletes and by entourage members at the Sochi 2014 Winter Olympic Games (WADA, 2016c). At the end of May 2016, WADA appointed Professor Richard McLaren as the independent person to head the investigation of the allegations made in relation to the Sochi 2014 Olympics (WADA, 2016d). The first report from the McLaren Investigation was published in July 2016 (WADA, 2016e) and the key findings were:

1   The Moscow laboratory operated, for the protection of doped Russian athletes, within a State-dictated failsafe system, described in the report as the Disappearing Positive Methodology;
2   The Sochi laboratory operated a unique sample swapping methodology to enable doped Russian athletes to compete at the Games; and
3   The Ministry of Sport directed, controlled and oversaw the manipulation of athlete's analytical results or sample swapping, with the active participation and assistance of the FSB, CSP, and both Moscow and Sochi Laboratories.

With respect to the sample swapping methodology, it was revealed that Russian secret service agents had developed ways of opening sample bottles and replacing their contents without intervention being detected. Urine samples from Russian athletes, containing prohibited substances, were removed from the testing facility through a "mouse hole", the tamperproof lids were removed in a manner which did not break the seal and the contaminated urine replaced with clean samples which were passed back through the mouse hole.

As a result of the overall findings from the McLaren Report, the WADA Executive Committee made wide-ranging recommendations, including a request for the IOC and IPC to consider declining entries for the Rio 2016 Olympic and Paralympic Games of all athletes submitted by the Russian Olympic Committee and the Russian Paralympic Committee (WADA, 2016f), a decision endorsed by WADA's Athlete Committee. Although the IPC accepted this recommendation and banned all Russian athletes from the Rio Paralympic Games, the IOC invested the decision as to which Russian athletes should compete at the Rio Olympic Games to individual International Federations (IOC, 2016), a decision acknowledged by WADA who expressed disappointment at the IOC decision (WADA, 2016g).

The McLaren Independent Person Second Report was published in December 2016 (WADA, 2016h). Key findings within this report included:

Institutionalised doping conspiracy and cover up

1   An institutional conspiracy existed across summer and winter sports athletes who participated with Russian officials within the Ministry of Sport and its infrastructure, such as RUSADA, CSP and the Moscow Laboratory, along with the FSB for the purposes of manipulating doping controls.
2   This systematic and centralised cover up and manipulation of the doping control process evolved and was refined over the course of its use at London 2012 Summer Games, Universiade Games 2013, Moscow IAAF World Championships 2013 and the Winter Games in Sochi in 2014.
3   The swapping of Russian athletes' urine samples further confirmed in this second report as occurring at Sochi, did not stop at the close of the Winter Olympics.
4   The key findings of the first report remain unchanged. The forensic testing, which is based on immutable facts, is conclusive.

The athlete part of conspiracy and cover up

Over 1,000 Russian athletes competing in summer, winter and Paralympic sports can be identified as being involved in or benefiting from manipulations to conceal positive doping tests.

In a response to the McLaren Reports, the Director General of WADA, Olivier Niggli, stated (WADA, 2016i):

"Today's Report represents the conclusion of the McLaren Investigation; and, yet again, more deeply troubling facts have emerged. While some progress has been made with RUSADA's efforts to regain compliance with the Code, there remain a number of challenges that must be addressed before that can happen. RUSADA must demonstrate that its processes are truly autonomous, independent from outside interference and properly resourced for the task of protecting clean athletes both in Russia and abroad. Only once RUSADA, and its governing structures, has successfully demonstrated that it can achieve such independence, will athletes and the broader public regain faith in Russian sport. To this end, WADA is resolutely focused on continuing to support their efforts."

15.5 Techniques for identifying chemical and physical manipulation

The most common method of manipulation used by athletes, as determined from WADA laboratory results, has involved sharing of urine samples between fellow athletes or using that from other individuals. In recent years, it has been possible to individualise urine specimens using steroid and metabolic profiling. An athlete steroid profile is made by recording ratios of various urinary steroid components repeatedly, each time the athlete is tested. These recordings are retained in the individual's Athlete Biological Passport. The steroidal ratios recorded include testosterone/epitestosterone (T/EpiT), andresterone/etiocholanolone (A/E), 5α-androstane-3α,17β-diol/5β-androstane-3α,17β-diol(Adiol/Bdiol) and androstane/testosterone (A/T) (Mareck et al., 2008). Any deviation from the individual's steroid profile will trigger further investigation into potential doping through steroid use or through urine manipulation.

The successful detection of manipulation by three weightlifters is described by Thevis et al. (2007a), who employed steroid profiling along with common drug testing approaches, including chromatographic and mass spectrometric assays as well as DNA typing.

Adulteration of urine samples with highly oxidative chemicals, which produce changes in endogenous steroid profile parameters, has been reported (Kuzhiumparambil and Fu, 2013). Cases involving athletes introducing protease granules into the urethra have been reported. When flushed out into the urine sample, protease enzymes digest urinary proteins, such as erythropoietin and insulins without affecting other urinary parameters. Testing regimes can detect increased levels of protease enzymes in the urine and also detect the absence of proteins normally excreted in the urine, such as albumin (Thevis et al., 2008). It is for this reason that WADA includes proteases as prohibited urine adulterants (see Table 15.1). Effective analytical procedures are available to detect the use of proteases (Thevis et al., 2007b)

Such strategies for combating drug misuse and sample manipulation require comprehensive out-of-competition testing and intelligent targeting of athletes.

In addition to biochemical laboratory urine testing, blood sampling and longitudinal monitoring of steroid profiles a further refinement involves performance profiling (Schumacher et al., 2009). Although sudden increases in performance can be induced by many factors, including improved training methods and nutrition regimes, performance profiling can identify suspicious athletes.

15.6 Summary

- Athletes who use prohibited substances and methods may employ various strategies to avoid detection of such practices at the time of testing.
- WADA classify these strategies/practices as chemical and physical manipulation.
- Many diverse methods have been attempted by athletes to avoid detection, either alone or in collaboration with others.
- Significant evidence for institutionalised manipulation of the doping control procedures was identified between 2014 and 2016.
- Effective techniques for identifying manipulation have been developed.

15.7 References

IOC (2016) Decision of the IOC Executive Board concerning the participation of Russian athletes in the Olympic Games Rio 2016. Available at: https://www.olympic.org/news/decision-of-the-ioc-executive-board-concerning-the-participation-of-russian-athletes-in-the-olympic-games-rio-2016 (Accessed January 2017).

Jaffee, W.B., Trucco, E., Levy, S. et al. (2007) Is this urine really negative? A systematic review of tampering methods in urine drug screening and testing. *Journal of Substance Abuse Treatment* 33: 33–42.

Kuzhiumparambil, U. and Fu, S. (2013) Effect of oxidising adulterants on human urinary steroid profiles. *Steroids* 78: 288–296.

Mareck, U., Geyer, H., Opfermann, G. et al. (2008) Factors influencing the steroid profile in doping control analysis. *Journal of Mass Spectrometry* 43: 877–891.

Schumacher, Y.O. and Pottgiesser, T. (2009) Performance profiling: A role for sport science in the fight against doping? *International Journal of Sports Physiology and Performance* 4: 129–133.

Squires, N. (2013) Italian athlete Devis Licciardi faces disciplinary action after using fake penis to beat doping test. Available at: http://www.telegraph.co.uk/sport/othersports/athletics/10330657/Italian-athlete-Devis-Licciardi-faces-disciplinary-action-after-using-fake-penis-to-beat-doping-test.html (Accessed January 2017).

Thevis, M., Geyer, H. and Mareck, U. (2007a) Detection of manipulation in doping control urine sample collection: A multidisciplinary approach to determine identical urine samples. *Analytical and Bioanalytical Chemistry* 388: 1,539–1,543.

Thevis, M., Maurer, J., Kohler, M. et al. (2007b) Proteases in doping control analysis. *International Journal of Sports Medicine* 28: 545–549.

Thevis, M., Kohler, M. and Schanzer, W. (2008) New drugs and methods of doping and manipulation. *Drug Discovery Today* 13(1/2): 59–66.

Thevis, M., Geyer, H., Sigmund, G. et al. (2012) Sports drug testing: Analytical aspects of selected cases of suspected, purported and proven urine manipulation. *Journal of Pharmaceutical and Biomedical Analysis* 57: 26–32.

WADA (2014) WADA announces details of Independent Commission. Available at: https://www.wada-ama.org/en/media/news/2014-12/wada-announces-details-of-independent-commission (Accessed January 2017).

WADA (2015a) WADA welcomes Independent Commission's Report into Widespread Doping in Sport. Available at: https://www.wada-ama.org/en/media/news/2015-11/wada-welcomes-independent-commissions-report-into-widespread-doping-in-sport (Accessed January 2017).

WADA (2015b) WADA Independent Commission Report #1. Available at: https://www.wada-ama.org/en/resources/world-anti-doping-program/independent-commission-report-1 (Accessed January 2017).

WADA (2015c) WADA takes immediate action on key recommendations of Independent Commission. Available at: https://www.wada-ama.org/en/media/news/2015-11/wada-takes-immediate-action-on-key-recommendations-of-independent-commission (Accessed January 2017).

WADA (2016a) Medical information to support the decisions of TUECs – intravenous infusion. Available at: https://www.wada-ama.org/en/resources/science-medicine/medical-information-to-support-the-decisions-of-tuecs-intravenous (Accessed January 2017).

WADA (2016b) WADA revokes accreditation of Moscow Laboratory. Available at: https://www.wada-ama.org/en/media/news/2016-04/wada-revokes-accreditation-of-moscow-laboratory (Accessed January 2017).

WADA (2016c) WADA to immediately probe new Russian doping allegations related to 2014 Sochi Olympics. Available at: https://www.wada-ama.org/en/media/news/2016-05/wada-to-immediately-probe-new-russian-doping-allegations-related-to-2014-sochi (Accessed January 2017).

WADA (2016d) WADA names Richard McLaren to Sochi Investigation Team. Available at: https://www.wada-ama.org/en/media/news/2016-05/wada-names-richard-mclaren-to-sochi-investigation-team (Accessed January 2017).

WADA (2016e) The Independent Person Report 18 July 2016. Available at: https://www.wada-ama.org/en/resources/doping-control-process/mclaren-independent-investigation-report-part-i (Accessed January 2017).

WADA (2016f) WADA Statement: Independent Investigation confirms Russian State manipulation of the doping control process. Available at: https://www.wada-ama.org/en/media/news/2016-07/wada-statement-independent-investigation-confirms-russian-state-manipulation-of (Accessed January 2017).

WADA (2016g) WADA acknowledges IOC decision on Russia, stands by Agency's Executive Committee recommendations. Available at: https://www.wada-ama.org/en/media/news/2016-07/wada-acknowledges-ioc-decision-on-russia-stands-by-agencys-executive-committee (Accessed January 2017).

WADA (2016h) The Independent Person 2nd Report. Available at: https://www.wada-ama.org/en/resources/doping-control-process/mclaren-independent-investigation-report-part-ii (Accessed January 2017).

WADA (2016i) WADA Statement regarding conclusion of McLaren Investigation. Available at: https://www.wada-ama.org/en/media/news/2016-12/wada-statement-regarding-conclusion-of-mclaren-investigation (Accessed January 2017).

Chapter 16

Gene doping

Dominic J. Wells

16.1 Introduction

Genetic manipulation is now a standard tool for biologists interested in understanding gene function in health and disease. This can take the form of adding genetic material to an organism (a transgene) or modifying the expression of endogenous genes (knockout or knockin experiments). The majority of such studies involve the modification of cells in culture or the modification of the reproductive cells of animals, mostly mice, so that the modification is expressed in all of the cells of a tissue-like muscle and the modification is heritable. However, it is also possible to modify non-reproductive (somatic) tissues in the mature animal. It is the latter technology, mostly intended for genetic therapies of inherited or acquired disease, which raises the possibility of genetic manipulation for increased sporting performance (gene doping).

The vast majority of drug treatments are given on an intermittent basis by mouth or by injection, for example weekly, daily or twice daily. As all drugs are removed from the body by metabolism or excretion, it is necessary to administer a large dose in order to maintain concentrations at or above the minimum effective dose in the target tissue(s) until the time of the next administration of drug. In the case of doping for increased athletic performance, such large doses increase the possibility of detection of the prohibited drug. In contrast, gene transfer generally leads to a continuous steady state expression which avoids the need for intermittent large doses. This is likely to make detection harder as the protein may only be close to the minimum therapeutic level. Secondly, as the protein is made within the body of the treated individual it is more likely to be indistinguishable from the normal endogenous protein. Finally, in many cases the gene and its product may remain within the treated tissue, for example skeletal muscle, and so are less likely to be detected by assays using urine or blood. Consequently gene doping may be harder to detect than conventional drug doping and so may be more likely to be adopted by athletes who are seeking to gain an unfair competitive advantage.

Detection of gene doping is likely to prove challenging and requires different methodologies compared to current strategies for detection of doping. The main targets, methods and detection of gene doping are reviewed in the following sections.

16.2 What is gene doping?

The potential of gene doping was first raised by experiments in mice that showed that increased expression of insulin-like growth factor 1 (IGF1) could aid repair and increase the performance of muscle. The key experiment was reported in 1998 when Barton-Davis and colleagues demonstrated that viral vector delivery of IGF-1 to the skeletal muscles of mice increased muscle mass and strength in both young and old mice. This was an important finding as it showed that it was possible to genetically enhance muscle in an adult animal by somatic gene transfer, a technology that should be applicable to man. The same group went on to demonstrate that gene transfer of IGf-1 can act synergistically with training to enhance muscle strength in rats (Lee et al., 2004) and others have noted that IGF-1 can improve the rate of muscle repair (Schertzer and Lynch, 2006) which further adds to the attractiveness of this form of performance enhancement.

There are now a large number of candidate genes that might be chosen for gene doping. Particularly important are those genes that (1) increase muscle mass, (2) modify the metabolic properties of muscle or (3) improve the performance of the cardiovascular system, either by increasing cardiac output or by increasing the carriage of oxygen in the blood. Well-known examples of genetic mutations conferring increased strength or endurance are the marked muscle hypertrophy reported in a myostatin null infant (Schuelke et al., 2004) and the Finnish cross country skier Eero Mantyranta whose natural mutation in his erythropoietin (Epo) receptor gene lead to high haemoglobin levels and so high endurance (de la Chapelle et al., 1993).

A number of genetic manipulations conferring an increased athletic performance have been tested only in laboratory animals and yet it is the result of these studies that has concerned the regulatory authorities. These include experiments in which the myostatin gene was removed or repressed. Myostatin is a negative regulator of muscle growth, acting to reduce muscle mass when the physical demand on the muscle is reduced. Mice lacking the myostatin gene (knockout) have muscles with both a greater number of muscle fibres (hyperplasia) and larger fibres (hypertrophy) than normal mice (McPherron et al., 1997). A number of natural myostatin mutants have been identified in dogs, cattle and sheep (Grobet et al., 1997; Mosher et al., 2007; Boman et al., 2009) and the human example quoted previously (Schuelke et al., 2004). Although the complete knockout of myostatin in mice has been linked to a decrease in specific force (Amthor et al., 2007), partial knockdown of myostatin due to a heterozygous genetic mutation has been clearly linked to improved muscle performance in the whippet (Mosher et al., 2007). A number of studies have shown that a partial knockdown of myostatin can be performed in normal animals using a variety of approaches including antibody blockade (Whittemore et al., 2003), blockade by use of a mutant propeptide (Qiao et al., 2008) and antagonism using follistatin or molecules derived from follistatin (Iezzi et al., 2004; Nakatani et al., 2008). Myostatin polymorphisms in racehorses have been linked to improved athletic performance at different distances (Hill et al., 2010). Further studies have shown that bone morphogenetic protein (BMP) signaling, acting through Smad1, Smad5 and Smad8 (Smad1/5/8), is the fundamental hypertrophic signal in mice (Sartori et al., 2013). This finding opens up additional potential routes to try to induce muscle hypertrophy through gene doping.

Our increasing understanding of the regulation of energy balance and fibre type determination in skeletal muscle has revealed a number of additional targets. Transgenic mice expressing peroxisome-proliferator-activated receptor-gamma (PPAR δ, sometimes called PPAR β/δ) have been shown to have double the running endurance compared to wild-type mice (Wang et al., 2004). Gene transfer of PPARδ into rat muscle by plasmid electroporation increased IIa and decreased IIb fibres following acute gene transfer (Lunde et al., 2007). Transgenic mice expressing the PPARγ co-activator alpha (PGC-1α) develop muscles comprised mostly of type I and demonstrate a high fatigue resistance (Lin et al., 2002) and improving aerobic performance (Calvo et al., 2008). Similar mice expressing PGC-1β develop muscles with a high proportion of type IIX fibres and have increased endurance at high work-loads (Arany et al., 2007). Finally, transgenic mice expressing phosphoenolpyruvate carboxykinase (PEPCK) show a substantially enhanced aerobic capacity (Hakimi et al., 2007). These findings correlate with observations in elite human athletes, for example mRNA expression of PPARα, PPARδ, PPARγ, PGC-1α and – PGC -1β is naturally increased in elite human cyclists, with an increased proportion of type I slow twitch, oxidative fibres, when compared with normally active subjects (Kramer et al., 2006).

It should be noted that apart from the study by Lunde et al. (2007) all the other experimental animal studies were performed in transgenic mice and therefore it is not certain that the same responses will follow gene transfer in the adult. In addition there are studies of the transgenic mice that show conflicting results. Although two reports showed improved performance in PGC-1α transgenic mice, Miura et al. found that over-expression of PGC-1α led to muscle atrophy (2006) and Choi et al. reported PGC-1α transgenics showed fat-induced insulin resistance in muscle similar to type 2 diabetics (2008). In contrast, the PPARδ agonist GW 1516 raised endurance levels by 75 per cent in normal exercising mice and the PPARδ-AMP-activated protein kinase (AMPK) agonist AICAR improved exercise performance by 44 per cent following four weeks' treatment without any training (Narkar et al., 2008), which demonstrates that these pathways can be effectively manipulated. Indeed such molecules are specified on the WADA Prohibited List.

A significant limitation to endurance in high performance athletes is the rate of delivery of oxygen to the muscle. This can be improved by increasing the proportion of red blood cells (hematocrit), and hence the oxygen carrying hemoglobin in the blood. Red blood cell production is governed by a hormone called erythropoietin (often shortened to Epo) that is produced in the kidney. Recombinant Epo has a long history of abuse in endurance events such as cross country skiing and cycling and a number of studies in animals have demonstrated the potential of gene transfer to boost circulating levels of Epo. Electroporation of plasmid encoding Epo into mouse and non-human primate muscle resulted in a raised hematocrit (Fattori et al., 2005), for example, and drug regulated expression of Epo has been demonstrated following intramuscular delivery of adeno-associated virus (AAV) encoding Epo into muscles of non-human primates (Rivera et al., 2005). In the latter study the hematocrit could be controlled by the administration of rapamycin thus avoiding the dangers associated with an excessively high hematocrit.

Finally, another paper described the role that alpha-calcitonin-gene-related peptide (aCGRP) plays in cardiac hypertrophy (Schuler et al., 2014). Cardiac hypertrophy occurs in response to exercise in order to be able to increase blood delivery to the skeletal muscle and this is mediated by the release of aCGRP from contracting skeletal muscles. Thus it is technically possible to accelerate cardiac hypertrophy through administration of aCGRP either from an exogenous source or from gene transfer into muscle. However, while this would initially be beneficial for delivery of oxygen to the muscle, it is uncertain what the health consequences of long-term exposure to elevated levels of aCGRP might be.

16.3 Clinical uses of gene therapy

There is concern that methods developed for genetic approaches to human disease (gene therapy) may be used for athletic enhancement (Fischetto and Bermon, 2013). Although there have been more than 2,463 human gene therapy trials approved in the past 25 years (http://www.wiley.co.uk/genmed/clinical/, as of April 2017), very few have shown clear efficacy and only two therapies (for lipoprotein lipase deficiency and for adenosine deaminase-deficient severe combined immunodeficiency, ADA-SCID) have been licensed in Europe (Kahlstein et al., 2013; Aiuti et al., 2017) for human use and two viral products for the treatment of cancer have been licensed in China (Kim et al., 2008).

Genetic manipulation of the early embryo can be used to produce transgenic animals in which additional gene(s) are added or where specific genes are inactivated in all cells of the body or in all cells of a specific cell type, for example skeletal muscle cells. Such germ-line genetic modification would pass on the modification to subsequent generations and so is not ethically acceptable in man. However in animals, particularly the mouse, the effects of such manipulations can be used to understand gene function and the potential consequences of genetic manipulation at the whole body level. This technology can be used to look at the ability of different forms of a therapeutic protein to prevent disease in a mouse model of human disease, for example testing different forms of dystrophin in the *mdx* mouse model of the lethal muscle wasting disease Duchenne muscular dystrophy (DMD; Phelps et al., 1995; Wells et al., 1995).

Genetic material can be delivered to cells both *in vitro* (cell culture) and *in vivo* (whole animal) using transfer systems called vectors. Modified viruses are the most common form of vectors as, during evolution, viruses have developed highly efficient systems for introducing their genomes into cells in order to complete their life cycle and generate more viruses. By deleting part or all of the viral genes from the modified viruses they can be rendered replication-deficient and so the introduction of genetic material into the cell is not followed by the normal cell damage associated with viral replication. This not only helps to prevent cell damage but also ensures that the spread of such modified viruses is limited. The production of replication deficient viral vectors is accomplished in specific cell lines where the genes for viral replication are introduced in a form that allows viral replication but does not allow these genes to be packaged into the viruses that are produced by the cells. The removal of viral genes from the virus also provides space for introduction of the gene(s) of choice together with the regulatory elements controlling their expression. The latter can be used to ensure that the genes are only expressed in the correct tissue, for example skeletal muscle.

A large number of viruses have been developed as viral vectors including adenoviruses, adeno-associated viruses (AAV), herpesviruses, retroviruses including lentiviruses and alphaviruses such as Semliki forest virus. The retroviruses have the particular property of inserting their genomes into the host genome and this leads to a permanent modification of the host cell. In contrast most of the other viruses exist as a non-integrated episome within the nucleus and can be lost with successive rounds of cell division. All viruses have viral proteins on their surface and these determine the cell types that the viruses are able to enter. This tropism can be modified by altering the viral proteins either by selecting different serotypes or by pseudotyping with proteins from other viruses. Advances in understanding AAV serotypes have identified minor changes in capsid protein sequences that dramatically alter the tissue targeting of the specific serotypes and these can be used to increase the efficiency and specificity of tissue targeting (Gao et al., 2002; Vandenberghe et al., 2009). Preclinical studies have shown that AAV is the viral vector of choice, particularly for targeting skeletal muscle. In rodents a number of studies have shown that it is possible to achieve body wide genetic modification of skeletal muscle in rodents and larger species using AAV vectors of several different serotypes (e.g. Gregorevic et al., 2004; Zhu et al., 2005; Denti et al., 2006;

Yue et al., 2008; Vitiello et al., 2009). However, a significant drawback with the use of viral vectors is that the presence of viral proteins on the surface leads to interaction with the acquired immune system that can neutralise and thus block any effects of repeated administration. In the case of people exposed to the wild-type virus such antibodies can effectively block the initial administration. Indeed, approximately 60 per cent of healthy people in France have neutralising antibodies to the most common form of AAV (Boutin et al., 2010). While it appears possible to use immunosuppression to modify the interaction with the immune system, this increases the risks associated with gene transfer. Plasmaphersis, which temporarily removes antibodies from the blood, has been used to allow successful administration of an AAV vector in non-human primates with pre-existing immunity to AAV (Chicoine et al., 2014). Removal of the antibodies causes a temporary immunosuppression but levels are restored rapidly.

Intramuscular injections of AAV carrying one of the alternatively spliced follistatin variants, FS344 (an antagonist of myostatin), increased muscle mass and strength in non-human primates (Kota et al., 2009) and more recently similar intramuscular injections have been shown to improve muscle performance in patients with Becker muscular dystrophy (Al-Zaidy et al., 2015) and inclusion body myositis (Mendell et al., 2017). However, intramuscular injections can only be used to treat a limited number of muscles and intravenous delivery would allow a global increase in muscle performance. Recent studies in dogs and man show that such a multi-muscle approach is not just limited to rodents. Clinically relevant increases in muscle function have been observed following such therapies in juvenile dogs affected with dystrophin deficient muscular dystrophy (Yue et al., 2015; Le Guiner et al., 2017) and juvenile dogs exhibiting myotubular myopathy (Mack et al., 2017). Critically, no immunosuppression was used in the two most recent trials (Le Guiner et al., 2017; Mack et al., 2017). Most impressively, a human clinical trial in human neonates with spinal muscular atrophy type 1 (SMA type 1) has shown remarkable results following administration of an AAV vector carrying an active version of the SMN1 gene (AveXis, 2017). Importantly, no adverse effects associated with the gene delivery were seen in either dog study or in the SMA type 1 patients.

An alternative to using viral vectors is to use plasmid DNA grown in bacteria. Plasmids are circular forms of DNA that replicate in bacteria separately from the bacterial genome. These can be isolated and highly purified so that the product is plasmid DNA without any protein contamination. When administered to animals the plasmid does not provoke an acquired immune response nor does it generate an auto-immune response. It does, however, activate the innate immune response, which produces an inflammatory reaction to DNA of bacterial origin. This inflammatory response can cause local swelling and transient non-specific flu-like symptoms but these do not prevent repeated administration of plasmid. Thus it is possible to top up the effects of previous treatments. The biggest problem with this approach is that the efficiency of cell entry is very poor. This can be improved by two methods. The first is to condense the plasmid which protects the DNA from degradation and enhances uptake by the cell. Specific ligands can be added to enhance cell uptake via receptor mediated pathways. This approach can work very efficiently in cell culture and moderately efficiently for some tissues *in vivo* (e.g. Midoux et al., 2008) but is not effective in skeletal muscle. The alternative method of enhanced delivery is to use a physical force to drive the plasmid across the cell membrane and into the cell, mostly commonly through transient micropores. This can be achieved using a high volume/high pressure (hydrodynamic, reviewed by Herweijer and Wolff, 2007), a set of electrical pulses (electroporation, reviewed by Trollet et al., 2008), firing the DNA into the cell/tissue (ballistic, reviewed by Wells, 2004) or using ultrasound, commonly in conjunction with contrast microbubbles (reviewed by Newman and Bettinger, 2007). It is therefore not feasible to consider efficient whole body treatment with non-viral vectors and these systems are better suited to local or regional, for example limb, treatment.

An alternative to the use of viral or non-viral vectors *in vivo* is to use cells modified *in vitro*. For example genetically modified cells can be used to aid the repair of damaged muscle or may be used as a platform for secreting proteins. In the latter case it is possible to encapsulate the cells in an inert capsule that can prevent the immune rejection of the cells. This has the advantage that such implants can be readily removed if they fail to express the protein of interest at appropriate levels and the coating means that the cells do not need to be those of the recipient (Ponce et al., 2006).

With all of the above techniques it is important to consider the regulation of gene expression. Where cells have been modified ex-vivo they can be assessed for the level of expression of the transferred gene prior to implantation. However for *in vivo* gene transfer the efficiency of gene transfer and hence the level of expression will be variable. In some cases excess expression carries significant health risks and may decrease performance. There are a range of drug inducible systems that would allow athletes to regulate the amount of gene expression. These include the tetracycline, rapamycin and tamoxifen regulated systems (e.g. Nordstrom, 2003; Rivera et al., 2005; Stieger et al., 2009). These not only allow control over any harm associated with excessive levels of expression but may also provide a method for avoiding doping detection in the case of systemically secreted proteins.

Temporary genetic modification can also be performed with the use of antisense sequences, either to reduce expression of a specific gene, most commonly using small interfering RNAs or by steric block oligonucleotides to inhibit translation or to modify splicing of the primary transcript. The latter have been extensively studied in the context of restoring the open reading frame in DMD and are in clinical trial at present. By preventing an exon from being spliced into the mature mRNA the reading frame can also be disrupted and this approach could conceivably be used to eliminate the open reading frame and thus prevent gene expression. A number of chemical modifications are available for oligonucleotide chemistry and such molecules can be highly gene-specific and may be difficult to identify unless the testing authorities suspect they are being used.

There are a number of small molecule drugs that are more or less gene specific and can be used to increase gene expression, for example by stabilising the mRNA or allowing the ribosomal apparatus to read through premature stop mutations, e.g. PTC 124 (Welch et al., 2007). This list can be expanded to include agonist or antagonists that act on the expression and function of specific genes, for example GW 1516, an agonist of PPARɣ, and AICAR, an agonist of AMPK (Narkar et al., 2008).

Finally, in the last few years a number of systems have been developed for specific targeted modifications of the genome including zinc finger nucleases (ZFN), transcription activator-like effector nucleases (TALEN) and clustered regularly interspaced short palindromic repeats (CRISPR)-Cas9 systems (Gaj et al., 2016). The most facile and potentially the most promising is the CRISPR-Cas9 system. This is derived from bacterial defense systems to combat integration of phage sequences into bacterial DNA and together with one or more sequence specific guide RNAs can be used to direct double stranded breaks at specific sites in the genome (Jinek et al., 2012). A number of recent papers have demonstrated that systemic delivery of CRISPR-Cas9 and guide RNAs using AAV vectors can result in successful gene modification in mouse muscles (Long et al., 2016; Nelson et al., 2016; Bengtsson et al., 2017). Given the current developments with the CRISPR-Cas9 system and optimised systemic delivery of AAV, it seems very likely that the efficiency of delivery and the genetic modification will only increase in the future. An obvious target would be to inactivate the myostatin gene leading to increased muscle mass which would likely benefit power athletes.

16.4 History of gene doping in sport

Gene doping was first added to the IOC/WADA list in 2003. In 2004 gene doping was included in the WADA Prohibited List with the following definition: "Gene or cell doping is defined as the non-therapeutic use of genes, genetic elements and/or cells that have the capacity to enhance athletic performance". To date there have been no recorded incidents of gene doping. However, anecdotal accounts exist of an attempt to procure gene doping and one laboratory reportedly offering gene doping services (Friedmann et al., 2010).

16.5 Action and use of gene doping in sport

Many of the impressive studies showing an increased athletic performance in experimental animals were performed with transgenic mice in which the genetic modification is made to the very early embryo. This is highly unlikely to be undertaken in humans due to the low efficiency of the procedures let alone the major ethical concerns that such manipulations raise. Relatively few of the genes in question have been modified by somatic gene transfer in adult animals and, until recently, most examples were in laboratory rodents. In these models, a single intramuscular injection is often sufficient to modify most, if not all, of one muscle. However, in larger animals the diffusion of gene transfer vectors from the site of treatment is very limited (O'Hara et al., 2001) and thus multiple intramuscular injections would be needed to modify human muscle. Systemic administration of AAV vectors have been effective in treating all muscles in mice but only very recently have high efficiencies been noted with studies in larger animals such as dogs (Mack et al., 2017). Regional perfusion in a limb temporarily isolated from the general circulation by a tourniquet has been quite successful in adult dogs (Arruda et al., 2005; Qiao et al., 2009; Le Guiner et al., 2014). Plasmid DNA can also be delivered hydrodynamically to the temporarily isolated limb although probably with a lower gene transfer efficiency than AAV (Hagstrom et al., 2004).

Intramuscular injection of either AAV or plasmid delivered by electroporation would probably be sufficient to boost the circulating Epo levels and would be quite practical using current technology. Alternatively, limbs could be perfused with AAV or plasmid. Although it would not be possible to target all of the muscle fibres in a limb, transfer of genes whose products work in an autocrine or paracrine fashion, such as IGF-1, might be sufficient to marginally improve performance. The production of plasmid DNA free of major contaminants, although not at a clinical grade acceptable for legal use in man, is relatively easy and would be within the capabilities of a small illegal laboratory. The production of large quantities of AAV is more difficult and currently would require specialist skills. However, as the methodologies continue to be refined it is becoming a more practical possibility for a well-equipped lab.

There are clear dangers associated with gene doping. Administration of large quantities of viral vectors or plasmids risks activating the innate immune system and in one trial in 1999 using an adenoviral vector led to disseminated intravascular coagulation, organ failure and death (Raper et al., 2003). Plasmid DNA can also activate the innate immune system via specific sequences that are recognised as bacterial and this leads to inflammation and fever. However, developments in non-viral vector design have largely removed these sequences, which significantly reduce interaction with the innate immune system and increases longevity of expression. The use of integrating viral vectors has been associated with oncogenesis in human clinical trials (Hacein-Bey-Abina et al., 2008) but the vectors that are more likely to be used for gene doping, AAV and plasmid, do not integrate at a significant rate and so this oncogenesis risk is relatively small. The use of CRISPR-Cas9 for gene editing appears sufficiently specific for use in man and to date off-target effects have not been shown to be a major problem based largely on cell culture based assays. However, there is a possibility that the Cas9 nuclease may activate the immune system in humans and that long-term expression may increase the incidence of off-target effects. Indeed, a very recent paper suggests that there may be a lot of off-target mutations *in vivo* (Schaefer et al., 2017).

Over-expression of genes may have harmful consequences. Excess Epo leads to polycythemia, an excess of red blood cells that makes the blood more viscous and thus puts greater load on the heart. This in turn can lead to blockage of the microcirculation and to stroke and heart failure. In addition, the production of Epo following gene transfer has been reported as causing autoimmune anaemia in macaques (Chenuaud et al., 2004; Gao et al., 2004). Over-expression of PGC-1a has been linked to a tendency to muscle atrophy and type II diabetes in some of the transgenic mouse studies (Miura et al., 2006; Choi et al., 2008). IFG-1 is a potent mitogen and has anti-apoptotic effects. Consequently, over-expression following gene transfer would imply an increased risk of oncogenesis (reviewed by Perry et al., 2006).

16.6 Gene doping and the WADA Prohibited List

WADA currently defines gene doping as (1) the transfer of polymers of nucleic acids or nucleic acid analogues or (2) the use of normal or genetically modified cells (WADA, 2017). The 2018 list will include genome engineering for precisely the reasons explained earlier so that gene doping will be defined as (1) the use of polymers of nucleic acids or nucleic acid analogues, (2) the use of gene editing agents designed to alter genome sequences and/or the transcriptional or epigenetic regulation of gene expression, or (3) the use of normal or genetically modified cells. While there is no evidence to date that athletes have practised gene doping, the threat of gene doping has lead to many laboratories working to develop systems to detect any possible gene doping.

Doping controls were originally developed to detect approved drugs and known methods of performance enhancement such as blood doping. However, there is increasing evidence of the use of non-clinically approved or designer drugs such as the anabolic steroid, Tetrahydrogestrinone (THG). Emerging drugs under development that could be used for doping were originally reviewed by Thevis et al. (2009) and have been updated annually (Thevis et al., 2017). The problems posed by designer drugs are more difficult and screening for a type of action rather than the specific drug will become an important part of the methodology, for example screening for androgenic activity in a mammalian cell bio-assay (Houtman et al., 2009). The diagnostic challenge posed by gene therapy may be even greater. Doping detection relies on urine and blood samples and it is not currently possible to take solid tissues which are most likely to give clear evidence of genetic manipulation.

Fortunately, products of gene doping that are secreted following gene transfer into ectopic sites show different patterns of post-translational modification, for example Epo secreted from muscle is demonstrably different from the endogenous Epo secreted from the kidney (Lasne et al., 2004).

It is possible to detect minute traces of gene transfer vectors using highly sensitive polymerase chain reaction based techniques. However, the window for detection of vector after administration is relatively small, particularly for non-viral vectors. A number of groups have developed quantitative methods for polymerase chain reaction (PCR) for viral and non-viral transgenes and have reported improved detection with a number of protocol modifications, for example (Baotina et al., 2013). An alternative is the use of a primer-internal, intron-spanning PCR approach (spiPCR, Beiter et al., 2008; Beiter et al., 2011) and a similar approach has been developed by another group (Baotina et al., 2010). Certified reference materials will be an important measurement tool to facilitate standardised, accurate and reliable genetic analysis in such applications (Baotina et al., 2016). Small interfering RNA (siRNA) has been shown to decrease gene expression for a number of targets and could be used to decrease genes that limit muscle mass such as myostatin (Takemasa et al., 2012). A liquid chromatography–high resolution/high accuracy mass spectrometry (LC-HRMS) method has been developed to detect such siRNA (Thomas et al., 2013).

Where regulated promoters are used it may be possible to detect the activating molecule such as tetracycline, rapamycin or tamoxifen, but each of these has another non-doping therapeutic action. Finally, it may be possible to detect evidence of prior administration of viral vectors by looking for evidence of an antibody response to the virus, but this could be explained by inadvertent exposure to the natural infectious virus.

An alternative approach is to use indirect techniques to detect gene doping by looking for the consequence of the genetic manipulation such as changes in patterns of target gene expression (transcriptomics), proteins (proteomics) or their metabolites (metabalomics). The transcriptomic approach has been reviewed (Rupert, 2009) and the use of the proteomics approach for detecting androgenic steroid abuse in racehorses is another example (Barton et al., 2009). However, these methods require the establishment of normal standards and some individuals are likely to fall outside of a normal range as a consequence of natural genetic variation. Indeed the problem of ethnic and individual variation has been highlighted with assessment of the metabolism of testosterone (Strahm et al., 2009). A solution to this problem would be the use of an athlete's endocrinological passport based on the results of repeated tests over time (Sottas et al., 2008) as has been done for "blood passports" for the detection of blood doping (Robinson et al., 2007). This would provide testers with a lifelong "biological fingerprint" of competitors to compare drug-test samples against.

16.7 Summary

The potential use of gene doping is critically dependent on our increasing understanding of the genetic modifiers of exercise physiology and the medical development of gene therapy systems that are highly efficient in man. It is now well established that in laboratory animals genes can be added to increase levels of specific proteins or manipulated with a range of technologies to decrease production of specific proteins.

A substantial number of candidate genes have been identified as possible targets for gene doping. As gene therapy using AAV vectors is being developed for clinical use in neuromuscular diseases, and given the rapid rise of genome engineering using CRISPR-Cas9, we are quickly moving towards the point where gene doping may become a reality. However, in many cases it is also likely that screening methods that have been developed will be able to detect many of the forms of gene doping.

16.8 References

Aiuti, A., Roncarolo, M.G. and Naldini, L. (2017) Gene therapy for ADA-SCID, the first marketing approval of an ex vivo gene therapy in Europe: Paving the road for the next generation of advanced therapy medicinal products. *EMBO Molecular Medicine* 9(6): 737–740.

Al-Zaidy, S.A., Sahenk, Z., Rodino-Klapac, L.R. et al. (2015) Follistatin gene therapy improves ambulation in Becker Muscular Dystrophy. *Journal of Neuromuscular Disease* 2(3): 185–192.

Amthor, H., Macharia, R., Navarrete, R. et al. (2007) Lack of myostatin results in excessive muscle growth but impaired force generation. *Proceedings of the National Academy of Sciences USA* 104: 1,835–1,840.

Arany, Z., Lebrasseur, N., Morris, C. et al. (2007) The transcriptional coactivator PGC-1beta drives the formation of oxidative type IIX fibers in skeletal muscle. *Cell Metabolism* 5: 35–46.

Arruda, V.R., Stedman, H.H., Nichols, T.C. et al. (2005) Regional intravascular delivery of AAV-2-F. IX to skeletal muscle achieves long-term correction of hemophilia B in a large animal model *Blood* 105: 3,458–3,464.

AveXis (2017): AveXis Presents Results from Phase 1 Trial of AVXS-101 in SMA Type 1 at the Annual Meeting of the American Academy of Neurology. Available at: http://investors.avexis.com/phoenix.zhtml?c=254285&p=irol-newsArticle&ID=2264492 (Accessed 1 December 2017).

Barton, C., Beck, P., Kay, R. et al. (2009) Multiplexed LC-MS/MS analysis of horse plasma proteins to study doping in sport *Proteomics* 9: 3,058–3,065.

Barton-Davis, E.R., Shoturma, D.I., Musaro, A. et al. (1998) Viral mediated expression of insulin-like growth factor I blocks the aging-related loss of skeletal muscle function *Proceedings of the National Academy of Sciences USA* 95: 15,603–15,607.

Baoutina, A., Alexander, I.E., Rasko, J.E. and Emslie, K.R. (2008) Developing strategies for detection of gene doping. *Journal of Genetic Medicine* 10: 3–20.

Baoutina, A., Bhat, S., Zheng, M. et al. (2016) Synthetic certified DNA reference material for analysis of human erythropoietin transgene and transcript in gene doping and gene therapy. *Gene Therapy* 23:708–717.

Baoutina, A., Coldham, T., Bains, G.S. and Emslie, K.R. (2010) Gene doping detection: Evaluation of approach for direct detection of gene transfer using erythropoietin as a model system. *Gene Therapy*, 17: 1,022–1,032.

Baoutina, A., Coldham, T., Fuller, B. and Emslie, K.R. (2013) Improved detection of transgene and nonviral vectors in blood. *Human Gene Therapy Methods* 24: 345–54.

Beiter, T., Zimmermann, M., Fragasso, A. et al. (2008) Establishing a novel single-copy primer-internal intron-spanning PCR (spiPCR) procedure for the direct detection of gene doping. *Exercise Immunology Review* 14: 73–85.

Beiter, T., Zimmermann, M., Fragasso, A. et al. (2011) Direct and long-term detection of gene doping in conventional blood samples. *Gene Therapy* 18: 225–231.

Bengtsson, N.E., Hall, J.K., Odom, G.L. et al. (2017) Muscle-specific CRISPR/Cas9 dystrophin gene editing ameliorates pathophysiology in a mouse model for Duchenne muscular dystrophy. *Nature Communications* 8: 14,454.

Boman, I.A., Klemetsdal, G., Blichfeldt, T. et al. (2009) A frameshift mutation in the coding region of the myostatin gene (MSTN) affects carcass conformation and fatness in Norwegian White Sheep (Ovis aries). *Animal Genetics* 40: 418–422.

Boutin, S., Monteilhet, V., Veron, P. et al. (2010) Prevalence of serum IgG and neutralizing factors against adeno-associated virus (AAV) types 1, 2, 5, 6, 8, and 9 in the healthy population implications for gene therapy using AAV vectors. *Human Gene Therapy* 21: 704–712.

Calvo, J.A., Daniels, T.G., Wang, X. et al. (2008) Muscle-specific expression of PPARgamma coactivator-1alpha improves exercise performance and increases peak oxygen uptake. *Journal of Applied Physiology* 104: 1,304–1,312.

Chenuaud, P., Larcher, T., Rabinowitz, J.E. et al. (2004) Autoimmune anemia in macaques following erythropoietin gene therapy. *Blood* 103: 3,303–3,304.

Chicoine, L.G., Montgomery, C.L., Bremer, W.G. et al. (2014) Plasmapheresis eliminates the negative impact of AAV antibodies on microdystrophin gene expression following vascular delivery. *Molecular Therapy* 22: 338–347.

Choi, C.S., Befroy, D.E., Codella, R. et al. (1995) Myogenic vector expression of insulin-like growth factor I stimulates muscle cell differentiation and myofiber hypertrophy in transgenic mice. *Journal of Biological Chemistry* 270: 12,109–12,116.

de la Chapelle, A., Träskelin, A.L. and Juvonen, E. (1993) Truncated erythropoietin receptor causes dominantly inherited benign human erythrocytosis. *Proceedings of the National Academy of Sciences USA* 90: 4,495–4,499.

Denti, M.A., Rosa, A., D'Antona, G. et al. (2006) Body-wide gene therapy of Duchenne muscular dystrophy in the *mdx* mouse model. *Proceedings of the National Academy of Sciences USA 103*: 3,758–3,763.

Fattori, E., Cappelletti, M., Zampaglione, I. et al. (2005) Gene electro-transfer of an improved erythropoietin plasmid in mice and non-human primates. *Journal of Genetic Medicine* 7: 228–236.

Fischetto, G. and Bermon, S. (2013) From gene engineering to gene modulation and manipulation: Can we prevent or detect gene doping in sports? *Sports Medicine* 43(10): 977–990.

Friedmann, T., Rabin, O. and Frankel, M.S. (2010) Ethics: Friedmann, T., Rabin, O Gene doping and sport. *Science* 327: 647–648.

Gaj, T., Sirk, S.J., Shui, S.L. and Liu, J. (2016) Genome-editing technologies: Principles and applications. *Cold Spring Harbour Perspectives in Biology* 8 pii: a023754.

Gao, G.P., Alvira, M.R., Wang, L. et al. (2002) Novel adeno-associated viruses from rhesus monkeys as vectors for human gene therapy. *Proceedings of the National Academy of Sciences USA* 99: 11,854–11,859.

Gao, G., Lebherz, C., Weiner, D.J. et al. (2004) Erythropoietin gene therapy leads to autoimmune anemia in macaques. *Blood* 103: 3,300–3,302.

Gregorevic, P., Blankinship, M.J., Allen, J.M. et al. (2004) Systemic delivery of genes to striated muscles using adeno-associated viral vectors. *Nature Medicine* 10: 828–834.

Grobet, L., Martin, L.J., Poncelet, D. et al. (1997) A deletion in the bovine myostatin gene causes the double-muscled phenotype in cattle. *Nature Genetics* 17: 71–74.

Hacein-Bey-Abina, S., Garrigue, A., Wang, G.P. et al. (2008) Insertional oncogenesis in 4 patients after retrovirus-mediated gene therapy of SCID-X1. *Journal of Clinical Investigation* 118: 3,132–3,142.

Hagstrom, J.E., Hegge, J., Zhang, G. et al. (2004) A facile nonviral method for delivering genes and siRNAs to skeletal muscle of mammalian limbs. *Molecular Therapy* 10: 386–398.

Hakimi, P., Yang, J., Casadesus, G. et al. (2007) Overexpression of the cytosolic form of phosphoenolpyruvate carboxykinase (GTP) in skeletal muscle repatterns energy metabolism in the mouse. *Journal of Biological Chemistry* 282: 32,844–32,855.

Herweijer, H. and Wolff, J.A. (2007) Gene therapy progress and prospects: hydrodynamic gene delivery. *Gene Therapy* 14: 99–107.

Hill E.W., Gu J., Eivers S.S. et al. (2010) A sequence polymorphism in MSTN predicts sprinting ability and racing stamina in thoroughbred horses. *PLOS ONE* 5: e8645.

Iezzi, S., Di Padova, M., Serra, C. et al. (2004) Deacetylase inhibitors increase muscle cell size by promoting myoblast recruitment and fusion through induction of follistatin. *Developmental Cell* 6: 673–684.

Jinek, M., Chylinski, K., Fonfara, I. et al. (2012) A programmable dual-RNA-guided DNA endonuclease in adaptive bacterial immunity. *Science* 337: 816–821.

Kastelein, J.J., Ross, C.J. and Hayden, M.R. (2013) From mutation identification to therapy: Discovery and origins of the first approved gene therapy in the Western world. *Human Gene Therapy* 24: 472–478.

Kim, S., Peng, Z. and Kaneda, Y. (2008) Current status of gene therapy in Asia. *Molecular Therapy* 16: 237–243.

Kota, J., Handy, C.R., Haidet, A.M. et al. (2009) Follistatin gene delivery enhances muscle growth and strength in nonhuman primates. *Science Translational Medicine* 1(6): 6ra15.

Krämer, D.K., Ahlsén, M., Norrbom, J. et al. (2006) Human skeletal muscle fibre type variations correlate with PPAR alpha, PPAR delta and PGC-1 alpha mRNA. *Acta Physiologica* 188: 207–216.

Lasne, F., Martin, L., de Ceaurriz, J. et al. (2004) Genetic doping with erythropoietin cDNA in primate muscle is detectable. *Molecular Therapy* 10: 409–410.

Lee, S., Barton, E.R., Sweeney, H.L. and Farrar, R.P. (2004) Viral expression of insulin-like growth factor-I enhances muscle hypertrophy in resistance-trained rats. *Journal of Applied Physiology* 96: 1,097–1,104.

Le Guiner, C., Montus, M., Servais, L. et al. (2014) Forelimb treatment in a large cohort of dystrophic dogs supports delivery of a recombinant AAV for exon skipping in Duchenne patients. *Molecular Therapy* 22: 1,923–1,935.

Le Guiner, C., Servais, L., Montus, M. et al. (2017) Long-term microdystrophin gene therapy is effective in a canine model of Duchenne muscular dystrophy. *Nature Communications.* 8: 16,105.

Lin, J., Wu, H., Tarr, P.T. et al. (2002) Transcriptional co-activator PGC-1 alpha drives the formation of slow-twitch muscle fibres. *Nature* 418: 797–801.

Long, C., Amoasii, L., Mireault, A.A. et al. (2016). Postnatal genome editing partially restores dystrophin expression in a mouse model of muscular dystrophy. *Science* 351: 400–403.

Lunde, I.G., Ekmark, M., Rana, Z.A. et al. (2007) PPAR{delta} expression is influenced by muscle activity and induces slow muscle properties in adult rat muscles after somatic gene transfer. *Journal of Physiology* 582: 1,277–1,287.

Mack, D.L., Poulard, K., Goddard, M.A. et al. (2017) Systemic AAV8-mediated gene therapy drives whole-body correction of myotubular myopathy in dogs. *Molecular Therapy* 25: 839–854.

McPherron, A.C., Lawler, A.M. and Lee, S.J. (1997) Regulation of skeletal muscle mass in mice by a new TGF-beta superfamily member. *Nature* 387: 83–90.

Mendell, J.R,, Sahenk, Z., Al-Zaidy, S. et al. (2017) Follistatin gene therapy for sporadic inclusion body myositis improves functional outcomes. *Molecular Therapy* 25(4): 870–879.

Midoux, P., Breuzard, G., Gomez, J.P. and Pichon, C. (2008) Polymer-based gene delivery: A current review on the uptake and intracellular trafficking of polyplexes. *Current Gene Therapy* 8: 335–352.

Miura, S., Tomitsuka, E., Kamei, Y. et al. (2006) Overexpression of peroxisome proliferator-activated receptor gamma co-activator-1alpha leads to muscle atrophy with depletion of ATP. *American Journal of Pathology* 169: 1,129–1,139.

Mosher, D.S., Quignon, P., Bustamante, C.D. et al. (2007) A mutation in the myostatin gene increases muscle mass and enhances racing performance in heterozygote dogs. *PLOS Genetics* 3: e79.

Nakatani, M., Takehara, Y., Sugino, H. et al. (2008) Transgenic expression of a myostatin inhibitor derived from follistatin increases skeletal muscle mass and ameliorates dystrophic pathology in *mdx* mice. *FASEB Journal* 22: 477–487.

Narkar, V.A., Downes, M., Yu, R.T. et al. (2008) AMPK and PPARdelta agonists are exercise mimetics. *Cell* 134: 405–415.

Nelson, C.E., Hakim, C.H., Ousterout, D.G. et al. (2016) In vivo genome editing improves muscle function in a mouse model of Duchenne muscular dystrophy. *Science* 351: 403–407.

Newman, C.M, and Bettinger, T. (2007) Gene therapy progress and prospects: Ultrasound for gene transfer. *Gene Therapy* 14: 465–475.

Nordstrom, J.L. (2003) The antiprogestin-dependent GeneSwitch system for regulated gene therapy. *Steroids* 68: 1,085–1,094.

O'Hara, A.J., Howell, J.M., Taplin, R.H. et al. (2001) The spread of transgene expression at the site of gene construct injection. *Muscle Nerve* 24: 488–495.

Perry, J.K., Emerald, B.S., Mertani, H.C. and Lobie, P.E. (2006) The oncogenic potential of growth hormone. *Growth Hormone IGF Research* 16: 277–289.

Petersen, K.F., Spiegelman, B.M. and Shulman, G.I. (2008) Paradoxical effects of increased expression of PGC-1alpha on muscle mitochondrial function and insulin-stimulated muscle glucose metabolism. *Proceedings of the National Academy of Sciences USA 105*: 19,926–19,931.

Phelps, S.F., Hauser, M.A., Cole, N.M. et al. (1995) Expression of full-length and truncated dystrophin mini-genes in transgenic *mdx* mice. *Human Molecular Genetics* 4: 1,251–1,258.

Ponce, S., Orive, G., Hernández, R.M. et al. (2006) *In vivo* evaluation of EPO-secreting cells immobilized in different alginate-PLL microcapsules. *Journal of Control Release* 116: 28–34.

Qiao, C., Li, J., Jiang, J. et al. (2008) Myostatin propeptide gene delivery by adeno-associated virus serotype 8 vectors enhances muscle growth and ameliorates dystrophic phenotypes in *mdx* mice. *Human Gene Therapy* 19: 241–254.

Qiao, C., Li, J., Zheng, H. et al. (2009) Hydrodynamic limb vein injection of AAV8 canine myostatin propeptide gene in normal dogs enhances muscle growth. *Human Gene Therapy* 20: 1–10.

Raper, S.E., Chirmule, N., Lee, F.S. et al. (2003) Fatal systemic inflammatory response syndrome in an ornithine transcarbamylase deficient patient following adenoviral gene transfer. *Molecular Genetic Metabolism* 80: 148–158.

Rivera, V.M., Gao, G.P., Grant, R.L. et al. (2005) Long-term pharmacologically regulated expression of erythropoietin in primates following AAV-mediated gene transfer. *Blood* 105: 1,424–1,430.

Robinson, N., Sottas, P.E., Mangin, P. and Saugy, M. (2007) Bayesian detection of abnormal hematological values to introduce a no-start rule for heterogeneous populations of athletes. *Haematologica* 92: 1,143–1,144.

Rupert, J.L. (2009) Transcriptional profiling: A potential anti-doping strategy. *Scandinavian Journal of Medicine and Sciences in Sports* 19: 753–763.

Sartori, R., Schirwis, E., Blaauw, B. et al. (2003) BMP signaling controls muscle mass. *Nature Genetics* 45 1,309–1,318.

Schaefer, K.A., Wu, W.H., Colgan, D.F. et al. (2017) Unexpected mutations after CRISPR-Cas9 editing in vivo. *Nature Methods* 14: 547–548.

Schertzer, J.D. and Lynch, G.S. (2006) Comparative evaluation of IGF-I gene transfer and IGF-I protein administration for enhancing skeletal muscle regeneration after injury. *Gene Therapy* 13: 1,657–1,664.

Schuelke, M., Wagner, K.R., Stolz, L.E. et al. (2004) Myostatin mutation associated with gross muscle hypertrophy in a child. *New England Journal of Medicine* 350: 2,682–2,688.

Schuler, B., Rieger, G., Gubser, M. et al. (2014) Endogenous α-calcitonin-gene-related peptide promotes exercise-induced, physiological heart hypertrophy in mice. *Acta Physiologica* 211: 107–121.

Sottas, P.E., Saudan, C., Schweizer, C. et al. (2008) From population- to subject-based limits of T/E ratio to detect testosterone abuse in elite sports. *Forensic Science International* 174: 166–172.

Stieger, K., Belbellaa, B., Le Guiner, C. et al. (2009) *In vivo* gene regulation using tetracycline-regulatable systems. *Advanced Drug Delivery* Review 61: 527–541.

Strahm, E., Sottas, P.E., Schweizer, C. et al. (2009) Steroid profiles of professional soccer players: An international comparative study. *British Journal of Sports Medicine* 43: 1,126–1,130.

Takemasa, T., Yakushiji, N., Kikuchi, D.M. et al. (2012) Fundamental study of detection of muscle hypertrophy-oriented gene doping by myostatin knock down using RNA interference. *Journal of Sports Science and Medicine* 11: 294–303.

Thevis, M., Thomas, A., Kohler, M. et al. (2009) Emerging drugs: Mechanism of action, mass spectrometry and doping control analysis. *Journal of Mass Spectrometry* 44: 442–460.

Thevis, M., Kuuranne, T., Geyer, H. and Schänzer, W. (2017) Annual banned-substance review: Analytical approaches in human sports drug testing. *Drug Testing and Analysis* 9(1): 6–29.

Thomas, A., Walpurgis, K., Delahaut, P. et al. (2013) Detection of small interfering RNA (siRNA) by mass spectrometry procedures in doping controls. *Drug Testing and Analysis* 5: 853–860.

Trollet, C., Scherman, D. and Bigey, P. (2008) Delivery of DNA into muscle for treating systemic diseases: Advantages and challenges. *Methods Molecular Biology* 423: 199–214.

Vandenberghe, L.H., Wilson, J.M. and Gao, G. (2009) Tailoring the AAV vector capsid for gene therapy. *Gene Therapy* 16: 311–319.

Vitiello, C., Faraso, S., Sorrentino, N.C. et al. (2009) Disease rescue and increased lifespan in a model of cardiomyopathy and muscular dystrophy by combined AAV treatments. *PLOS ONE* 4: e5051.

WADA (2017): Prohibited List 2017. Available at: https://www.wada-ama.org/en/resources/science-medicine/prohibited-list-documents (Accessed 1 December 2017).

Wang, Y.X., Zhang, C.L., Yu, R.T. et al. (2004) Regulation of muscle fiber type and running endurance by PPARdelta. *PLOS Biology* 2: e294.

Welch, E.M., Barton, E.R., Zhuo, J. et al. (2007) PTC124 targets genetic disorders caused by nonsense mutations. *Nature* 447: 87–91.

Wells, D.J., Wells, K.E., Asante, E.A. et al. (1995) Expression of human full-length and minidystrophin in transgenic *mdx* mice Implications for gene therapy of Duchenne muscular dystrophy. *Human Molecular Genetics* 4: 1,245–1,250.

Wells, D.J. (2004) Gene therapy progress and prospects: Electroporation and other physical methods. *Gene Therapy* 11: 1363–1,369.

Whittemore, L.A., Song, K., Li, X. et al. (2003) Inhibition of myostatin in adult mice increases skeletal muscle mass and strength. *Biochemical and Biophysical Research Communications* 300: 965–971.

Yue, Y., Ghosh, A., Long, C. et al. (2008) A single intravenous injection of adeno-associated virus serotype-9 leads to whole body skeletal muscle transduction in dogs. *Molecular Therapy* 16: 1,944–1,952.

Yue, Y., Pan, X., Hakim, C.H. et al. (2015). Safe and bodywide muscle transduction in young adult Duchenne muscular dystrophy dogs with adeno-associated virus. *Human Molecular Genetics* 24: 5,880–5,890.

Zhu, T., Zhou, L., Mori, S. et al. (2005) Sustained whole-body functional rescue in congestive heart failure and muscular dystrophy hamsters by systemic gene transfer. *Circulation* 112: 2,650–2,659.

Chapter 17

Stimulants

David R. Mottram

17.1 Introduction

The class of substances referred to as stimulants encompasses a group of drugs with diverse pharmacological activity. There are limited applications for the use of these drugs as therapeutic agents but many are used in a "recreational" context. Statistics, reported annually by World Anti-Doping Agency (WADA) laboratories, reveal that the annual number of adverse analytical findings (AAFs) for stimulants is second only to anabolic agents. It is claimed that many of these adverse findings were a result of inadvertent use, not associated with deliberate performance enhancement. This fact is reflected by the complex WADA anti-doping regulations associated with this class of drugs.

17.2 Types of stimulants and their modes of action

Figure 17.1 shows inter-relationships between the various nervous systems of the body.

Overall control of body function lies with the Central Nervous System (CNS). The CNS receives information about the body's environment, such as sight, sound, touch and taste, through Sensory Nerves. The CNS then relays information through either the Motor Nervous System, to the skeletal muscles or through the Autonomic Nervous System (ANS) to the parts of the body that are not under conscious control, such as the heart, blood vessels, respiratory tract, gastro-intestinal tract and various glands. The ANS is divided into the Parasympathetic Nervous System (PNS), which controls function under times of rest, and the Sympathetic Nervous System (SNS) which controls function under times of stress. Under extreme stress conditions, the SNS is augmented by secretion of the hormone adrenaline (epinephrine) from the adrenal medulla.

There are numerous neurotransmitters released from neurones within the CNS and ANS, including adrenaline, noradrenaline, dopamine and 5-hydroxytryptamine. Stimulants either mimic the effects of these neurotransmitters or elevate the levels of the transmitters at their site of action by increasing their release, preventing re-uptake or reducing metabolism (Jones, 2008).

The original, 1967, IOC Prohibited List classified stimulants as:

- sympathomimetic amines;
- psychomotor stimulants; and
- central nervous system (CNS) stimulants.

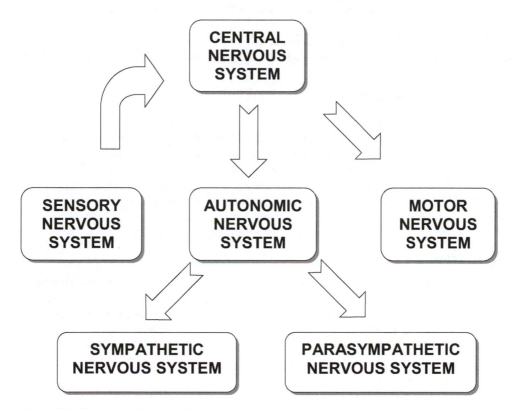

Figure 17.1 The inter-relationship between the various nervous systems of the body

Sympathomimetic amines

Sympathomimetic amines mimic or potentiate the effects of the SNS through its principal neurotransmitter noradrenaline (norepinephrine). Sympathomimetics, such as ephedrine, methylephedrine, pseudoephedrine and cathine, are structurally related to amphetamine and exert their effect by displacing noradrenaline and other monoamine transmitters from their storage sites or by acting on the same receptors as noadrenaline to potentiate its effect. They also exhibit some central stimulant properties. Other sympathomimetics, including phenylephrine, phenylpropanolamine and synephrine, are permitted in sport, although their use by athletes is recorded through the WADA Monitoring Program (https://www.wada-ama.org/en/resources/science-medicine/monitoring-program).

Ephedrines occur naturally in the plant genus Ephedra and have been a component of ancient Chinese medicine for many centuries. This, and other herbal sources of stimulants, has been reviewed by Bucci (2000). Ephedrine is similar in structure and function to amphetamine but is reported to have a 25-fold lower biological potency (Robergs et al., 2003). The effects of ephedrines are produced within 40 minutes after administration and can last up to three hours.

Adverse effects of ephedrines are, most commonly, tachycardia, hypertension, headache and dizziness. These drugs may cause anorexia, insomnia, irritability and nervousness at low to medium doses, whereas high doses are associated with mania and a psychosis similar to that occasionally seen with amphetamine.

Cathine is derived from the plant Khat, which contains a number of active constituents, the most potent of which is cathinone, which has amphetamine-like actions (Kalix, 1992).

Psychomotor stimulants

Psychomotor stimulants have a number of effects related to mental function and behaviour. They can induce excitement and euphoria, increase motor activity or reduce fatigue. Psychomotor stimulants include amphetamines, cocaine and methylxanthines, such as caffeine.

A large number of stimulants are listed on the WADA Prohibited List (see Table 17.3). A review of the pharmacology of these different types of stimulants is provided by Docherty (2008). Some of the stimulants that are more commonly misused within sport are described below.

Amphetamines (Amfetamines)

Several structurally related drugs are known as "amphetamines" and include dextroamphetamine, fenfluramine, methamphetamine, methylphenidate, phenmetrazine and phentermine. Amphetamine was first synthesised in 1920. It was originally prescribed for the treatment of nasal congestion. In 1935, amphetamine was used to treat the neurological condition narcolepsy, and its use in the treatment of depression, anxiety and hyperactivity in children followed from this. Amphetamine was used widely during the Second World War to reduce fatigue and increase alertness.

Amphetamines are readily absorbed, mainly from the small intestine and the peak plasma concentration occurs 1–2 hours following administration. Absorption is usually complete in 2.5–4 hours and is accelerated by food intake.

THE EFFECT OF AMPHETAMINES ON HUMAN MOOD AND PERFORMANCE

Although there is considerable inter-individual variation in the effects of amphetamine on mood the general effects are of positive mood enhancement. These effects include an increase in physical energy, mental aptitude, talkativeness, restlessness, vigour, excitement and good humour. Subjects taking amphetamine also report that they feel confident, efficient and ambitious, and that their food intake is reduced. Many athletes report that they feel most aggressive when taking amphetamines and are unlikely to report or complain of injuries (Laties and Weiss, 1981). Methamphetamine is a powerful, positive reinforcing agent in humans (Hart et al., 2001).

The effects of amphetamine on judgement are uncertain (Brookes, 1985). There is general agreement that amphetamines cause a mild distortion of time perception, which may lead to misjudgement in planning manoeuvres or in manipulations such as driving a car.

ADVERSE EFFECTS OF AMPHETAMINES

Peripheral side effects of amphetamines include sweating, palpitations, dilation of the pupil and rapid breathing, hypertension, tachycardia, tremors, muscle and joint pain.

Amphetamines also produce a number of centrally-mediated side effects including anxiety, indifference, slowness in reasoning, irresponsible behaviour, irritability, restlessness and insomnia. There is much evidence to show that amphetamines induce drug dependence and the amphetamine-dependent person may become psychotic, aggressive and anti-social. Withdrawal of amphetamines is associated with mental and physical depression. The rapid development of tolerance to amphetamine and the occurrence of dependence have led to the drug being withdrawn from clinical use.

Cocaine

Cocaine is derived from leaves of the coca plant (Erythroxylam coca). Cocaine first became available commercially in the 1880s. Sigmund Freud took the drug to try to cure his own bouts of depression and suggested it as a "cure all" for others. The drug fell out of medical use by the 1920s, only to reappear in the 1960s, as a major drug of abuse. "Crack" cocaine is a highly purified form of freebase cocaine. The name derives from the cracking sound produced when the freebase of cocaine is heated.

Cocaine affects the brain in a complex way. The most obvious initial effects are a decrease in fatigue, an increase in motor activity and an increase in talkativeness, coupled with a general feeling of euphoria and well-being. These mood changes soon subside and are replaced by a dysphoria (mood lowering). The mechanism by which cocaine produces these effects is not known fully. Cocaine is a powerful "reinforcer" and rewarding agent. It stimulates elements of the brain's pleasure and reward "centres" (Fibiger et al., 1992).

CNS stimulants

CNS stimulants have relatively little effect on mental function but increase the activity of the respiratory and vasomotor centres of the CNS or increase reflex excitability. Few CNS stimulants are misused in sport, although strychnine, a drug that has been used as a doping agent for over one hundred years, remains on the Prohibited List, as do nikethamide, crotethamide and cropropamide.

17.3 The use of stimulants in sport

Stimulants have a long history of use as potential performance-enhancing agents in sport, with cases involving the use of strychnine dating back to the end of the nineteenth century. Amphetamines, first developed in the 1920s, were frequently used by athletes in many sporting disciplines. Consequently, stimulants, along with narcotic analgesics, were the first classes of drugs to be included on an IOC list of prohibited substances, in 1967.

It can be seen from the statistics, released by WADA-accredited laboratories, that in recent years the annual number of AAFs for stimulants has been second only to that for anabolic agents. The most frequently used stimulants are shown in Table 17.1

The modern day use of stimulating agents in sport is clearly widespread and the health consequences of athletes using stimulants is a prime concern (Angell et al., 2013).

Athletes may take stimulants under a variety of circumstances, which may be classed as:

Table 17.1 Statistics from WADA-accredited laboratories for adverse analytical findings (AAFs) for substances classed as stimulants (2008–2015)

	2008	2009	2010	2011	2012	2013	2014	2015
Methylhexaneamine[+]	1	31	123	283	320	169	76	56
Amphetamine	166	27	112	133	58	47	70	80
Methylphenidate[+]	40	31	73	59	47	66	71	96
Cocaine	77	60	65	40	59	52	46	70
Oxilofrine (Methylsynephrine) [+]	3	6	7	14	3	22	27	22
Ephedrine[+]	54	44	32	33	12	10	25	19
Sibutramine[+]	17	11	25	14	14	20	18	15
Tuaminoheptane[+]	5	1	5	16	15	15	14	12
Methamfetamine (D-)	5	9	6	29	31	7	11	13
Phentermine	8	6	5	32	3	7	11	11
Fonturacetam	10	8	10	7	12	10	12	9
Pseudoephedrine[*+]	–	–	17	9	13	7	8	9
Others	86	91	94	49	112	98	85	116
Total	472	325	574	718	697	530	474	528

* Pseudoephedrine was removed from the WADA Prohibited List and placed on a monitoring list in 2004 and was returned to the Prohibited List in 2010.
+ Specified substances – those prohibited substances that are more likely to have been consumed by an athlete for a purpose other than enhancement of sport performance.

- Deliberate doping for performance enhancement;
- Treatment of medical conditions through:

  o   Prescribed medications; and
  o   Self-medication;

- Recreational use; and
- Supplement use.

Use of stimulants in deliberate doping for performance enhancement

Stimulants may be used by athletes to reduce tiredness and to increase alertness, competitiveness and aggression (Avois et al., 2006). They are more likely to be used within competition but may also be used during training to increase the intensity of the training session. WADA regulations only prohibit the use of stimulants in-competition. The potential benefit with respect to performance enhancement is variable depending on the class of stimulant being used.

Deliberate doping with ephedrine and other sympathomimetics

Ephedrine is closely related in structure to metamphetamine, although CNS effects are much less potent though longer acting than those of amphetamines (Avois et al., 2006). Peripheral effects of ephedrine mimic, to a lesser degree, those of adrenaline and noradrenaline and include increase in heart rate and thereby cardiac output, constriction of peripheral arteries leading to a rise in blood pressure, and bronchodilation. Ephedrine has therefore been perceived as having potential use as a performance-enhancing drug. However, research has shown that the isolated use of ephedrine and related drugs at usual dosages has an inconsistent, and probably insignificant, ergogenic benefit for power, endurance, strength or speed (Avois et al., 2006).

With respect to weight loss due to ephedrine, a review by Shekelle et al. (2003) revealed that ephedrine can promote modest weight loss in the short term, for up to 6 months, but that the differences in the parameters used to measure performance within the various trials mean that conclusive evidence for performance enhancement could not be perceived. Robergs et al. (2003) advised exercise physiologists and dieticians not to recommend the use of ephedrines or other stimulants for increased weight loss as they expose the user to unacceptable health risks relative to the minimal weight loss or ergogenic potential.

Serious side effects, such as a significant increase in blood pressure, may arise following the use of ephedrine (Jacobs et al., 2003). Shekelle et al. (2003) showed that ephedrine was associated with a two- to three-fold increase in adverse effects, including heart palpitations, and the risk of psychiatric and upper gastrointestinal symptoms.

In recent years, significant attention has been directed towards the sympathomimetic, pseudoephedrine. Pseudoephedrine was removed from the WADA Prohibited List in 2004 but reintroduced in 2010, due to the substantial increase in its use by athletes both in terms of the number of athletes and the dosages of drug being used (Deventer et al., 2011). WADA introduced a pseudoephedrine threshold level of 150 micrograms per millilitre. Research evidence regarding the performance-enhancing effects of pseudoephedrine is inconclusive, with improvements being reported in some studies (Hodges et al., 2006; Betteridge et al., 2010; Pritchard-Peschek et al., 2010) and little or no improvement in others (Berry and Wagner, 2012; Pallarés et al., 2015).

Deliberate doping with amphetamines

In a review of CNS stimulants, Avois et al. (2006) concluded that amphetamines may improve reaction time when fatigued; increase muscular endurance and strength; increase aerobic endurance capacity and stimulate metabolism by inducing a loss of body fat. A review by Conlee (1991) reported on a considerable inconsistency of amphetamine effects in humans particularly with regard to ergogenicity.

Since no significant improvement in performance is associated with amphetamine use, why does it continue to be taken? The answer could be an effect on mental attitude in terms of improved mood, greater confidence and optimism and increased alertness. Amphetamines could be abused for different reasons by different athletes. Thus, baseball and football players may use them to increase alertness and concentration, whereas runners or swimmers use them to increase energy and endurance (Smith and Perry, 1992). The effect of amphetamine on the psychological state of athletes might be a result of the athlete expecting to perform better and be more alert.

Adversely, Golding (1981) reported that the euphoriant effects of amphetamines rendered the takers unaware of the errors and misjudgements they were making on the field of play. Adverse effects of amphetamine use in sport has largely focussed on CNS effects, however, significant cardiovascular events are associated with their use with long-term atherosclerotic risk, even with moderate usage (Angell et al., 2013).

Some important side effects of amphetamine have been revealed in individuals undertaking extremely arduous training or sporting schedules. One of the most widely publicised side effects of amphetamine, from which a number of fatalities have occurred, is heatstroke.

This has been most prominent in cyclists owing to the intensity of their exercise, the endurance required and the high ambient temperatures at which the exercise frequently occurs. Amphetamines cause a redistribution of blood flow away from the skin, thus limiting the cooling of the blood. As a result, two cyclists (Knud Jenson and Tommy Simpson) who had both been taking amphetamine died of heatstroke and cardiac arrest respectively during gruelling road races. The former occurred in the intense summer heat of Rome, the latter during the 1967 Tour de France.

Box 17.1   Tommy Simpson (1967)

Tommy Simpson, the British cyclist, died of heatstroke and cardiac arrest whilst climbing the infamous Mont Ventoux during the 13th Stage of the 1967 Tour de France. Simpson was trying to make up time lost in earlier stages, resulting from the fact that he had been suffering from a stomach complaint. The post mortem found that Simpson had taken amphetamines and alcohol. The effect of these drugs was compounded by the fact that the temperatures on the mountain were extremely high on that day, the upper slopes of the mountain offer no shade from the sun and, in those days, the Tour organisers limited the fluid intake of riders during each stage, the effects of dehydration being poorly understood at that time.

Deliberate doping with cocaine

Despite the popular myth, cocaine does not appear to enhance performance in any sphere, including sport (Avois et al., 2006). Several studies have shown that cocaine has no beneficial effect on running times and reduces endurance performance. A more serious aspect of cocaine use in sport relate to its use as a recreational drug. This is discussed later in this chapter.

The use of stimulants in sport for the treatment of medical conditions

Although the clinical uses for stimulants are limited, it must be noted that their use by athletes for the treatment of valid medical conditions may be subject to Therapeutic Use Exemption regulations.

Stimulants in prescribed medications

ATTENTION DEFICIT HYPERACTIVITY DISORDER (ADHD)

ADHD is a common neuropsychiatric disorder with an estimated prevalence of 5–10% of school-age children and adolescents (Kreher, 2012). Symptoms of ADHD may persist into adulthood and in some cases be lifelong.

ADHD is characterised by the inability to maintain attention span and focus concentration at a normal developmental level (Kutcher, 2011; Kreher, 2012). The condition results from a dysfunction of catecholamines (adrenaline and noradrenaline) and dopamine. Hence, psychostimulant drugs, such as methylphenidate and amphetamine derivatives, are effective in treating symptoms of ADHD. These drugs have a number of side effects, which include sleep disturbances, appetite suppression, tachycardia, tremor anxiety and irritability, all of which may adversely affect athletic performance. Alternative treatment for ADHD includes non-prohibited drugs, such as atomoxetine, which is the preferred first-line treatment in some countries.

Clearly, athletes who are diagnosed with ADHD and who require treatment with prohibited stimulants would need to apply for a Therapeutic Use Exemption (TUE). WADA provide comprehensive guidance regarding the medical information to support the decisions of TUE Committees with respect to ADHD in children and adults (WADA, 2014). Due to the chronic nature of ADHD, a TUE in the case of well-documented, long-standing diagnosis of ADHD can be granted for up to four years at a time. An initial application for a newly diagnosed ADHD patient may be more appropriately approved for 12 months, until a stable dose is achieved. Evidence of yearly reviews by the treating clinician must accompany a TUE reapplication for ADHD.

A review by Reardon and Factor (2016) published arguments for and against the use of stimulants to treat ADHD in adult athletes. They concluded that stimulants may be a reasonable option for school-aged athletes with ADHD but that they make less sense at the elite or professional level.

CENTRALLY-ACTING APPETITE SUPPRESSION

Sibutramine was added to the WADA Prohibited List in 2006 since when it has been frequently detected through WADA-accredited laboratories (see Table 17.1). Sibutramine reduces food intake in individuals by enhancing the physiological response to the feeling of fullness following ingestion of food (Heal et al., 1998). It has been used clinically to treat obesity (McNeely and Goa, 1998). Although it is unlikely that athletes would require treatment for obesity, AAFs for this drug may have been related to the presence of sibutramine in slimming products, whose labels did not disclose the presence of the drug (Geyer et al., 2008). Other stimulant drugs that possess anti-obesity activity and which appear on the WADA Prohibited List include fenfluramine, dexamphetamine and phentermine.

SLEEP DISORDERS

Excessive episodes of daytime sleepiness associated with narcolepsy, sleep apnoea/hypopnoea syndrome and shift work sleep disorders may be treated with modafinil, a psychostimulant claimed to be non-addictive (Daventer et al., 2011). In 2003, a case involving the use of modafinil, by an elite athlete, was reported (Kaufman, 2005).

Box 17.2   Kelli White (2003)

Kelli White tested positive for modafinil at the World Athletics Championships in 2003. She claimed that her physician was prescribing modafinil for narcolepsy. Arising from the 2003 BALCO investigation, the US Anti-Doping Agency also found evidence for the use of tetrahydrogestrinone (THG) and erythropoietin (EPO). Kelli White was banned for two years and stripped of her medals. The athlete had also claimed that modafinil was not on the Prohibited List. However, although not specifically cited on the list of examples of stimulants, modafinil was banned as it had the pharmacological properties of a stimulant and fell under the umbrella phrase of "and related substances".

The approval to grant a TUE for modafinil or other stimulants for narcolepsy requires expert opinion from a consultant physician in sleep medicine plus a comprehensive investigation, including a positive multiple sleep latency test (Fitch, 2012).

ANAPHYLAXIS

Severe, life-threatening hypersensitivity reactions may be induced by poorly controlled asthma, insect bites, allergy to certain foods or by medicinal products. On rare occasions anaphylaxis may be exercise-induced (Huynh, 2015). First-line treatment for such anaphylactic reactions includes the emergency administration of adrenaline.

DENTAL ANAESTHESIA

Adrenaline is widely used with dental anaesthetics, such as lidocaine, in order to restrict the area of anaesthesia through vasoconstriction at the site of injection.

BRONCHODILATION

Ephedrine will produce bronchodilation and has been used to relieve symptoms of asthma, however, ephedrine is less suitable for conditions requiring this treatment than selective beta-2 agonists.

Stimulant use for self-medication

There is evidence to support a causal link between intense exercise and the incidence of upper respiratory tract (URT) infection (Nieman et al., 1990; Heath et al., 1991). In the case of male endurance runners, there appears to be a dose-related effect of exercise training on the risk of URT infection (Heath et al., 1991; Nieman et al., 1990; Peters and Bateman, 1983). This relationship is highlighted by the "J" curve model proposed by Nieman et al. (1993) whereby the risk of URT infection is reduced below that of sedentary individuals when engaged in mild to moderate intensity exercise training and increased when engaged in high intensity, high volume exercise training. However, a direct link between infection and disturbed immune function in athletes has not been fully established. There is evidence that there are important cofactors in the immune response to exercise including diet, lifestyle and stress (König et al., 2000).

Conditions that affect the URT whose symptoms can be managed through the use of over-the-counter (OTC) preparations, include viral or bacterial infections such as the common cold, influenza, pharyngitis, laryngitis, sinusitis and allergic reactions such as seasonal allergic rhinitis. Symptoms are a consequence of an immune response to the infection or allergic reaction and at the very least are viewed as a nuisance. However symptoms may be an important part of recovery from infection and whether symptomatic treatment using OTC preparations affects the recovery time course of URT infection is unclear (Eccles, 2005).

The number of OTC medications available for the treatment of symptoms associated with URT conditions is vast. Sales of OTC cough, cold and sore throat preparations in the UK during the year 2015/16 amassed over £415 million (Proprietary Association of Great Britain, 2016). Sales of OTC products in the UK for the specific treatment of hay fever symptoms amounted to over £104 million in the year 2015/16 (Proprietary Association of Great Britain, 2016).

NASAL CONGESTION

Sympathomimetic stimulants, such as ephedrine, methylephedrine, pseudoephedrine, met-amphetamine and cathine reduce nasal congestion through vasoconstriction in the nasal passages. These prohibited stimulants are available to purchase, without a prescription, in over-the-counter (OTC) products for the treatment of conditions such as nasal congestion associated with the common cold or allergies. There have been cases where AAFs for these substances have caused significant problems for athletes.

Box 17.3 Andreea Raducan (2000)

At the 2000 Olympic Games, in Sydney, the gymnast Andreea Raducan tested positive for the drug pseudoephedrine, which was present in an OTC cough and cold product that the gymnast had taken (Dikic et al., 2013). Despite the fact that she had taken the drug on advice from her team doctor, strict liability rules prevailed and she was stripped of her gold medal. Her physician was also sanctioned, being expelled from the Games and barred from Olympic Games for four years (Hilderbrand et al., 2003).

Box 17.4 Alain Baxter (2002)

Alain Baxter won a bronze medal in the Men's Slalom Skiing event at the Salt Lake City Winter Olympic Games in February 2002. He then tested positive for meth-amphetamine and was stripped of his bronze medal. Baxter had used an American product (Vicks Vapour Inhaler) as a nasal decongestant to treat a cold. This product contains Levmetamfetamine, the levo isomer of methamphetamine, a relatively inactive isomer compared with the dextro isomer. Baxter claimed that he was unaware that the product contained a banned substance since the medicine looked the same as a similar Vicks product that Baxter had used in the UK, which did not contain Levmetamfetamine. The International Ski Federation (ISF) accepted that Baxter had taken the drug inadvertently but imposed a ban of three months from all competitions. This ban was lifted by the Court of Arbitration in Sport, which accepted that Baxter "did not intend to obtain a competitive advantage". However, the IOC refused to overturn the medal disqualification. A subsequent study on the effects of inhaled levmetamfetamine on athlete performance showed that modest doses of the drug did not improve performance (Dufka et al., 2009).

These, and other similar cases, led WADA, in 2004, to remove most of the OTC stimulants from the Prohibited List. These drugs were placed on the Monitoring Program and their use by athletes continues to be monitored by WADA (https://www.wada-ama.org/en/resources/science-medicine/monitoring-program). Evidence suggests that athletes do not fully understand the status and function of these OTC medicines and many consider that they should be returned to the Prohibited List (Mottram et al., 2008). Indeed, pseudoephedrine was returned to the WADA Prohibited List in 2010. The current, 2017, WADA regulations with respect to the stimulants that remain on the prohibited list and are subject to threshold limits is shown in Table 17.2.

Athletes should be made aware that alternative drugs, such as xylometazoline and ipratropium, that are not prohibited in sport are a safer alternative treatment for nasal congestion in athletes.

Recreational use of stimulants in sport

Recreational use of drugs in society is a growing concern, worldwide. This wider societal trend in recreational drug use is reflected in sport, where a study on enquiries made via an online drug information database for athletes showed that 10.4 per cent of enquiries were for drugs categorised as recreational (Petróczi and Naughton, 2009). Substances that are commonly used recreationally include alcohol, cannabis and the prohibited stimulants, amphetamines and cocaine.

Cocaine is highly addictive and the abuser may experience acute psychotic symptoms. Chronic symptoms include a paranoid psychosis similar to that induced by amphetamine, coupled with spells of delirium and confusion. Other CNS side effects include stimulation of epileptic seizures.

Cocaine may be administered by injection, orally, intra-nasally or by inhalation. Oral administration produces peak effects at variable times with behavioural changes lasting up to one hour. The most popular route, for recreational use, is via nasal "snorting", which produces peak effects from 5–15 mins lasting for an hour. Effects of the drug such as increases in heart-rate and blood pressure are longer-lasting via the oral compared to the intravenous (iv) route (Smith et al 2001). Cocaine is mainly metabolised, by plasma and liver cholinesterases, to benzoyl ecgonine and ecgonine methyl ester which are excreted in the urine. Cocaine and its metabolites may remain within the body for significant periods after consumption. Since stimulants are only prohibited in-competition, athletes may believe that using these recreational drugs out-of-competition would be safe. This has led to a number of cases involving the claim by athletes of the inadvertent use of cocaine.

Box 17.5   Martina Hingis (2007)

Urine samples taken from Martina Hingis at the 2007 Wimbledon Tennis Championships showed a positive result for cocaine. She was banned from competition for two years but announced her retirement from tennis in November 2007. Hingis claimed that she had never used cocaine and independently submitted a hair sample for testing, which was negative for drugs. Furthermore she argued that the urine samples must have been handled improperly. However she stated that she did not wish to contest the finding or the two-year ban.

Box 17.6   Richard Gasquet (2009)

On 28 March 2009, the French tennis player Richard Gasquet submitted a urine sample at a tournament in Florida which tested positive for cocaine. Gasquet was charged with a doping offence and banned from competition. An independent Anti-Doping Tribunal appointed by the International Tennis Federation (ITF) held a hearing on 29/30 June 2009, at which Gasquet claimed his positive result was a result of cocaine entering his body when he kissed a girl who had been using cocaine at a night club. The tribunal stated that since the amount of cocaine found in Gasquet's system was "about the size of a grain of salt", he was cleared to return to competition. On 6 August 2009, the ITF and WADA announced that they were appealing to the Court of Arbitration for Sport (CAS) against the tribunal's decision. However, in December 2009, the CAS dismissed the appeal and Gasquet returned to competitive tennis.

Box 17.7   Frankie Dettori (2012)

The jockey Frankie Dettori was given a six-month ban from racing after testing positive for a banned substance, at Longchamp, in September 2012. It was later revealed that the substance was cocaine.

There have been cases in which athletes have claimed inadvertent use of cocaine due to passive inhalation of cocaine when smoked by others. Yonamine et al. (2004) have reviewed the literature on this issue and concluded that only individuals exposed to cocaine smoke under "extremely harsh conditions" would eliminate cocaine metabolites in the urine.

There have been reports of athletes combining cocaine abuse with other drugs such as alcohol. McCance-Katz et al. (1998) reported that cocaine and alcohol taken together have additive deleterious effects, that simultaneous consumption of alcohol and cocaine leads to the formation of cocaethylene, and that although cocaethylene is less potent than cocaine it is eliminated more slowly and could thus accumulate during or following an alcohol/cocaine binge. This may well have been the ultimate cause of death of the Canadian ice-hockey player John Kordic who abused cocaine, alcohol and anabolic steroids. His downfall has been chronicled in detail by Scher (1992) and included frequent fights on the pitch with opponents, team mates and officials.

Stimulants in supplements

The WADA draws athletes' attention to the risks that athletes face when using supplements:

> Extreme caution is recommended regarding supplement use. The use of dietary supplements by athletes is a concern because in many countries the manufacturing and labeling of supplements may not follow strict rules, which may lead to a supplement containing an undeclared substance that is prohibited under anti-doping regulations. A significant number of positive tests have been attributed to the misuse of supplements and taking a poorly labeled dietary supplement is not an adequate defense in a doping hearing.
>
> (WADA, 2017)

Numerous nutritional and dietary supplements, promoted for performance enhancement, stimulating effects and weight loss, contain stimulant drugs. Many contain caffeine, a stimulant that was removed from the WADA Prohibited List in January 2004. Some products contain extracts of the plant, guarana, which also contains caffeine. The relationship between caffeine and sport is reviewed extensively in Chapter 25 of this book.

Of more concern to athletes are those supplements that contain prohibited substances, whose use, deliberate or inadvertent, may result in an AAF during doping control procedures. Some of the prohibited stimulants that are more commonly found in supplements are shown in Table 17.2.

Prohibited stimulants may be present within supplements as a component of the product and declared on the label, as a component but undeclared on the label or as a contaminant present through poor, unregulated manufacturing processes (Baume et al., 2006). Even in cases where the component of the supplement is declared on the label, it may be a different name from that on the Prohibited List (e.g. ephedrine listed as ephedra or methylhexaneamine listed as geranamine). The risk to athletes who use supplements is further compounded by the fact that the amount of stimulant that manufacturers include within products may vary widely over time (Attipoe et al., 2016).

One of the oldest medicinal herbs is Ephedra or Ma Huang (*Ephedra sinica*) which contains six active ephedrine alkaloids. Today, herbal supplements containing parts of Ephedra sinica are frequently promoted for their performance-enhancing effects or their possible effects on weight reduction (Deventer et al., 2011). Some of these supplements contain much higher concentrations of ephedrines than can be expected from a "natural" source, suggesting the addition of ephedrines into the herbal product (Geyer et al., 2008; van der Merwe and Grobbelaar, 2004; Gurley et al., 2000). Serious side effects due to ephedrine within dietary supplements, such as seizures, stroke and even death, have been reported by Haller et al. (2000). The stimulant phentermine is also used in supplements that promote appetite suppression and therefore weight loss. Many AAFs for sibutramine can be related to its presence in slimming products (Geyer et al., 2008), for example, there has been a report that sibutramine has been detected in "pure herbal" Chinese slimming products (Vidal and Quandte, 2006).

Table 17.2 Stimulants that appear on the WADA Prohibited List and which are commonly found in supplements

Prohibited stimulant	Classified as specified or non-specified* for anti-doping regulations	Urinary threshold concentration
Ephedrine	Specified	10 micrograms per milliliter
Methylephedrine	Specified	10 micrograms per milliliter
Pseudoephedrine	Specified	150 micrograms per milliliter
Phentermine	Non-specified	
Cocaine	Non-specified	
Sibutramine	Specified	
Methylhexamine	Specified	

* Specified substances are considered to be potentially consumed by an athlete for a purpose other than enhancement of sport performance.

Although the principal reason for AAFs resulting from cocaine is probably related to its use as a recreational drug, cocaine may be present in a variety of supplements. Cocaine is used in several regions of South America, to alleviate the effects of high altitude. It may be ingested through direct chewing of leaves from the coca plant (*Erythroxylon coca*) or through drinking traditional coca teas such as Mate de Coca (Turner et al., 2005).

In recent years, one of the highest annual records of AAFs for the stimulant class of prohibited substances has been for methylhexaneamine (see Table 17.1), following its addition to the WADA Prohibited List in 2009. This probably reflects both the widespread inclusion of methylhexaneamine within supplements and the complex array of names for this drug that are used by companies when listing the ingredients for such supplements.

Methylhexaneamine is classed as a stimulant due to its effect of releasing the neurotransmitter noradrenaline from its nerve endings. It is listed on the 2017 WADA Prohibited List as 4-methylhexan-2-amine. It was originally patented as a nasal decongestant (Forthane); however, it is now marketed within supplements under many names including: dimethylpentylamine (DMP), 2-amino-4-methylhexane; 1,3-dimethylamine (DMAA), forthane, geranamine and geranium oil or root extract, and many more. A study by Lisi et al. (2011) suggests that geranium oils do not contain methylhexaneamine and that products labelled as containing geranium oil, but which contain methylhexaneamine, can only arise from the addition of synthetic material. The supplements in which methylhexaneamine appears are marketed for a wide variety of reasons but mainly focus on potential benefits for fat loss or increase in energy.

There have been a significant number of AAFs relating to methylhexaneamine, involving high profile athletes. The Syrian hurdler Ghafran Almouhamad provided an AAF for methylhexaneamine at the London 2012 Olympic Games, from which she was disqualified. Three further cases relating to the use of methylhexaneamine were recorded at the Sochi Winter Olympic Games in February 2014.

Box 17.8   Vitalijs Pavlovs, William Frullani and Evi Schenbacher-Stehle (2014)

The International Olympic Committee (IOC) announced that men's ice hockey player Vitalijs Pavlovs of Latvia, Italian bobsleigher William Frullani and biathlete Evi Sachenbacher-Stehle of Germany had been excluded from the XXII Olympic Winter Games in Sochi. All had tested positive for methylhexaneamine (dimethylpentylamine).

There have been reports of significant acute toxicity associated with the use of methylhexaneamine, including association with the death of a marathon runner (Archer et al., 2015). Attempts have been made in some countries to remove supplements containing methylhexaneamine from the market.

A recent report has identified, within dietary supplements, a structurally related analogue of methylhexaneamine, namely, 1,3-dimethylbutylamine (DMBA) (Cohen et al., 2015).

Oxilofrine, another prohibited stimulant that appears frequently on the list of AAFs, has been shown to be a common constituent of dietary supplements (Cohen et al., 2017). A high profile case involving oxilofrine was reported in 2013.

> ## Box 17.9   Asafa Powell (2013)
>
> The world of athletics was rocked in July 2013 by the revelation that Asafa Powell had been given an 18-month ban for testing positive for oxilofrine at the Jamaican national championships in June 2013. He claimed that the drug was present as a contaminant in a supplement that he had been provided with by one of his physical therapists. Following an appeal to the Court of Arbitration for Sport, his ban was reduced to six months.

17.4 Stimulants and the WADA Prohibited List

Stimulants have the potential to enhance performance at the time of competing and are therefore only banned by WADA in-competition. Out-of-competition testing for stimulants is not considered necessary, thereby saving resources. This decision has been supported through a study by Boghosian et al. (2011) who investigated data from 11 WADA-accredited laboratories to determine whether athletes were using stimulants during the training phase (out-of-competition). Results showed that there was no significant prevalence (0.36% of positive findings), suggesting that this does not pose a challenge to the fight against doping.

The WADA (2017) regulations relating to stimulants are shown in Table 17.3.

Table 17.3 WADA (2017) regulations regarding stimulants

All stimulants, including all optical isomers, e.g. d- and l- where relevant, are prohibited. Stimulants include:

a: Non-specified stimulants:

Adrafinil;
Amfepramone;
Amfetamine;
Amfetaminil;
Amiphenazole;
Benfluorex;
Benzylpiperazine;
Bromantan;
Clobenzorex;
Cocaine;
Cropropamide;
Crotetamide;
Fencamine;
Fenetylline;
Fenfluramine;
Fenproporex;
Fonturacetam [4-phenylpiracetam (carphedon)];
Furfenorex;
Lisdexamfetamine;
Mefenorex;
Mephentermine;
Mesocarb;
Metamfetamine(d-);
p-methylamphetamine;

Modafinil;
Norfenfluramine;
Phendimetrazine;
Phentermine;
Prenylamine;
Prolintane.
A stimulant not expressly listed in this section is a specified substance.

b: Specified stimulants:
Including, but not limited to:
4-Methylhexan-2-amine(methylhexaneamine);
Benzfetamine;
Cathine**;
Cathinone and its analogues e.g. mephedrone,
    methedrone and α- pyrrolidinovalerophenone;
Dimethylamphetamine;
Ephedrine***;
Epinephrine**** (adrenaline);
Etamivan;
Etilamfetamine;
Etilefrine;
Famprofazone;
Fenbutrazate;
Fencamfamin;
Heptaminol;
Hydroxyamfetamine (parahydroxyamphetamine);
Isometheptene;
Levmetamfetamine;
Meclofenoxate;
Methylenedioxymethamphetamine;
Methylephedrine***;
Methylphenidate;
Nikethamide;
Norfenefrine;
Octopamine;
Oxilofrine (methylsynephrine);
Pemoline;
Pentetrazol;
Phenethylamine and its derivatives;
Phenmetrazine;
Phenpromethamine;
Propylhexedrine;
Pseudoephedrine*****;
Selegiline;
Sibutramine;
Strychnine;
Tenamfetamine (methylenedioxyamphetamine);
Tuaminoheptane;
and other substances with a similar chemical structure or similar biological effect(s).

Except:

- Clonidine;
- Imidazole derivatives for topical/ophthalmic use and those stimulants included in the 2017 Monitoring Program*.

(continued)

Table 17.3 (continued)

*	Bupropion, caffeine, nicotine, phenylephrine, phenylpropanolamine, pipradrol, and synephrine: These substances are included in the 2017 Monitoring Program, and are not considered prohibited substances.
**	Cathine: Prohibited when its concentration in urine is greater than 5 micrograms per milliliter.
***	Ephedrine and methylephedrine: Prohibited when the concentration of either in urine is greater than 10 micrograms per milliliter.
****	Epinephrine (adrenaline): Not prohibited in local administration, e.g. nasal, ophthalmologic or co-administration with local anaesthetic agents.
*****	Pseudoephedrine: Prohibited when its concentration in urine is greater than 150 micrograms per milliliter.

The list of prohibited stimulants is extensive, however, they are sub-classed as Specified or Non-specified.

Classification of stimulants as "Specified" and "Non-specified"

In 2009, WADA introduced the categorisation of substances on the Prohibited List as "Specified" or "Non-specified". The move was made to align the 2009 Prohibited List with the more flexible sanctions set forth in the revised World Anti-Doping Code (WADC) of 2009 (WADA, 2009). The objective of more flexible sanctions was to allow enhanced sanctions for deliberate doping offenders and reduced sanctions for inadvertent cheaters or for athletes who can unequivocally establish that the substance involved was not intended to enhance performance. This policy was endorsed and expanded in the 2015 WADC (WADA, 2015).

As can be seen in Table 17.3, the majority of prohibited stimulants are classed as Specified, reflecting the likelihood of their being taken as a result of self-medication or supplement use. With respect to cathine, ephedrine, methylephedrine and pseudoephedrine, WADA specify urinary threshold limits, below which no sanctions are applied.

Stimulants on the WADA Monitoring Program

The 2015 WADC states: "WADA, in consultation with signatories and governments, shall establish a monitoring program regarding substances which are not on the Prohibited List, but which WADA wishes to monitor in order to detect patterns of misuse in sport". The Monitoring Program was introduced in 2004 and since that date selected stimulants have been listed each year. The list of stimulants included on the 2017 Monitoring Program were: bupropion, caffeine, nicotine, phenylephrine, phenylpropanolamine, pipradol and synephrine.

Up to 2004, caffeine had been included on the IOC Prohibited List subject to a threshold urinary level of 12 micrograms per millilitre. Following its removal from the Prohibited List in 2004, monitoring has revealed that it has been used extensively by athletes. A study by del Coso et al. (2011) reported that three out of four athletes had consumed caffeine before or during sports competition but only a small proportion (0.6%) had a urine concentration higher than 12 micrograms per millilitre. Caffeine is perceived as a performance-enhancing substance by many athletes (see Chapter 25).

Few reports exist regarding the use of bupropion by athletes. One study, in 2012, suggested limited improvement in performance in the heat but only at the maximum therapeutic dose of bupropion (Roelands et al., 2012).

Synephrine is marketed within supplements as a fat-burner, sometimes under the name "bitter orange". However, a recent study found that acute consumption of 3 milligrams per kilogram of p-synephrine was ineffective to increase performance in competitive sprint athletes (Gutiérrez-Hellin et al., 2016).

The effects of nicotine may be beneficial in a wide variety of sports and it has been suggested that nicotine is abused by athletes (Martinsen & Sundgot-Borgen, 2012; Pesta et al., 2013). A study by Pyšný et al. (2015) suggested that nicotine may be useful to help athletes relax, lower stress, increase motivation, improve concentration or mask fatigue but that short-term athletic performance is not influenced by nicotine consumption. A study by Mündel et al. (2017) concluded that the evidence for performance-enhancing effects of nicotine is limited and that more research and continued monitoring of the use of this drug, by athletes, is required.

17.5 Summary

- Stimulants are a broad class of drugs, many of which are abused recreationally.
- Stimulants are one of the classes of drugs that appear most frequently on WADA's statistics on AAFs.
- The potential benefit of many stimulants as performance enhancing agents is equivocal.
- The WADA regulations for stimulants, including Therapeutic Use Exemption are complex.

17.6 References

Angell, P.J., Chester, N., Sculthorpe, N. et al. (2013) Performance enhancing drug abuse and cardiovascular risk in athletes: Implications for the physician. *British Journal of Sports Medicine* 46(Suppl 1): i78–i84.

Archer, J.R.H., Dargan, P.I., Lostia, A.M. et al. (2015) Running an unknown risk: A marathon death associated with the use of 1,3-dimethylamylamine (DMAA). *Drug Testing Analysis* 7: 433–438.

Attipoe S., Cohen, P.A., Eichner, A. and Deuster, P.A. (2016) Variability of stimulant levels in nine sports supplements over a 9-month period. *International Journal of Sport Nutrition and Exercise Metabolism* 26: 413–420.

Avois, L., Robinson, N., Saudan, C., et al. (2006) Central nervous system stimulants and sport practice. *British Journal of Sports Medicine*, 40(Suppl 1): i16–i20.

Baume, N., Mahler, N., Kamber, M. et al. (2006) Research of stimulants and anabolic steroids in dietary supplements. *Scandanavian Journal of Medical Sciences in Sports* 16: 41–48.

Berry, C. and Wagner, D.R. (2012) Effect of pseudoephedrine on 800-m-run times of female collegiate track athletes. *International Journal of Sports Physiology and Performance* 7: 237–241.

Betteridge, S., Mündel, T. and Stannard, S. (2010) The effect of pseudoephedrine on self-paced endurance cycling performance. *European Journal of Sports Science* 10(1): 53–58.

Boghosian, T., Mazzoni, I., Barroso, O. et al. (2011) Investigating the use of stimulants in out-of-competition sport samples. *Journal of Analytical Toxicology* 35: 613–616.

Brookes, L.G. (1985) Central Nervous System stimulants. In S.D. Iverson (ed.) *Psychopharmacology: Recent Advances and Future Prospects*. Oxford, Oxford University Press, 264–277.

Bucci, L.R. (2000) Selected herbals and human performance. *Americam Journal of Clinical Nutrition* 72: 624S-636S

Cohen, P.A., Avula, S., Venhuis, B. et al. (2017) Pharmaceutical doses of the banned stimulant oxilofrine found in dietary supplements sold in the USA. *Drug Testing and Analysis* 9(1): 135–142.

Cohen, P.A., Travis, J.C. and Venhuis, B.J. (2015) A synthetic stimulant never tested in humans, 1,3-dimethylbutylamine (DMBA), is identified in multiple dietary supplements. *Drug Testing and Analysis* 7: 83–87.

Conlee, R.K. (1991) Amphetamine, caffeine and cocaine. In D.R. Lamb and M.H. Williams (eds) *Perspectives in Exercise Science and Sports Medicine 4*. New York, Brown and Benchmark, 285–328.

Del Coso, J., Muñoz, G. and Muñoz-Guerra, J. (2011) Prevalence of caffeine use in elite athletes following its removal from the World Anti-Doping Agency list of banned substances. *Applied Physiology and Nutritional Metabolism* 36: 555–561.

Deventer, K., Roels, K., Delbeke, F.T. et al. (2011) Prevalence of legal and illegal stimulating agents in sport. *Annals of Bioanalytical Chemistry* 401: 421–432.

Dikic, N., McNamee, M., Günter, H. et al. (2013) Sports physicians, ethics and antidoping governance: Between assistance and negligence. *British Journal of Sports Medicine* 47: 701–704.

Docherty, J.R. (2008) Pharmacology of stimulants prohibited by the World Anti-Doping Agency (WADA). *British Journal of Pharmacology* 154: 606–622.

Dufka, F., Galloway, G., Baggott, M. et al. (2009) The effects of inhaled L-methamphetamine on athlete performance while riding a stationary bike, a randomised placebo-controlled trial. *British Journal of Sports Medicine* 43: 832–835.

Eccles R. (2005) Understanding the symptoms of the common cold and influenza. *Lancet* 5: 718–725.

Fibiger, H.C., Phillips, A.G. and Brown, E.E. (1992) The neurobiology of cocaine-induced reinforcement. In G.E.W. Wolstenholme (ed.) *Cocaine: Scientific and Social Dimensions. Ciba Foundation Symposium 166*. Chichester, John Wiley, 96–124.

Fitch, K. (2012) Proscribed drugs at the Olympic Games: Permitted use and misuse (doping) by athletes. *Clinical Medicine* 12(3): 257–260.

Geyer, H. Parr, M.K., Koehler, K. et al. (2008) Nutritional supplements cross-contaminated and faked with doping substances. *Journal of Mass Spectrometry* 43: 892–902.

Golding, L.A. (1981) Drugs and hormones. In W.P. Morgan (ed.) *Ergogenic Aids and Muscular Performance*. New York, Academic Press, 368–397.

Gurley, B.J., Gardner, S.F. and Hubbard, M.A. (2000) Content versus label claims in ephedra-containing dietary supplements. *American Journal of Health-System Pharmacy* 57(10): 963–969.

Gutiérrez-Hellin, J., Salinero, J.J., Abían-Vicen, J. et al. (2016) Acute consumption of p-synephrine does not enhance performance in sprint athletes. *Applied Physiology and Nutritional Metabolism* 41: 63–69.

Haller, C.A. and Benowitz, N.L. (2000) Adverse cardiovascular and central nervous system events associated with dietary supplements containing ephedra alkaloids. *New England Journal of Medicine* 343(25): 1,833–1,838.

Hart, C.L., Ward, A.S., Harvey, M. et al. (2001) Methamphetamine self-administration by humans. *Psychopharmacology* 57: 75–81.

Heal, D.J., Aspley, S., Prow, M.R. et al. (1998) Sibutramine: A novel anti-obesity drug. A review of the pharmacological evidence to differentiate it from d-amphetamine and d-fenfluramine. *International Journal of Obesity* 22 Suppl 1: S18–S28.

Heath, G.W., Ford, E.S., Craven, T.E. et al. (1991) Exercise and the incidence of upper respiratory tract infections. *Medicine and Science in Sports Exercise* 23: 152–157.

Hilderbrand, R.L., Wanninger, R. and Bowers, L.D. (2003) An update on regulatory issues in antidoping programs in sport. *Current Sports Medicine Reports* 2: 226–232.

Hodges, K., Hancock, S., Currell, K. et al. (2006) Pseudoephedrine enhances performance in 1500-m runners. *Medicine and Science in Sports and Exercise* 38: 329–333.

Huynh, P.N. (2015) Exercise-induced anaphylaxis. Available at: http://emedicine.medscape.com/article/886641-overview (Accessed January 2017).

Jacobs, I., Pasternak, H. and Bell, D.G. (2003) Effects of ephedrine, caffeine and their combination on muscular endurance. *Medicine and Science in Sports and Exercise* 35(6): 987–994.

Jones, G. (2008) Caffeine and other sympathomimetic stimulants: Modes of action and effects on sports performance. *Drugs and Ergogenic Aids to Improve Sport Performance* 44: 109–123.

Kalix, P. (1992) Cathinone, a natural amphetamine. *Pharmacological Toxicology* 70: 77–86.

Kaufman, K.R. (2005) Modafinil in sports: Ethical considerations. *British Journal of Sports Medicine* 39: 241–244.

König, D, Grathwohl, D., Weinstock, C. et al. (2000) Upper respiratory tract infection in athletes: Influence of lifestyle, type of sport, training effort and immunostimulant intake. *Exercise Immunology Review* 6: 102–120.

Kreher, J.B. (2012). Attention Deficit/Hyperactivity Disorder (ADHD) in athletes. *International Journal of Athletic Therapy and Training* 17(3): 15–19.

Kutcher, J.S. (2011) Treatment of Attention-Deficit Hyperactivity Disorder in athletes. *Current Sports Medicine Reports* 10(1): 32–36.

Laties, V.G. and Weiss, B. (1981) The amphetamine margin in sports. *Federation Proceedings* 40: 2,689–2,692.

Lisi, A., Hasick, N., Kazlauskas, R. et al. (2011) Studies of methylhexaneamine in supplements and geranium oil. *Drug Testing and Analysis* 3: 873–876.

Martinsen, M. and Sundgot-Borgen, J. (2012) Adolescent elite athletes' cigarette smoking, use of snus and alcohol. *Scandanavian Journal of Medicine and Science in Sports* 24(2): 439–446.

McCance-Katz, E.F., Kosten, T.R. and Jatlow, P. (1998) Concurrent use of cocaine and alcohol is more potent and potentially more toxic than use of either alone: A multi-dose study. *Biological Psychiatry* 44: 250–259.

McNeely, W. and Goa, K.L. (1998) Sibutramine: A review of its contribution to the management of obesity. *Drugs* 56(6): 1,093–1,124.

Mottram, D., Chester, N., Atkinson, G. et al. (2008) Athletes' knowledge and views on OTC medication. *International Journal of Sports Medicine* 29: 851–855.

Mündel, J., Machal, M., Cochrane, D.J. and Barnes, M.J. (2017) A randomised, placebo-controlled, crossover study investigating the effects of nicotine gum on strength power and anaerobic performance in nicotine naïve active males. *Sports Medicine – Open* 3(1): 5.

Nieman, D.C., Johanssen, L.M., Lee, J.W. et al. (1990) Infectious episodes in runners before and after the Los Angeles Marathon. *Journal of Sports Medicine and Physical Fitness* 30: 316–328.

Nieman, D.C., Henson, D.A. and Gusewitch, G. (1993) Physical activity and immune function in elderly women. *Medicine and Science in Sports and Exercise* 25: 823–831.

Pallarés, J.G., López-Samanes, A., Fernández-Elias, V.E. et al. (2015) Pseudoephedrine and circadian rhythm interaction on neuromuscular performance. *Scandanavian Journal of Medicine and Science in Sports* 25: e603–e612.

Pesta, D.H., Angadi, S.S., Burtscher, M. and Roberts, C.K. (2013) The effects of caffeine, nicotine, ethanol and tetrahydrocannabinol on exercise performance. *Nutrition and Metabolism* 10: 71–86.

Peters, E.M. and Bateman, E.D. (1983) Ultramarathon running and upper respiratory tract infections. *South African Medical Journal* 64: 582–584.

Petróczi, A. and Naughton, D.P. (2009) Popular drugs in sport: Descriptive analysis of the enquiries made via the Drug Information Database (DID). *British Journal of Sports Medicine* 43: 811–817.

Pritchard-Peschek, K.R., Jenkins, D.G., Osborne, M.A. et al. (2010). Pseudoephedrine ingestion and cycling time-trial performance. *International Journal of Sports Nutrition and Exercise Metabolism* 20: 132–138.

Proprietary Association of Great Britain (2016) Annual Review 2015–16. Available at: https://www.pagb.co.uk/content/uploads/2016/06/PAGB_Annual-Review_210mm-x-210mm_24pp_Web.pdf (Accessed on 28 July 2017).

Pyšny, L., Petrů, D. Pyšná et al. (2015) The acute effect of nicotine intake on aerobic exercise performance. *Journal of Physical Exercise and Performance* 15(1): 103–107.

Reardon, C.L. and Factor, R.M. (2016) Consideration in the use of stimulants in sport. *Sports Medicine* 46: 611–617.

Robergs, R.A., Boone, T. and Lockner, D. (2003) Exercise physiologists should not recommend the use of ephedrine and related compounds as ergogenic aids or stimulants for increased weight loss. *Journal of Exercise Physiology* 6(4): 42–52.

Roelands, B., Watson, P., Cordery, P. et al. (2012) A dopamine/noradrenaline reuptake inhibitor improves performance in the heat, but only at a maximum therapeutic dose. *Scandinavian Journal of Medicine and Science in Sports* 22: e95–e98.

Scher, J. (1992) Death of a goon. *Sports Illustrated* 76: 112–116.

Shekelle, P.G., Hardy, M.L., Morton, S.C. et al. (2003) Efficacy and safety of ephedra and ephedrine for weight loss and athletic performance: A meta analysis. *Journal of the American Medical Association* 289(12): 1,537–1,545.

Smith B.J., Jones, H.E., and Griffiths, R.R. (2001). Physiological, subjective and reinforcing effects of oral and intravenous cocaine in humans. *Psychopharmacology* 156: 435–444

Smith, D.A. and Perry, P.J. (1992). The efficacy of ergogenic agents in athletic competition Part II: Other performance-enhancing agents. *Annals of Pharmacotherapy* 26: 653–659.

Turner, M., McCrory, P. and Johnston, A. (2005) Time for tea, anyone? *British Journal of Sports Medicine* 39(10): e37.

van der Merwe and Grobbelaar, E. (2004) Inadvertent doping through nutritional supplements is a reality. *Sports Medicine* 16(2): 3–7.

Vidal, C. and Quandte, S. (2006) Identification of a sibutramine metabolite in patient urine after intake of a "pure herbal" Chinese slimming product. *Therapeutic Drug Monitoring* 28(5): 690–692.

WADA (2009) World Anti-Doping Code 2009 Available at http://www.wada-ama.org (Accessed 1 December 2017).

WADA (2014) Medical Information to Support the Decisions of TUE Committees Attention Deficit Hyperactivity Disorder (ADHD) In Children And Adults. Available at: https://www.wada-ama.org/sites/default/files/resources/files/WADA-MI-ADHD-5.0.pdf (Accessed January 2017).

WADA (2017) Dietary and nutritional supplements Available at: https://www.wada-ama.org/en/questions-answers/dietary-and-nutritional-supplements (Accessed January 2017).

Yonamine, M., Garcia, P.R. and de Moraes Moreau, R.L. (2004) Non-intentional doping in sports. *Sports Medicine* 34(1): 697–704.

Chapter 18

Narcotics

David R. Mottram

18.1 Introduction

The use of certain drugs by athletes is prohibited because there is the potential for achieving enhanced levels of performance. With some drugs, the potential to induce serious harm to the user is of prime importance. In most countries, worldwide, the use of certain drugs for "recreational" purposes is against the law. All three of these criteria apply to the class of drugs known as narcotics.

18.2 What are narcotics?

In the strict sense of the word, narcotics are drugs that can induce narcosis, which can be defined as a state of insensibility. In addition, this class of drugs possesses significant analgesic activity, in which context they are frequently referred to as narcotic analgesics or opioid analgesics as they were originally derived from the opium poppy (*Papaver somniferum*). The active constituents of the poppy, of which morphine is the most potent, are extracted from the latex that exudes from incisions made in the unripe capsule of the flowering head. Opium has been used by humans for thousands of years. Morphine was first isolated in 1806 and named after the Greek god of dreams, Morpheus.

The potency of morphine can be significantly enhanced by acetylation to diamorphine (heroin), which has the convenience of greater solubility. Codeine (3-methylmorphine) has only a fifth of the potency of morphine but is more reliably absorbed from the gastrointestinal system. Dihydrocodeine is similar in potency to codeine when given orally though is about twice its potency when injected.

Morphine-like drugs are not just analgesics. They exhibit multiple activities including respiratory depression, emesis and smooth muscle relaxation. In addition they have profound CNS effects on perception. It can be argued that their analgesic effect is more to do with a change in concern about pain than in a "physical" reduction of pain. Euphoria is a common experience too.

18.3 Clinical uses of narcotic analgesics

Narcotics are drugs which are able to change psychic and physical status of humans through a wide range of symptoms from sleep to euphoria and excitation.

Analgesia

Pain is a subjective phenomenon the scale of which is dependent on many factors apart from the severity of an injury. Pain is notoriously difficult to measure.

Narcotic analgesics have a number of clinical uses, the most significant of which is the alleviation of pain. Non-opioid analgesics, such as aspirin, paracetamol (acetaminophen) and non-steroidal anti-inflammatory drugs (NSAIDs), including ibuprofen and diclofenac, are suitable for the relief of pain in musculoskeletal conditions. Opioid (narcotic) analgesics are more appropriate for the relief of moderate to severe pain, particularly of visceral origin.

In the 1970s, it was discovered that the body produces neuropeptides called endorphins which stimulate neural receptors resulting in a reduction of nociception and inducing a sense of well-being (Kosterlitz and Hughes, 1977; Simantov and Snyder, 1976). Narcotic analgesics stimulate the same receptors inducing similar or more profound levels of analgesia and euphoria. Narcotic analgesics relieve most types of pain, including that associated with traumatic injuries.

Other clinical uses for narcotics

Acute diarrhoea

There are a number of types of medicines that can be used to manage cases of acute diarrhoea. The primary goal should be to counter the dehydrating effects of this condition using oral rehydration preparations. However, gut motility can be controlled using anti-motility drugs including the opioids codeine and low doses of morphine. These medicines can be purchased over-the-counter, without a prescription.

Cough suppression

Cough may result from a number of causes, such as irritation to the respiratory epithelium due to an infection, exposure to environmental pollutants or as a symptom of another underlying disorder. A cough may be productive, with mucous, or non-productive. For most cases of cough, particularly a productive cough, the use of a cough suppressant is ill-advised. However, for a dry, non-productive cough it may be appropriate to use a cough suppressant, of which mild opioids, such as codeine and pholcodine are used, widely.

Side effects of narcotic analgesics

Significant differences exist in the extent and severity of side effects between the milder and the more potent examples of this class of drugs, the most common of which are:

- Nausea, vomiting and constipation;
- Sweating;
- Mental confusion and drowsiness; and
- Enhanced libido, but depressed sexual drive and performance.

More serious side effects are experienced if opioids are taken in overdose. These may affect the cardiovascular, respiratory and central nervous systems. Tolerance and psychic and physical dependence occur when narcotics are used regularly. Tolerance is the need for an increased dose of the drug to produce the same pharmacological effect. Psychic dependence is characterised by the continued desire or craving for a substance, whilst physical dependence is observed when a substance is no longer administered and physical withdrawal symptoms are experienced. Dependence is a compulsion to take a substance regularly, which may lead to impairment of physical, mental and behavioural actions. The user is compelled to take the drug in order to feel good and to avoid withdrawal symptoms.

Opioid dependence is common, particularly if the drug is taken for long periods of time. Users become tolerant to the pleasurable effects, which leads to the use of increased doses in order to regain these pleasurable effects. Opioid withdrawal syndrome, sometimes referred to as "cold turkey" results in serious adverse effects. Methadone is frequently prescribed to substitute for opioids.

It is for these reasons that the possession and use of the more potent narcotics is controlled by legislation in most countries.

18.4 The history of narcotics in sport

Classification of narcotics on IOC/WADA Prohibited Lists

Narcotic analgesics were one of the four classes of drugs listed on the first IOC Prohibited List, published in 1967 (see Chapter 2). The mild narcotic analgesic, codeine, was removed from the IOC Prohibited List in 1993 following frequent cases of inadvertent use as a result of athletes taking over-the-counter self-medication. The first Prohibited List drawn up by WADA, in 2004, designated narcotics as a class of drugs prohibited only within competition.

Prevalence of narcotics use in sport

There have been few cases of adverse analytical findings (AAFs) for narcotics reported by the WADA-accredited laboratories. However, the numbers reported annually have been consistent (Table 18.1).

The figures include cases where therapeutic use exemption may have applied.

Cases involving narcotics

Some cases relate to serial use of narcotics by athletes within teams.

Box 18.1   "Pot Belge"

Cycling has been a sport in which narcotic abuse cases have been reported. To be successful in long-distance cycling races it is necessary for the cyclist to be able to overcome significant pain barriers. A mixture of drugs including a narcotic analgesic, such as heroin, stimulants such as amphetamines and cocaine was nicknamed the Belgian Mix or "Pot Belge". Its use has certainly not been limited to cyclists in Belgium, where cycling is a very popular sport, but it is this country which may well have been its original source.

Table 18.1 WADA statistics for the number of adverse analytical findings for substances classed as narcotics (2006–2015)

	2006	2007	2008	2009	2010	2011	2012	2013	2014	2015
Morphine	11	19	21	17	6	11	14	25	9	7
Methadone	3	–	2	–	2	6	1	5	2	1
Hydromorphone	1	–	2	–	2	1	–	–	–	–
Oxycodone	–	–	–	4	3	2	6	6	6	7
Pethidine	1	–	–	–	–	–	–	1	–	–
Heroin	–	–	–	–	–	–	–	–	–	–
Buprenorphine	–	–	–	1	2	–	–	2	4	2
Hydrocodone	–	–	–	–	–	–	–	–	–	–
Pentazocine	–	–	–	–	–	–	–	–	–	–
Oxymorphone	–	–	–	–	–	–	–	–	–	3
Diamorphine	–	–	–	–	–	–	–	–	–	–
Fentanyl and its derivatives	–	–	–	–	1	–	5	4	3	1
Total	16	21	28	24	20	20	26	43	26	21

Results on narcotics include adverse findings for which the athlete may have been granted Therapeutic Use Exemption under WADA regulations

Box 18.2   Festina affair (1998)

In the 1998 Tour de France, the Festina team was suspended when its physiotherapist, Willy Voet, was found to have a large number of drugs, including narcotics, in his possession.

Box 18.3   Cahors affair (2005)

Perhaps the most significant case involving the use of narcotics in cycling was the infamous "Cahors Affair". Emanating from cases in the year 2004, the trial opened in 2005 and culminated in 2006 with 23 convictions relating to the illicit use of performance enhancing drugs including "Pot Belge". These convictions included some custodial sentences. Those testifying and those mentioned in testimonies could read like a who's who of European cycling. The former French professional cyclist, Laurent Roux, intimated that some teams spent more on "doctors" than on riders.

Other cases relating to narcotics are attributable to use by individual athletes.

Box 18.4   Christophe Brandt (2004)

The Belgian cyclist Christophe Brandt tested positive for methadone in the 2004 Tour de France. Methadone is a drug which shares many of the properties of morphine, however it is principally used as a heroin substitute for heroin addicts in some countries.

Endurance events, other than cycling, have also had cases involving narcotic usage.

Box 18.5   Ambesse Tolossa (2007)

The Ethiopian runner, Ambesse Tolossa, who had already experienced success in other marathon events (San Diego and Tokyo), was the winner of the December 2007 Honolulu race. He was subsequently disqualified because of a positive test for morphine and his prize money of $40,000 withheld. He also received a two-year ban.

As a measure of the seriousness with which governing bodies take illegal drug abuse, one only has to consider the case of British runner Kate Reed.

> ## Box 18.6   Kate Reed (2008)
>
> Kate, who was part of the 2008 Beijing Olympics team, had been suffering from an injury to her leg, and had apparently joked with team mates about taking morphine for the pain. Shortly afterwards, her room was searched for drugs by British Olympic Association officials! Of course, none were found and she duly passed a doping test.

18.5 The action and use of narcotics in sport

Inflammation is a key response to sports injuries, a component of which is pain. Pain is an important, protective cue to the individual that all is not well. It is a stimulus which should promote rest, an important adjunct to recovery. It is also associated with a learning process which encourages the individual to avoid a repetition of the incident. Pain is also unpleasant and at a moderate to severe level frequently requires alleviation.

Pain and inflammation associated with a sports injury are usually treated with non-steroidal anti-inflammatory drugs. In some circumstances, however, the level of pain associated with a serious injury will require the use of more powerful analgesic drugs such as the narcotic analgesic drugs (possibly in association with anti-inflammatory drugs).

Given that one of the barriers to optimal performance is pain, there has been much speculation over many years as to whether powerful analgesic drugs could raise levels of performance. There is no convincing evidence that narcotics can provide such an enhancement but they are nevertheless banned substances in competition. The therapeutic use of narcotic analgesics is permissible outside of competition periods.

An interesting investigation by Benedetti et al. (2007) looked at opioid-medicated placebo responses to boost pain endurance and physical performance. After repeated administration of morphine in the pre-competition training phase, its replacement with a placebo on the day of competition induced opioid-mediated effects. However, questions were raised about the ethical acceptability of this type of procedure or whether they have to be considered as doping procedures.

WADA recognise the need for Therapeutic Use Exemption (TUE) with respect to the use of narcotics to treat neuropathic pain (WADA, 2016). Neuropathic pain arises from a lesion or any disease that causes dysfunction of the somatosensory system. Athletes with musculoskeletal injury have a higher incidence of neuropathic pain. Such pain may interfere with effective participation in sport. For neuropathic pain, current clinical practice guidelines typically recommend that narcotic analgesics are used as a second-line treatment, or in combination with other classes of medication in the management of chronic, refractory neuropathic pain. Use is often long-term, therefore a TUE would be required and may be granted for periods of one to four years. However, an annual review of the status of the athlete-patient by a relevant specialist is recommended to ensure that the on-going treatment remains appropriate (WADA, 2016).

Equestrian sport

The abuse of narcotics is not restricted to humans. Twenty British-owned or -trained racehorses tested positive for morphine. The most celebrated horse involved in this scandal was

Be My Royal, winner of the 2002 Hennessy Cognac Gold Cup at Newbury. Despite appeals by the trainer, Willie Mullins, the horse was disqualified from the race. It was claimed that the horse was fed with contaminated feed.

18.6 Narcotics and the WADA Prohibited List

The current WADA regulations regarding narcotics are shown in Table 18.2.

Nicomorphine was added to the list as it is an opioid analgesic which is converted to morphine following administration.

With respect to morphine, WADA-accredited laboratories declare a test result as an adverse analytical finding if the urinary concentration of morphine exceeds 1µg/ml (WADA, 2013). This limit is used because morphine is one of the metabolites of codeine, a narcotic which is permitted in sport.

Monitoring Program

The WADA Code states that a Monitoring Program should be established regarding substances that are not on the Prohibited List but which WADA wishes to monitor in order to detect patterns of misuse in sport.

The first Monitoring Program, in January 2004, listed narcotics particularly related to in-competition morphine/codeine ratios, in order to monitor the use of these by athletes. In 2012, the narcotics hydrocodone and tramadol were added to the Monitoring Program, with tapentadol being added in 2013 and mitragynine in 2014. In 2016, hydrocodone, morphine/codeine ratio and tapentadol were removed from the Monitoring Program; however, codeine was re-inserted into the Monitoring Program for 2017.

Recreational use of narcotics

As previously discussed, narcotics are a class of drugs that is misused recreationally. Although drug abuse in society is increasing, it is drugs other than narcotics that are mainly implicated. Nonetheless, athletes who indulge in recreational drug use risk an adverse analytical finding for narcotics, as well as for other prohibited drugs such as amphetamines, cocaine and cannabinoids.

Inadvertent use of narcotics

In addition to inadvertent use through OTC self-medication, athletes should be aware of the risk of poppy seed ingestion through food products which may trigger an adverse analytical finding for morphine (Lachenmeier et al., 2010), although the likelihood of this is low (Anderson, 2011).

Table 18.2 WADA (2017) Prohibited List regulations with respect to in-competition use of narcotics

The following are prohibited:

Buprenorphine, dextromoramide, diamorphine (heroin), fentanyl and its derivatives, hydromorphone, methadone, morphine, nicomorphine, oxycodone, oxymorphone, pentazocine, pethidine.

18.7 Summary

- Narcotics possess significant analgesic activity. For this reason they are used both clinically and as a performance aid in sport.
- These drugs exhibit serious side effects including the onset of dependence which may lead to addiction.
- The annual number of adverse analytical findings for narcotics is low. However, narcotics represent a potent class of pharmacological agents with consequences for their use in sport.

18.8 References

Anderson, J.M. (2011) Evaluating the athlete's claim of an unintentional positive urine drug test. *Nutrition and Ergogenic Aids* 10(4): 191–196.

Benedetti, F., Pollo, A. and Colloca, L. (2007) Opioid-mediated placebo responses to boost pain endurance and physical performance: Is it doping in sport competition? *The Journal of Neuroscience* 27(44): 11.934–11.939.

Kosterlitz, H.W. and Hughes, J. (1977) Peptides with morphine-like action in the brain. *The British Journal of Psychiatry* 130: 298–304.

Lachenmeier, D.W., Sproll, C., Musshoff, F. (2010) Poppy seed foods and opiate drug testing: Where are we today? *Therapeutic Drug Monitoring* 32: 11–18.

Simantov, R. and Snyder, S.H. (1976) Morphine-like peptides in mammalian brain: Isolation, structure elucidation, and interactions with the opiate receptor. *Proceedings of the National Academy of Sciences USA* 73(7): 2,515–2,519.

WADA (2013) Decision limits for the confirmatory quantification of threshold substances. Available at: https://www.wada-ama.org/en/resources/science-medicine/td2014-dl (Accessed December 2016).

WADA (2016) Medical information to support the decisions of TUECs: Neuropathic pain. Available online at: https://www.wada-ama.org/en/resources/medical-information-to-support-the-decisions-of-tuecs-neuropathic-pain (Accessed January 2017).

Cannabinoids

David R. Mottram

19.1 Introduction

Cannabinoids are derived from cannabis, which is taken, commonly, as a "recreational" drug. Although the pharmacological effects of cannabinoids are more likely to produce performance deterioration, rather than enhancement, cannabinoids are one of the more frequently detected classes of drugs during anti-doping tests conducted through World Anti-Doping Agency (WADA) laboratories. It has been suggested by some that cannabinoids should be removed from the WADA Prohibited List. These issues will be explored within this chapter.

19.2 What are cannabinoids?

The source of cannabinoids

Cannabinoids are defined, chemically, as aryl-substituted meroterpenes. They are derived principally from the plant *Cannabis sativa*. This plant contains more than 400 chemical constituents. Cannabis includes more than 80 different cannabinoids and terpenes, many of which have different and even contradictory effects (Izzo et al., 2009; Russo et al., 2011) and whose potency varies from one strain to another. The most potent of these cannabinoids, that which produces psychoactive effects, is Δ^9-tetrahydrocannabinol (Δ^9-THC). Other plant cannabinoids include cannabinol and cannabidiol which, along with other cannabinoids, produce complex pharmacological actions and interactions when herbal cannabis is smoked (Ashton, 2001).

The Δ^9-THC content varies to a great extent depending on the source of the plant and how the drug is taken (Ashton, 2001). New varieties of cannabis plant have been bred in recent years leading to more potent products than those that were available in the 1960s and 1970s (Ashton, 1999).

The cannabis plant, when used for recreational purposes, is processed in various ways in order to derive the effects of the active constituents. The two most common are cannabis resin (hashish) and marijuana which is normally associated with the dried and ground leaves, flower and other parts of the plant prepared for smoking (Campos et al., 2003; NIH, 2016). When inhaled, in addition to the cannabinoids, the smoke from cannabis contains many of the constituents of tobacco smoke (Ashton, 1999).

Tetrahydrocannabinol-like derivatives, such as dronabinol and nabilone, have been synthesised and are prescribed in some countries to treat weight loss and nausea and vomiting associated with cancer therapy (Campos et al., 2003).

Mode of action of cannabinoids

Specific receptors for cannabinoids have been identified in humans. These are termed CB_1 and CB_2 receptors and are located in the membrane of nerve endings in the brain. Stimulation of these receptors inhibits transmitter release, particularly acetylcholine within the hippocampus, the area of the brain responsible for learning and memory, and noradrenaline in the cerebral cortex and cerebellum, responsible for alertness and motor coordination (Pertwee, 1997). They are amongst the most numerous receptors in the brain. The CB_2 receptors are mainly found peripherally in association with the immune system.

The discovery of cannabinoid receptors led to a search for endogenous mediators, of which a number have been identified. The two well-established endocannabinoids are anandamide and 2-arachidonoyl glycerol (Porter and Felder, 2001). Anandamide has a high affinity for CB_1 receptors and has most of the actions of Δ^9-THC (Ashton, 2001).

The effects of cannabinoids are perceived within minutes, when cannabis is smoked. Oral cannabis results in absorption of around 25–30 per cent of the amount of cannabinoids obtained by smoking. The onset of effects is around 30 minutes to two hours, although the duration of action may be more prolonged by the oral route (Maykut, 1985). Following absorption, cannabinoids are rapidly and widely distributed throughout the body. They tend to accumulate in fatty tissue from where they are slowly released over extended periods of time. Complete elimination from the body may take as long as 30 days (Huestis et al., 1995), which may have consequences with respect to dope testing. Another reason for the extended period of elimination is that the metabolites are only partially excreted in the urine (approximately 25%) whereas most (65%) are excreted into the gastrointestinal tract from where they are re-absorbed into the body, a process that continues over a considerable period of time (Ashton, 2001).

Effects and side effects of cannabinoids

Cannabinoids produce both physical and psychological effects, the extent of which will vary depending on patterns of use. Therefore, isolated or infrequent use can lead to mild intoxication, drowsiness and sedation, slower reaction times and memory deficiency. Regular consumption can lead to social detachment and psychological dependence (Saugy et al., 2006).

Cannabinoids affect almost any system in the body and combine many of the properties of alcohol, tranquillisers, opiates and hallucinogens. They are therefore anxiolytic, sedative, analgesic and psychedelic in their action (Ashton, 2001).

The main central effects of cannabinoids are impairment of short-term memory, learning tasks and motor coordination along with catalepsy, hypothermia, analgesia, an increase in appetite and an anti-emetic action. The main peripheral effects are tachycardia, bronchodilation, vasodilation and a reduction of intra-ocular pressure (Rang et al., 2007). Users of cannabis develop a mild form of tolerance and dependence to the drug.

The incidence of serious, acute toxic side effects due to cannabinoids is low and no deaths directly attributable to acute cannabis use have been reported (Ashton, 1999). However, Ashton (1999 and 2001) reviews a number of significant adverse effects of cannabinoids on the cardiovascular and respiratory systems as well as on the central nervous system.

Cannabis use in society

There is no doubt that cannabis use as a recreational drug in society is widespread, with figures up to 16 per cent being quoted for use by young adults in Europe and the USA (Saugy et al., 2006). It is not, therefore, surprising that this trend is reflected in the use by athletes (Mottram, 1999). Cannabinoids are amongst the more frequently detected substances, according to the annual statistics from WADA-accredited laboratories (WADA, 2016a).

Synthetic marijuana (cannabimimetics)

Synthetic marijuana is a cannabis substitute in which herbs or other leafy materials are sprayed with laboratory-synthesised liquid chemicals to mimic the effect of tetrahydrocannabinol. Synthetic marijuana is also known by the name "spice" or "K2". These products are frequently marketed as "legal" cannabinoids and cannabinomimetics (Hilderbrand, 2011). Laboratory-synthesised cannabinoid compounds that have been found in synthetic marijuana include HU-210, CP 47,497, JWH-018, JWH-073, JWH-398, JWH-250 and oleamide (EMCDDA, 2016). These synthetic compounds can bind more strongly to cannabinoid receptors than regular marijuana and may lead to more unpredictable effects. A review of these cannabimimetics is provided by Hilderbrand (2011).

Cannabimimetics are included on the WADA Prohibited List within the class of Cannabinoids. Like marijuana, the active ingredients in Spice/K2 can remain in the body for long periods of time, a fact of importance with respect to anti-doping testing in sport.

Cannabinoid use to treat medical conditions

Apart from their recreational use, cannabinoids are increasingly being investigated for use as therapeutic agents to treat epilepsy and obesity (Izzo et al., 2009) pain, particularly in palliative care (Peat, 2010), chemotherapy-induced nausea and vomiting (Delmás, 2010) and spasticity in multiple sclerosis (Rog, 2010).

WADA recognise the need for Therapeutic Use Exemption (TUE) with respect to the use of "medicinal marijuana" to treat neuropathic pain (WADA, 2016b). Neuropathic pain arises from a lesion or any disease that causes dysfunction of the somatosensory system. Athletes with musculoskeletal injury have a higher incidence of neuropathic pain. Such pain may interfere with effective participation in sport.

The most common medicinal use of cannabinoids is for the management of neuropathic pain. Its use is often long-term and necessitates regular monitoring. A TUE would be required and may be granted for periods of one to four years. However, an annual review of the status of the athlete-patient by a relevant specialist is recommended to ensure that the ongoing treatment remains appropriate (WADA, 2016b).

It is recognised that the use of medicinal marijuana may have a negative impact on the ability to participate effectively in sports requiring dexterity and rapid coordination. In addition, due caution should be exercised in the prescription of cannabinoids, especially for an athlete with a history of substance abuse, psychosis, poorly controlled mood or anxiety disorders.

Evidence on the medical benefit of cannabis is under constant review, occasionally leading to the decriminalisation or legislation of cannabis use (Hanson, 2014).

19.3 History of cannabis in sport

Addition to the Prohibited List

The International Olympic Committee (IOC) first included cannabis on its list of prohibited substances in 1989. At that time, the decision was left to the governing international sports federation as to whether cannabinoids were prohibited in their respective disciplines and whether anti-doping tests for cannabinoids should be conducted. This led to confusion within sport and in the minds of athletes, as to whether they considered cannabis to be performance enhancing or not (Venema et al., 1999). WADA, in 2004, placed cannabinoids on their Prohibited List for all athletes in all sports, within competition. Whether that decision was rational remains open to debate.

Case studies relating to cannabinoids

A number of high profile case studies have been reported in which cannabinoids have been involved.

Box 19.1   Ross Ribagliati (1998)

Ross Ribagliati, a Canadian snowboarder, won the inaugural men's giant slalom event at the 1998 Winter Olympic Games in Nagano. Immediately after the event, he tested positive for cannabinoids and was stripped of his Gold Medal. He claimed that he had not taken marijuana himself but that he was a victim of passive smoking (Hilderbrand, 2011). Regardless of the veracity of this claim, he had his medal re-instated three days later. Although the IOC had marijuana on its Prohibited List, Rebagliati's governing body, the International Ski Federation, did not prohibit the use of the drug at that time. This landmark case further highlighted the inconsistency in the application of rules between sporting organisations that eventually led to harmonisation through the establishment of WADA.

Despite the introduction of a harmonised approach to the application of rules for doping violations, cases involving cannabinoids have been treated very differently.

Box 19.2   Tomas Enge (2002)

In August 2002, the Czech motor racing driver Tomas Enge tested positive for cannabinoids after a Formula 3000 race in Hungary. He was conditionally suspended from racing for 12 months by his governing body, the International Automobile Federation (Campos et al., 2003).

Box 19.3   Michael Phelps (2009)

A photograph of Michael Phelps, at that time a holder of 14 Olympic Gold Medals, smoking marijuana at a party in South Carolina was published by a British newspaper in January 2009. Although this incident was not the subject of a dope test violation, USA Swimming decided to suspend Michael Phelps for three months, under its code of conduct.

A case involving cannabinoids was reported at the London 2012 Olympic Games.

Box 19.4   Nicholas Delpopolo (2012)

At the London 2012 Olympic games, Nicholas Delpopolo was disqualified by the IOC after metabolites of cannabis were identified in a urine sample. The athlete insisted that it was the result of eating food containing the banned substance, however this was not deemed a sufficient defence. It should be noted that, at that time, the period designated "in-competition" for Olympic Games began from the time when the Games Athlete Village opened and applied to anywhere that the athlete may have been living or training.

Some sports bodies recognise the problem faced by athletes with respect to recreational drug use.

Box 19.5   Jake Humphries (2016)

Humphries received a five-month ban by the UK Football Association (FA) having tested positive for carboxy-THC. In addition to his suspension, the player was required to undertake and complete a bespoke course of assessment, counselling, treatment and/or rehabilitation, as determined by the FA in conjunction with the Professional Footballers' Association (http://ukad.org.uk/news/article/fa-suspends-jake-humphries-for-five-months/).

19.4 Cannabinoids in sport

The use of cannabinoids within sport

There are few studies that have been undertaken relating to the use of cannabinoids in athletes.

A study on college student athletes, reported that 28.4 per cent of US National Collegiate Athletic association students used marijuana (Green et al., 2001). A later investigation, in 2012, looking at cannabis use in 20,474 college athletes from 23 different sports in more than 1,000 institutions, found that 22.6 per cent of college athletes reported using cannabis in the past year (NCAA, 2012).

An investigation by Lorente et al. (2005), involving French university sports students, suggested that around 12 per cent of students had used cannabis in an attempt to enhance "performance". The authors noted that using cannabis to enhance performance in a recreational manner can, ultimately, lead to attempts to enhance sporting performance. These authors also showed that cannabis use to enhance sport performance was positively related to the level of competition and to particular sports such as "sliding sports" (skiing, snowboarding, surfing, windsurfing and sailing).

Results from an analysis of elite athletes tested at the Italian Anti-Doping Laboratory between 2000 and 2009 showed, among positive results, there was a high prevalence of stimulants and drugs of abuse, of which cannabis was the most frequently found (Rossi and Botrè, 2011). However, a systematic literature review of selective risk behaviour among young athletes revealed high alcohol use but low recreational drug use, particularly with marijuana (Diehl et al., 2012).

Are cannabinoids performance enhancing?

The balance of evidence suggests that cannabinoids, in most sports, are ergolytic rather than ergogenic (Eichner, 1993; Pesta et al., 2013). Recreationally, cannabis use produces a feeling of euphoria and reduces anxiety. These properties may be beneficial in alleviating the stress induced through competition, either pre- or post-event. However, cannabis smoking impairs cognition and psychomotor and exercise performance (Saugy et al., 2006). When compared with control subjects, marijuana was shown to reduce maximal exercise performance (Renaud and Cornier, 1986).

There is evidence that cannabis reduces pain, muscle spasms, stiffness and inflammation in humans (Borgelt et al., 2013), a potential benefit to athletes. Gillman et al. (2015) stated that there are common anecdotal reports that cannabis decreases motivation, including motivation to exercise. Nonetheless, other reports say that cannabis is used prior to exercise. However, there is little scientific evidence to support either one of these opposing lay perspectives. A study of US college athletes indicated that a small minority of those athletes using cannabis claimed that it helped to improve sport performance (0.5 per cent) or to deal with sport related injuries (0.7 per cent) (NCAA, 2012).

Adverse effects of cannabinoids in sport

The adverse effects of cannabinoids on physical and psychological function means that cannabis consumption can be dangerous in sports that rely on clear thinking, quick reactions and split-second timing (Campos et al., 2003). Particular adverse effects include somnolence, dizziness, euphoria and feelings of paranoia. Anxiety and tachycardia may also occur. All these effects are incompatible with most athletic endeavours (Campos et al., 2003).

Hilderbrand (2011) observed that, whilst impairment of response or inappropriate decision making as a result of cannabis use may be compensated by individuals this does not apply to elite sport as in competitive sport the athlete cannot afford compensating actions.

A review by Brisola-Santos et al. (2016) expresses surprise that enhancement of sport performance is a common rationale for the use of cannabis by athletes. Furthermore, the authors concluded that cannabis confers considerable risk for sub-groups of athletes in specific types of sport.

The consequences of cannabinoid use for other competitors

Does cannabinoid use pose a threat to fellow competitors? This probably depends on the sport. Menetrey et al. (2005) have assessed driving capability under the influence of cannabinoids, concluding they have a negative effect which would impair alertness and reflexes in motor sports, leading to danger for both the user and their fellow competitors.

19.5 Cannabinoids and the WADA Prohibited List

WADA regulations with respect to cannabinoids

WADA have included cannabinoids on their prohibited list since they undertook responsibility for the list in 2003. In 2010, WADA first included synthetic cannabinoids on the Prohibited List. In 2011, marijuana-like substances (cannabimimetics) were included. The current WADA Prohibited List (WADA, 2017) prohibits the following cannabinoids:

S8. Cannabinoids

Prohibited:

- Natural, e.g. cannabis, hashish and marijuana, or synthetic $\Delta 9$-tetrahydrocannabinol (THC).
- Cannabimimetics, e.g. "Spice", JWH-018, JWH-073, HU-210.

Cannabinoids are prohibited in all sports but an adverse analytical finding is only reported if a positive urine sample is detected in-competition. Furthermore cannabinoids are classed as "Specified Substances", which allows for more flexible sanctions to be applied in the case of an inadvertent adverse finding. WADA laboratories undertake urine analysis, using gas chromatography/mass spectrometry, of 11-nor-delta 9-tetrahydrocannabinol-9-carboxylic acid (THC-COOH), the principal metabolite of Δ^9-THC, in either its free or conjugated form. If the sum of the concentration of free and conjugated THC-COOH is greater than 15ng/ml an adverse analytical finding is reported by the laboratory (WADA, 2013).

Prevalence of adverse findings for cannabinoids

Statistics from WADA-accredited laboratories, between 2003 and 2015 (WADA, 2016c), show that cannabinoids constitute between 15.7 per cent and 2.0 per cent of all adverse analytical findings (see Figure 19.1).

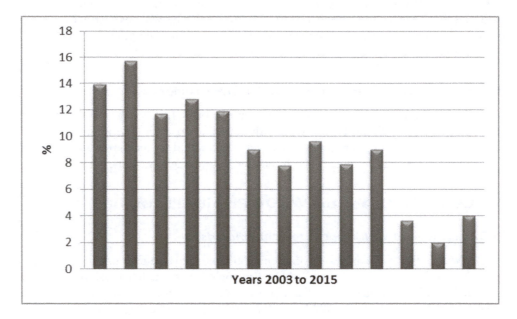

Figure 19.1 Percentage of all adverse analytical findings from WADA anti-doping testing figures that relate to cannabinoids, for the years from 2003 to 2015

These percentages placed cannabinoids as the second or third most reported prohibited substance in each of the years up to and including 2012. From 2013 to 2015 cannabinoids were placed sixth, eighth and sixth, respectively. The trend indicates that fewer athletes are testing positive for cannabinoids in-competition. Whether this is indicative of a reduced use of cannabinoids by athletes or a more enlightened approach to its pharmacokinetics and the WADA regulations is open to debate. Figure 19.2 shows the sports within which AAFs for cannabinoids were most frequently recorded in 2015.

It is worth noting that because cannabinoids are only tested in-competition, any positive results found in urine samples taken out-of-competition are not reported by the laboratory. The extent of cannabis use by athletes could therefore be significantly higher than that indicated by the WADA statistics.

Passive ingestion of cannabinoids

The WADA Anti-Doping Code states that urinary levels of THC-COOH must exceed a threshold of 15ng/ml in order to trigger an adverse analytical finding (WADA, 2016c). This has been established in part to distinguish between active consumers of cannabinoids and those athletes who may have been exposed, passively, to cannabis smoke (Campos et al., 2003).

Several studies have been conducted to determine the likelihood of passive inhalation of cannabinoids sufficient to trigger an adverse analytical finding (Yonamine et al., 2004). The extent of passive inhalation depends on factors such as the size of the room and the effectiveness of the ventilation within the room as well as the number of marijuana cigarettes being

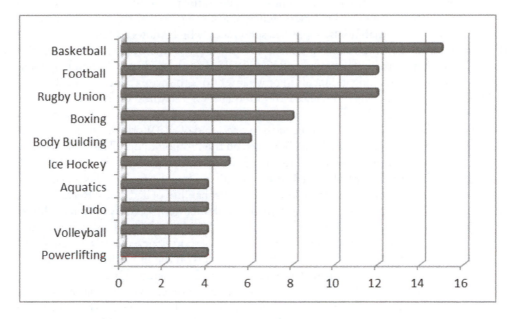

Figure 19.2 The sports within which AAFs for cannabinoids were most frequently recorded in 2015

smoked and the concentration of Δ^9-THC within the cigarettes. The conclusion reached was that an individual could produce urinary levels of THC-COOH sufficient to exceed the 15ng/ml threshold only after "extremely severe" conditions of passive exposure to marijuana smoke (Yonamine et al., 2004; Anderson, 2011).

Hilderbrand (2011) suggests that the concept of "strict liability" applies in sport and one can safely say that the presence of THC-COOH in urine at any level approaching the 15ng/ml confirmation threshold could not occur without the knowledge of the athlete.

The threshold limit also reduces the chance of an adverse test result after the consumption of food products which may contain traces of cannabinoids (Saugy et al., 2006). In this context, there has been an increase in the sale of hemp-containing products, such as cakes, cookies and brownies or of hemp seed oil products (Yonamine et al., 2004). However, research into the chances of exceeding urinary threshold levels when consuming such products reveals very variable and inconsistent results (Cone et al., 1988; Bosy and Cole, 2000; Leson et al., 2000).

Should cannabinoids be on the WADA Prohibited List?

There are arguments for and against removing cannabinoids from the WADA Prohibited List. The US Anti-Doping Agency (USADA, 2016) provide cogent reasons why marijuana and cannabinoids meet the criteria for inclusion on the WADA Prohibited List. Arguments for removing cannabinoids from the Prohibited List include the fact that, in most countries, the possession and consumption of cannabis products is illegal. Is it therefore appropriate for WADA to impose a further level of legislation? Of course, this argument is flawed since the laws relating to cannabis use are not universally in place or rigorously applied.

Other arguments for removing cannabinoids relate to the possibility of passive consumption, although this is countered by the presence of a threshold level for THC-COOH and the classification of cannabinoids as specified substances, which allows athletes to prove that they had not intended to use cannabinoids for performance enhancing purposes. It should be noted, however, that the elimination of THC-COOH from the body is a slow and individually variable process, making it difficult to prove intent or otherwise (Saugy et al., 2006).

Huestis et al. (2011) have reviewed the rationale for retaining cannabinoids on the WADA Prohibited List by relating the pharmacological and sociological implications of cannabinoid use to the three criteria specified in Section 4 of the World Anti-Doping Code to determine whether substances should be placed on the Prohibited List. The Code specifies that only two of the three criteria need to be fulfilled. The authors argue that cannabinoids have the potential for health risks, not only for the athlete but also for their fellow competitors as a result of impaired decision making and the probability of accidents. Regarding the second criterion, cannabinoids can be performance enhancing, albeit only for some athletes in certain sport disciplines. Thirdly, considering the ethical and societal aspects of using a "recreational" drug, cannabinoids contravene the spirit of sport. Consequently, Huestis et al. conclude that the WADA decision to retain cannabinoids on the Prohibited List is correct, a view supported by Bergamaschi and Crippa (2013) and Hilderbrand (2011).

The international anti-doping community generally consider that the role model that athletes portray in society is intrinsically incompatible with the use of cannabinoids. It can therefore be argued that cannabinoids should be banned by WADA both within competition, as at present, but also out-of-competition.

19.6 Summary

- Cannabinoids produce a wide range of effects in the body, most of which would not be classed as performance enhancing.
- Despite this, cannabinoids are one of the most frequently detected prohibited classes of substances in athletes, according to WADA laboratory statistics.
- This high frequency of detection in athletes probably reflects their use as recreational drugs.
- Although it has been argued that cannabinoids should be removed from the WADA Prohibited List, balance of opinion is that they should remain.

19.7 References

Anderson, J.M. (2011) Evaluating the athlete's claim of an unintentional positive drug test. *Current Sports Medicine Reports* 10(4): 191–196.

Ashton, C.H. (1999) Adverse effects of cannabis and cannabinoids. *British Journal of Anaesthesia* 83(4): 637–649.

Ashton, C.H. (2001) Pharmacology and effects of cannabis: A brief review. *British Journal of Psychiatry* 178: 101–106.

Bergamaschi, M.M. and Crippa, J.A.S. (2013) Why should cannabis be considered doping in sports? *Frontiers in Psychiatry* 4: 1–2.

Borgelt, L.M., Fransom, K.L., Nussbaum, A.M. et al. (2013) The pharmacological and clinical effects of medicinal cannabis. *Pharmacotherapy* 33(2): 195–209.

Bosy, T.Z. and Cole, K.A. (2000) Consumption and quantititation of Δ^9-tetrahydrocannabinol in commercially available hemp seed oil products. *Journal of Analytical Toxicology* 24: 562–566.

Brisola-Santos, M.B., Guilherme de Melloe e Galliarno, J., Gil, F. et al. (2016) Prevelance and correlates of cannabis use among athletes: A systematic review. *The American Journal of Addictions* 25: 518–528.

Campos, D.R., Yonamine, M. and de Moraes Moreau, R.L. (2003) Marijuana as doping in sports. *Sports Medicine* 33(6): 395–399.

Cone, E.J., Johnson, R.E., Paul, B.D. et al. (1988) Marijuana-laced brownies: Behavioural effects, physiologic effects and urinalysis in humans following ingestion. *Journal of Analytical Toxicology* 12: 169–175.

Delmás, M.D. (2010) Preliminary efficacy and safety of an oromucosal standardized cannabis extract in chemotherapy-induced nausea and vomiting. *British Journal of Clinical Pharmacology* 70: 656–663.

Diehl, K., Thiel, A., Zipfel, S. et al. (2012) How healthy is the behaviour of young athletes? A systematic literature review and meta-analysis. *Journal of Sports Science and Medicine* 11: 201–220.

Eichner, E.R. (1993) Ergolytic drugs in medicine and sport. *American Journal of Medicine* 94(2): 205–211.

EMCDDA (2016) European Monitoring Centre for Drugs and Drug Addiction. Synthetic cannabinoids and "Spice" drug profile. Available online at: http://www.emcdda.europa.eu/publications/drug-profiles/synthetic-cannabinoids (Accessed January 2017).

Gillman, A.S., Hutchison, K.E. and Bryan, A.D. (2015) Cannabis and exercise science: A commentary on existing studies and suggesting future directions. *Sports Medicine* 45: 1,357–1,363.

Green, G.A., Uryasz. F.D., Petr, T.A., et al. (2001) NCAA study of substance use and abuse habits of college student-athletes. *Clinical Journal of Sports Medicine* 11(1): 51–56.

Hanson, K. (2014) State medical marijuana laws. National conference of state legislatures. Available online at: http://www.ncsl.org/research/health/state-medical-marijuana-laws.aspx (Accessed January 2017).

Hilderbrand, R.L. (2011) High performance sport, marijuana and cannabimimetics. *Journal of Analytical Toxicology* 35: 624–637.

Huestis, M.A., Mitchell, J.M. and Cone, E.J. (1995) Detection times of marijuana metabolites in urine by immunoassay and GC-MS. *Journal of Analytical Toxicology* 19(6): 443–449.

Huestis, M.A., Mazzoni, I. and Rabin, O. (2011) Cannabis in sport: Anti-doping perspective. *Sports Medicine* 41(11): 949–966.

Izzo, A.A., Borrelli, F., Capasso, R. et al. (2009) Non-psychotropic plant cannabinoids: New therapeutic oppoxrtunities from an ancient herb. *Trends in Pharmacological Sciences* 30(10): 515–527.

Leson, G., Pless, P., Grotenhermen, F. et al. (2000) Evaluating the impact of hemp food consumption on workplace drug tests. *Journal of Analytical Toxicology* 25: 691–698.

Lorente, F.O., Peretti-Watel, P. and Grelot, L. (2005) Cannabis use to enhance sportive and non-sportive performances among French sport students. *Addictive Behaviours* 30: 1,382–1,391.

Maykut, M.O. (1985) Health consequences of acute and chronic marijuana use. *Progress in Neuropsychopharmacology and Biological Psychiatry* 9: 209–238.

Menetrey, A., Augsburger, M., Favrat, B. et al. (2005) Assessment of driving capability through the use of clinical and psychomotor tests in relation to blood cannabinoids levels following oral administration of 20mg dronabinol or of a cannabis decoction made with 20 or 60mg delta 9-THC. *Journal of Analytical Toxicology* 29: 327–338.

Mottram, D.R. (1999) Banned drugs in sport: Does the International Olympic committee (IOC) list need updating? *Sports Medicine* 27(1): 1–10.

NCAA (2012) National study of substance use trends among NCAA college student-athletes. Available online at: http://www.ncaapublications.com/productdownloads/SHAS09.pdf (Accessed January 2017).

NIH (2016) Marijuana. Available at: http://www.drugabuse.gov/drugs-abuse/marijuana (Accessed January 2017).

Peat, S. (2010) Using cannabinoids in pain and palliative care. *International Journal of Palliative Nursing* 16: 481–485.

Pertwee, R.G. (1997) Pharmacology of cannabinoid CB1 and CB2 receptors. *Pharmacological Therapeutics* 74(2): 129–180.

Pesta, D.H., Angadi, S.S., Burtscher, M. and Roberts, C.K. (2013) The effects of caffeine, nicotine, ethanol and tetrahydrocannabinol on exercise performance. *Nutrition and Metabolism* 10: 71–86.

Porter, A.C. and Felder, C.C. (2001) The endocannabinoid nervous system: Unique opportunities for therapeutic intervention. *Pharmacological Therapeutics* 90: 45–60.

Rang, H.P., Dale, M.M., Ritter, J.M. et al. (2007) Cannabinoids. In H.P. Rang, M.M. Dale, J.M. Ritter and R.J. Flower (eds) *Rang and Dale's Pharmacology*, 6th edition. London, Churchill Livingstone, 248–255.

Renaud, A.M. and Cornier, Y. (1986) Acute effects of marijuana smoking on maximal exercise performance. *Medicine and Science in Sports and Exercise* 18(6): 685–689.

Rog, D.J. (2010) Cannabis-based medicines in multiple sclerosis: A review of clinical studies. *Immunobiology* 215: 658–672.

Rossi, S.S. and Botrè, F. (2011) Prevalence of illicit drug use among the Italian athlete population with special attention on drugs of abuse: A 10-year review. *Journal of Sports Sciences* 29(5): 471–476.

Russo, E.B. et al. (2011) Taming THC: Potential cannabis synergy and phyto-cannabinoid-terpinoid entourage effects. *British Journal of Pharmacology* 163(7): 1,344–1,364.

Saugy, M., Avois, L., Saudan, C. et al. (2006) Cannabis and sport. *British Journal of Sports Medicine* 40(Suppl 1): i13–i15.

USADA (2016) Marijuana and cannabinoids: Frequently asked questions. Available online at: http://www.usada.org/substances/marijuana-faq/ (Accessed 1 December 2017).

Venema, H., de Boer, D., Horta, L. et al. (1999) Different anti-doping policies of International Sport Federations towards the ban of the use of cannabis. Fifth World Congress of Sports Sciences: Book of abstracts. Canberra, Sports Medicine Australia, 218.

WADA (2013) WADA Laboratory Standards. Available at www.wada-ama.org (Accessed January 2013).

WADA (2016a) Anti-doping testing figures. Available at: https://www.wada-ama.org/en/resources/laboratories/anti-doping-testing-figures (Accessed January 2017).

WADA (2016b) Medical information to support the decisions of TUECs: Neuropathic pain. Available at: https://www.wada-ama.org/en/resources/medical-information-to-support-the-decisions-of-tuecs-neuropathic-pain (Accessed January 2017).

WADA (2016c) Decision limits for the confirmatory quantification of threshold substances. Available at: https://www.wada-ama.org/sites/default/files/resources/files/2016-12-13_td2017dl.pdf (Accessed January 2017).

WADA (2017) Prohibited List. Available at: https://www.wada-ama.org/sites/default/files/resources/files/2016-09-29_-_wada_prohibited_list_2017_eng_final.pdf (Accessed January 2017).

Yonamine, M., Garcia, P.R. and de Moraes Moreau, R.L. (2004) Non-intentional doping in sports. *Sports Medicine* 34(11): 697–704.

Chapter 20

Glucocorticoids

Nick Wojek

20.1 Introduction

Glucocorticoids (also referred to as corticosteroids) are adrenal steroid hormones with diverse physiological effects that can be anti-inflammatory, immunosuppressive and metabolic in nature. They also affect central nervous system function and the activity of other endogenous hormones. Glucocorticoids are regulated by a negative feedback loop involving the hypothalamic-pituitary-adrenal (HPA) axis (Figure 20.1). Cortisol is the main hormone secreted from the adrenal cortex following the activation of the HPA axis and is released during stressful situations such as when encountering emotional stress, infection, trauma and exercise. In addition to responding to stress stimuli, endogenous cortisol is released in an hourly pulsatile manner and exhibits a circadian rhythm with peak concentrations occurring at the onset of the daily activity period (Young et al., 2004; Son et al., 2011).

Glucocorticoids exert their multiple actions through genomic and non-genomic mechanisms. In genomic mediated mechanisms, glucocorticoids bind primarily to intracellular glucocorticoid receptors (GR) which translocate into the cell nucleus following a conformational change in the GR. In the nucleus, this GR-glucocorticoid complex regulates gene transcription and consequently protein synthesis by either binding to glucocorticoid response elements (GRE) in the promoter region of genes or by inhibiting the activity of other transcription factors such as activator protein-1 and nuclear factor-κB (Czock et al., 2005; Stahn et al., 2007). In non-genomic mediated mechanisms, glucocorticoids exert rapid actions that cannot be explained by genomic mechanisms. Non-genomic modes of action may involve the binding of glucocorticoids with cell membrane-bound GRs, binding with intracellular GRs or through physiochemical interactions with cell membranes (Czock et al., 2005; Stahn et al., 2007).

The two isoforms of the intracellular GR, GR-alpha (α) and GR-beta (β) are widely expressed in almost all tissues, explaining why glucocorticoids have such diverse physiological effects. However, glucocorticoids only bind with GR-α, which is expressed at much higher levels than GR-β in most tissues (Oakley et al., 1997; Pujols et al., 2002). Instead, GR-β is thought to affect GR-α gene transcription by acting as a dominant negative inhibitor of GR-α signalling (Oakley et al., 1996; Charmandari et al., 2005) or by independently regulating genes not controlled by GR-α (Lewis-Truffin et al., 2007; Kino et al., 2009).

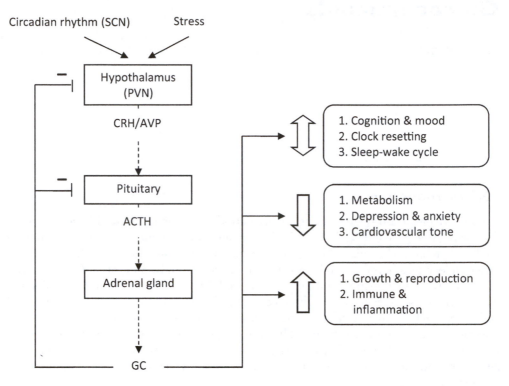

Circadian rhythm (SCN)   Stress

Hypothalamus
(PVN)

CRH/AVP

1. Cognition & mood
2. Clock resetting
3. Sleep-wake cycle

Pituitary

ACTH

1. Metabolism
2. Depression & anxiety
3. Cardiovascular tone

Adrenal gland

1. Growth & reproduction
2. Immune &
   inflammation

GC

Figure 20.1 Simplified scheme of the synthesis, secretion and actions of glucocorticoids

20.2 Clinical uses, side effects and mode of action

Synthetic glucocorticoids are administered by systemic (i.e. oral, rectal, intravenous, intramuscular) or local routes (e.g. inhalation, intranasal, intraarticular, peritendinous, topical), and are often used in a multitude of clinical applications despite not having a reparative function to resolving injury or illness.

Systemic glucocorticoids are used for their potent anti-inflammatory and immunosuppressive effects in the treatment of allergies (e.g. urticaria), gastrointestinal disorders (e.g. inflammatory bowel disease), autoimmune diseases (e.g. systemic lupus erythematosus), respiratory diseases (e.g. exacerbation of asthma), rheumatologic diseases (e.g. arthritis), musculoskeletal injuries (e.g. hamstring injuries) and in emergency medicine (e.g. anaphylactic reactions; Czock et al., 2005; Nichols, 2005; Dvorak et al., 2006). They also possess analgesic properties that alleviate post-operative pain (Romundstad et al., 2004; De Oliveira et al., 2011). Prednisolone is the most commonly prescribed systemic glucocorticoid in the UK (Fardet et al., 2011); other types include dexamethasone, budesonide, methylprednisolone, hydrocortisone and triamcinolone.

In contrast, local glucocorticoids target specific sites of inflammation in an attempt to reduce the side effects that are often associated with systemic administration. Inhaled preparations are the mainstay of asthma treatment; topically applied preparations are routinely used to treat skin conditions such as eczema; and intranasal preparations help to reduce nasal inflammation and symptoms associated with allergic rhinitis.

Local glucocorticoids are also frequently administered by intraarticular and peritendinous injections to treat athletic musculoskeletal injuries such as tendinopathies, soft-tissue and over-use injuries. It is thought that by reducing inflammation and alleviating pain associated with the injury, glucocorticoid use in turn improves motion and function around the site of injury to hasten an athlete's return to competition. Although there is a rationale for their use in sport, there is little published evidence supporting the benefit of local glucocorticoid use in this way over the risk of complications to health (Harmon and Hawley, 2003; Nichols, 2005; Dvorak et al., 2006). Long-term complications may include tendon rupture, loss of tensile strength in ligaments and cartilage degeneration (Brukner and Nicol, 2004; Nichols, 2005).

Systemic glucocorticoids have many other side effects that limit their clinical use, especially when used for long durations. In particular, long-term use may adversely affect bone (osteoporosis, increased bone fracture risk), muscle (wasting, weakness), the skin (thinning, delayed wound healing), the eyes (glaucoma, cataract), the immune system (increased risk of infection), metabolism and the endocrine system (insulin resistance, redistribution of fat), and the central nervous system (disturbances in mood, behaviour, memory and cognition) (Schäcke et al., 2002; Buttgereit et al., 2005).

The withdrawal of glucocorticoids can also lead to abnormalities in HPA axis function characterised by a reduction in adrenal cortisol release. Abnormalities in HPA axis function arise since glucocorticoids provide negative feedback to the hypothalamus and pituitary glands attenuating the release of corticotrophin-releasing hormone and adrenocorticotropic hormone (ACTH), respectively (Figure 20.1). The reduction in ACTH levels ultimately leads to atrophy of the adrenal cortex and the appearance of secondary adrenal insufficiency when the withdrawal of the glucocorticoid occurs. This effect is evident at rest (Petrides et al., 1997; Marquet et al., 1999) and occurs during exercise where the normal increase in pituitary release of ACTH and dehydroepiandrosterone is blunted (Arlettaz et al., 2006; Collomp et al., 2008; Le Panse et al., 2009).

Suppression of the HPA axis seems to be temporary as adrenal function returns to normal in most individuals within two to four weeks after short-term ($\leq$ 7 days) glucocorticoid treatment has ended (Streck and Lockwood, 1979; Henzen et al., 2000; Jollin et al., 2010; Habib et al., 2014). However, suppression can occur for much longer if treatment continues for longer than seven days (Henzen et al., 2000) and ultimately depends on the dose, frequency of use, route of administration, and type of glucocorticoid (Johnston, et al., 2015). The risk of adrenal insufficiency has also been found to be apparent following one-off intraarticular and epidural injections in elite cyclists (Duclos, 2007; Guinot et al., 2007) and within the general population (Borresen et al., 2015; Johnston et al., 2015).

The effect of adrenal insufficiency on athletic performance has not been studied to any great extent but appears to be underestimated as atypical forms of adrenal crisis such as hypoglycaemia, sudden exhaustion and feelings of faintness could possibly explain some of the unusual decreases in performance observed in athletes following glucocorticoid treatment (Duclos, 2007). The etiology of these symptoms may well go unrecognised by the athlete and their medical support staff, particularly in a sporting context where symptoms could be mistaken as fatigue related to overtraining.

Mode of action: anti-inflammatory

The anti-inflammatory effects associated with glucocorticoids are mediated mainly via genomic modes of action as outlined in the introduction to this chapter. There are two genomic modes of action: transrepression and transactivation.

Glucocorticoids primarily inhibit the synthesis of inflammatory proteins through the suppression of the genes that encode them (transrepression). In the cell nucleus, the interaction of GR-glucocorticoid complexes with transcription factors such as activator protein-1 and nuclear factor-κB leads to the inhibition of their transcriptional activity. This inhibition prevents the expression of pro-inflammatory proteins such as cytokines (extracellular signalling proteins that induce cellular responses), chemokines (attract inflammatory cells to the site of inflammation), adhesion molecules (bind inflammatory cells to the site of inflammation) and inflammatory enzymes (mediators of the inflammatory response), which are known to be involved in the inflammatory process (Czock et al., 2005; Barnes, 2006).

Glucocorticoids also switch on genes with anti-inflammatory effects through the binding of GR-glucocorticoid complexes with GREs (transactivation). This interaction leads to an increase in the transcription of genes coding for anti-inflammatory proteins such as lipocortin-1 (inhibits the inflammatory enzyme phospholipase A2), interleukin-10 (inhibits the activity of various pro-inflammatory cytokines) and interleukin-1 receptor antagonist (blocks the action of the pro-inflammatory chemokine interleukin-1; Schäcke et al., 2002; Czock et al., 2005; Barnes, 2006). In addition, glucocorticoids increase the transcription of the mitogen-activated protein kinase phosphatase-1 (MKP-1) gene which inhibits signal transduction of the mitogen-activated protein kinase pathways (Barnes, 2006). These pathways would normally activate pro-inflammatory transcription factors leading to inflammation.

20.3 Physiological and pharmacological effects

The physiological effects of glucocorticoids suggest that they could enhance performance and therefore appeal to athletes for non-therapeutic reasons. This section outlines why glucocorticoids have the potential to be misused in sport focussing on their effects on metabolism and the central nervous system. Speculative modes of action will also be described particularly in relation to weight loss.

Central nervous system effects

One-off and short-term (≤ 14 days) glucocorticoid intake moderately increases vigour and reduces feelings of fatigue at rest in patients (Swinburn et al., 1988) and healthy individuals (Plihal et al., 1996; Tops et al., 2006). There is no research that exists to confirm whether glucocorticoids exert similar ergogenic effects during exercise. However, such an effect seems likely at low to moderate exercise intensities since high serum cortisol levels, induced by a single ACTH injection, delays the onset of fatigue during submaximal (Soetens et al., 1995) but not maximal exercise (Soetens et al., 1995; Baume et al., 2008), and has a positive influence on mood by increasing vigour following successive days of exercise (Soetens et al., 1995).

It is difficult to determine the significance of how these central effects translate into performance gains based on the limited research. Nevertheless, experiencing an increase in vigour and a reduction in the feelings of fatigue even at submaximal exercise intensities may convince athletes of the in-competition benefits of glucocorticoids. These central effects may especially appeal to athletes in sports involving prolonged exertion where exercise is not maximal throughout or in sports where repetition of performance over several successive days is required.

Mode of action: central nervous system

The central effects described above are likely to occur through glucocorticoid-induced activation of the mesolimbic dopaminergic transmission pathway; the area of the brain that is associated with reward and desire. It is evident that both acute and short-term glucocorticoid administration stimulates an increase in extracellular dopamine (the neural substrate for reward) in the nucleus accumbens of rats and leads to an increase in wheel running activity (Piazza et al., 1996b; Duclos et al., 2009). Glucocorticoid treatment also restores dopamine levels in the nucleus accumbens of adrenalectomised rats, which further demonstrates its stimulatory effect on the mesolimbic dopaminergic pathway (Piazza et al., 1996a).

The precise mechanism by which glucocorticoids stimulate increases in extracellular dopamine is unknown. Nevertheless, glucocorticoids are likely to exert their central effects through the inhibition of dopamine reuptake at presynaptic dopaminergic neurons and through inhibiting monoamino oxidase activity to reduce dopamine degradation (Piazza et al., 1996b). GRs are likely to be involved in this mechanism as they are largely expressed on dopaminergic neurons that project to the mesolimbic areas of the brain (Harfstrand et al., 1986).

Dopamine also inhibits the secretion of prolactin from the anterior pituitary gland. Prolactin is considered to reflect alterations in 5-hydroxytryptamine (serotonin) and dopaminergic activity in the brain and is used as a marker of central fatigue (Davis, 1995). Prolactin remains suppressed during submaximal exercise following a short-term course of a glucocorticoid, which may be a contributing factor to delaying the perceived onset of fatigue in time to exhaustion protocols (Arlettaz et al., 2007; Le Panse et al., 2009).

Metabolic effects

Glucocorticoids play a key role in accelerating carbohydrate, lipid and protein metabolism (McMahon et al., 1988; Del Corral et al., 1998). These metabolic effects are apparent during exercise as both glucocorticoid and ACTH administration increase plasma glucose (Soetens et al., 1995; Arlettaz et al., 2007; Collomp et al., 2008), free fatty acid (Gorostiaga et al., 1988; Soetens et al., 1995), and amino acid levels (Thomasson et al., 2011), increasing the availability of these substrates for energy ahead of glycogen stores. Following endurance exercise, hypercortisolemia may also assist metabolic recuperation as glucocorticoid intake enhances muscle and liver glycogen store content in insulin-resistant rats (Gorostiaga et al., 1988; Ruzzin and Jensen, 2005); this recovery effect has yet to be studied in humans.

In addition, acute and short-term ($\leq$ 7 days) glucocorticoid intake seems to increase energy expenditure and shift substrate utilisation from carbohydrate towards lipid at rest (Brillon et al., 1995; Qi et al., 2004) and during submaximal exercise (Arlettaz et al., 2008b). These effects coupled with the catabolic, energy mobilising effects of high circulating glucocorticoid levels suggests that glucocorticoid intake may induce weight loss in individuals undertaking high volume, low to moderate intensity endurance training on calorie-maintained diets. This proposed alteration in body composition may be specific to fat loss as low-intensity exercise training seems to also negate the catabolic effects of glucocorticoids on muscle glycogen and protein in rat and human skeletal muscle (Horber et al., 1985; Pinheiro et al., 2009; Barel et al., 2010).

Indeed, new animal data suggests that transient or moderate exposure to glucocorticoids may mediate a metabolic gene program in skeletal muscle, whereby the direct activation of the metabolic transcription factor Kruppel-like factor-15 dissociates the metabolic effects of glucocorticoids from the metabolic pathways that are responsible for causing muscle wasting (Morrison-Nozik et al., 2015).

Mode of action: substrate utilisation

Glucocorticoids increase the transcription of enzymes involved in gluconeogenesis, lipolysis and proteolysis through binding to GRs located in the liver, adipose tissue and muscle. Glucocorticoids exert their metabolic effects through the following actions (Sarpolsky et al., 2000; Vegiopoulos and Herzig, 2007):

1   They stimulate hepatic gluconeogenesis by increasing the expression of phosphoenolpyruvate carboxykinase (PEPCK) and glucose-6-phosphatase (G6Pase) enzymes, which are normally rate limiting steps in the gluconeogenic pathway. This leads to an increase in glucose production from non-hexose substrates such as amino acids and glycerol.
2   They stimulate lipolysis in peripheral adipose tissue by increasing the expression of hormone sensitive lipase and decreasing the expression of lipoprotein lipase (key enzyme in the formation of triglycerides) and PEPCK (key enzyme in glyceroneogenesis). This leads to the release of FFAs (substrate for β-oxidation) and glycerol (substrate for gluconeogenesis).
3   They stimulate proteolysis through inhibiting the protein kinase b (Akt)/mammalian target of rapamycin (mTOR) signalling pathway in muscle. This pathway normally promotes protein synthesis and decreases protein degradation. Glucocorticoids inhibit the transcription of PI3-kinase (phosphoinositide 3-kinase) or AKt, which removes the inhibition of the adenosine-tri-phosphate (ATP) dependent ubiquitin-proteasome proteolysis pathway allowing an increase in protein degradation to occur. This increase in proteolysis leads to the mobilisation of amino acids (substrate for gluconeogenesis).

Body composition effects

An athlete's power-to-weight ratio is an important factor that contributes to success in weight bearing endurance sports. Testimonies from road cyclists who were caught doping during their careers or admitted to doping following retirement have described how they misused glucocorticoids out-of-competition, in part, to control for body weight. A report on doping in Danish Cycling between 1998 and 2015 revealed that many riders interviewed reported a performance enhancing effect of cortisone, primarily through increased weight loss and pain relief, and that these effects of the drug were perceived to increase endurance during competition (Anti-Doping Denmark, 2015).

David Millar, a former British road cyclist, was banned for two years in 2004 after admitting to doping following an investigation by the French authorities into the doping practices of his professional cycling team Cofidis. Millar has since become an advocate of clean sport and in a 2016 interview with the *New York Times* disclosed that he used a 20–40 milligram intramuscular dose of Kenacort (triamcinolone) ahead of the 2002 Vuelta a España and 2003 Tour de France. This was followed by a 10–20 milligram top up dose approximately ten days later to prolong its effects and to avoid adrenal insufficiency during both races. Millar remarked that it was the lightest he had been in his career, yet he didn't lose power, which is often the penalty when a rider sheds weight (Millar, 2016).

Thomas Dekker, a former Dutch road cyclist, was a user of cortisone during the 2007 Tour de France whilst riding for Rabobank (*The Times*, 2017). Dekker described how he and a teammate used betamethasone (Diprofos) injections every other day to stay "nice and skinny" and to help dig deeper during the race. He also remarked that he had never been so thin (68 kilograms), especially when considering his height (6 feet 2 inches).

Information taken from such sources require careful interpretation as the "feeling of lightness" described by some cyclists could in fact be attributable to the neuro-stimulatory effects of glucocorticoids. The observations of weight loss and preserved muscle mass could also be accounted for by the concomitant use of other prohibited substances such as testosterone, human growth hormone or insulin, which were known to have been misused during this era of cycling. Despite these explanations, anecdotal reports do seem to suggest that a short period of glucocorticoid use may induce weight loss in the region of 4–5 kilograms over three to four weeks when combining with long duration, low to moderate intensity exercise.

Mode of action: body composition

Such dramatic weight loss outlined in the above section could be the result of glucocorticoid induced increases in circulating plasma free fatty acid (FFA) levels, which are then preferentially utilised as the predominant fuel source if an athlete trains at a relatively low to moderate intensity for long durations. Recent studies on mitochondrial functioning show that high rates of FFA uptake by skeletal and cardiac muscle activates the nuclear transcription factor, peroxisome proliferator-activated receptor alpha (PPARα). PPARα activation not only increases the expression of fatty acid oxidation enzymes but also up-regulates the expression of uncoupling protein-3, peroxisome proliferator-activated receptor γ co-activator 1α and mitochondria thioesterase-1 (Stavinoha et al., 2004; Murray et al., 2005; Turner et al., 2007; Cole et al., 2011), which are indicators of mitochondria uncoupling.

This combination of increased fatty acid oxidation and mitochondria uncoupling raises metabolic rate. This means that the mitochondria consume a higher amount of oxygen to produce the same amount of ATP, which ultimately may lead to the observed reduction in adipose tissue. Moreover, glucocorticoid administration over five days has been shown to decrease the efficiency of oxidative phosphorylation in rat liver mitochondria (Roussel et al., 2004), which in principle supports the theory of a glucocorticoid induced decrease in the metabolic efficiency of mitochondria.

Summary of studies measuring performance

No consensus exists regarding whether the ergogenic effects of glucocorticoids on metabolism, the central nervous system or on body composition outlined in this chapter translate into performance gains. Short-term glucocorticoid use (5–7 days) increases time to exhaustion during cycling at $\leq 75\%$ VO_{2max} (Arlettaz et al., 2008b; Collomp et al., 2008; Le Panse et al., 2009), but not at exercise intensities of $> 75\%$ VO_{2max} (Marquet et al., 1999). In contrast, acute glucocorticoid use does not improve submaximal cycling or high-intensity intermittent running (Petrides et al., 1997; Arlettaz et al., 2006 and 2008a), although acute supratherapeutic doses have yet to be explored at exercise intensities of $\leq 75\%$ VO_{2max}. Acute ACTH administration also fails to improve maximal exercise (Soetens et al., 1995) or time-trial performance (Baume et al., 2008).

These inconsistent findings may be attributable to the dose, duration or type of glucocorticoid used; and the duration, intensity and type of exercise protocols selected. Performance indicators such as VO_{2max}, maximal heart rate, ventilatory threshold and maximal blood lactate may be inappropriate to confirm the ergogenic effects of glucocorticoids in comparison to other central and metabolic variables that may indirectly enhance performance. Furthermore, the ergogenic effects of glucocorticoids on prolonged exercise tests lasting 3–4 hours, sport-specific intermittent exercise tests or one-off sprint tests following a fatiguing protocol are unknown (Duclos, 2010). It seems that an ergogenic effect at least occurs at submaximal exercise intensities following short-term use of a systemic glucocorticoid.

20.4 Anti-doping regulations

All glucocorticoids are prohibited in-competition when administered by oral, intravenous, intramuscular or rectal routes but are not prohibited out-of-competition (WADA, 2017). This means that athletes should not have a synthetic glucocorticoid present in their urine following an in-competition drug test even when the administration of a systemic dose has occurred out-of-competition. The only exception to this rule is when an athlete has obtained a therapeutic use exemption (TUE) to authorise such use.

All glucocorticoids administered by "local injection" routes (e.g. epidural, intraarticular, intradermal, periarticular, peritendinous) or by inhalation are permitted at all times regardless of if administered in- or out-of-competition. Topical preparations when used for auricular, buccal, dermatological, gingival, nasal, ophthalmic and perianal disorders are also permitted at all times.

The interpretation of analysed urine samples showing the presence of a glucocorticoid is complicated by this mix of regulations. Consequently, WADA-accredited laboratories are directed to only report urinary concentrations if the parent compound is detected in-competition above the minimum required performance limit (MRPL) of 30ng/mL (WADA, 2015). This strategy seems to assume that a low concentration is more likely to be due to legitimate therapeutic use of a glucocorticoid via a permitted route of administration rather than systemic use for non-therapeutic reasons close to competition.

However, it is difficult to accurately discriminate between the urinary levels of glucocorticoids received by a permitted "local injection" and prohibited systemic administration. Glucocorticoids may be systemically absorbed after an intra-articular injection (Duclos, 2007; Habib et al., 2014), and the degree of absorption can depend on the size and type of joint, vascularisation around the joint, the preparation of glucocorticoid used, its esterification, the dosage and the frequency of injections (Johnston et al., 2015; Freire and Bureau, 2016). It is also conceivable for a doctor to inadvertently mischaracterise the site of a local injection in the absence of radiological or ultrasound guidance leading to an increase in systemic absorption. Indeed, there are instances at the Olympic Games where urinary glucocorticoid concentrations in excess of 30ng/ml have resulted from a local route of administration (Fitch, 2016).

It is apparent that further research is warranted regarding investigating the pharmacokinetics and detection of glucocorticoids. One area that could be examined in more detail is the appropriateness of the 30ng/mL universal reporting limit on all glucocorticoids. Substance specific reporting limits may be more appropriate as the potency of glucocorticoids varies depending on if they are short-acting (e.g. cortisone and hydrocortisone), intermediate-acting (e.g. prednisolone and triamcinolone), or long-acting (e.g. betamethasone and dexamethasone; Collomp et al., 2016; Freire and Bureau, 2016).

Identifying differences in the urinary excretion of glucocorticoids for permitted and prohibited routes of administration have started to be explored. The identification of 6β-hydroxy-budesonide as a metabolite of budesonide (Matabosch et al., 2012 and 2013a) has led to its adoption by WADA as a discriminator to determine when systemic budesonide administration has occurred (WADA, 2015). Similar research is ongoing to discover and characterise the metabolites of betamethasone (Matabosch et al., 2015a), methylprednisolone (Pozo et al., 2012; Matabosch et al., 2013b), prednisolone (Matabosch et al., 2015b) and triamcinolone (Matabosch et al., 2014a and 2015c). Identifying such metabolites may even extend the window of detection if differences in the urinary excretion of glucocorticoid metabolites can first be established to help better discriminate between local and systemic routes of administration.

Anti-doping statistics

Table 20.1 summarises the number of adverse analytical findings (AAFs) reported by WADA-accredited laboratories between 2009 and 2015 for the in-competition presence of a glucocorticoid (WADA Anti-Doping Testing Figures 2009–2015). Of all AAFs reported in these years, glucocorticoid detection ranges between 5 and 8 per cent of the proportion of substances detected per Prohibited List category, and in most years, is the fourth most detected category. Since 2014, a notable decrease in budesonide AAFs has been observed; this is attributable to the introduction of the mandatory requirement to detect 6β-hydroxy-budesonide to determine the administration of budesonide via a systemic route (WADA, 2014).

Nevertheless, these statistics are likely to include many AAFs from athletes who have been either granted a TUE or received glucocorticoid treatment via a permitted route of administration. This means that these statistics are not necessarily an accurate reflection of the number of athletes to have incurred an anti-doping rule violation because of glucocorticoid misuse. Indeed, UK TUE data revealed that 48 per cent of all TUE approvals between 2010 and 2015 were for the use of systemic glucocorticoids (unpublished UK Anti-Doping findings).

Summary of medical policies that control for glucocorticoid use in sport

The Union Cycliste Internationale (UCI) introduced new medical rules in 2011 to prohibit the use of needles, unless the purpose for the injection is medically appropriate and fulfils a series of strict medical criteria (UCI, 2015). This policy is often referred to as the "no needles'" policy and includes a rule requiring an athlete to rest for two days following a glucocorticoid injection (local or systemic). The policy was introduced to (1) address the concerns of widespread glucocorticoid misuse within cycling that were not being effectively addressed by the current anti-doping regulations; and (2) to help reduce the pressure put on doctors by athletes and their entourage (such as coaches) to inject glucocorticoids and other injectable substances in circumstances that were medically inappropriate. In 2015, the UCI revised its rules extending the period of rest following any glucocorticoid injection from two to eight days for athlete welfare reasons.

Glucocorticoid misuse is less of a concern in sports where use is not beneficial to performance but widely occurs for legitimate therapeutic reasons. Misuse in these sports

Table 20.1 Incidences of glucocorticoids reported as adverse analytical findings by WADA-accredited laboratories from 2009–2015 (taken from WADA Anti-Doping Testing Figure reports)

Type	2009	2010	2011	2012	2013	2014	2015
16a-hydroxyprednisolone	1	0	0	0	0	0	0
Betamethasone	39	27	25	30	35	34	31
Budesonide	120	111	113	157	135	74	7
Deflazacort	0	3	1	0	0	1	4
Desonide	6	0	0	0	0	0	0
Dexamethasone	17	8	21	18	18	12	19
Fluticasone propionate	0	1	2	1	2	0	5
Methylprednisolone	9	7	16	15	14	14	19
Prednisolone	16	16	19	67	58	56	60
Prednisolone + Prednisone	41	39	40	0	0	0	0
Prednisone	3	9	19	60	55	44	52
Triamcinolone	12	6	2	1	1	1	1
Triamcinolone Acetonide	1	7	16	16	12	16	17
Total (proportion per drug category)	265 (5%)	234 (4%)	274 (5%)	365 (8%)	330 (6%)	252 (8%)	215 (6%)

is likely to be due to inappropriate medical practices. The international federations for rowing (FISA) and gymnastics (FIG) have adopted their own versions of the "no needles" policy to cover the period of international regattas and gymnastic competitions but both exclude the rule requiring athletes to rest following the use of a glucocorticoid. Similarly, the IOC adopted a "needles" policy for all participating athletes at the Rio Olympic Games (IOC, 2016).

20.5 Summary

- Glucocorticoids are adrenal steroid hormones with diverse physiological effects that are regulated by a negative feedback loop involving the hypothalamic-pituitary-adrenal axis.
- They are widely used in medicine for their potent anti-inflammatory and immunosuppressive effects.
- Glucocorticoids exert their multiple actions primarily through genomic mechanisms in which they bind to intracellular glucocorticoid receptors that regulate the transcription of key proteins that are involved in inflammation, metabolism and the activation of the central nervous system.
- Glucocorticoids have deleterious effects that can cause several side effects that limit their clinical use, especially when used for long durations.
- The ergogenic effects of short-term systemic glucocorticoid use have been observed at rest and at exercise intensities of $\leq 75\%$ VO_{2max} but no higher. Anecdotal evidence from athlete testimonies in cycling suggest that performance may be indirectly enhanced through a glucocorticoid-induced weight loss mechanism in sports where power-to-weight ratio is a performance limiting factor. Therefore, glucocorticoid misuse seems to be most likely to be a risk in endurance based sports.
- Athletes using glucocorticoids for doping purposes appear to limit their use to only a few days or times per year. Use is therefore likely to revolve around key competitions to avoid the well-known catabolic effects on skeletal muscle, which are associated with long-term use.
- Glucocorticoids are currently only prohibited in-competition when administered by systemic routes. Further discussion is warranted regarding whether the systemic use of glucocorticoids should be prohibited in- and out-of-competition, especially in sports where out-of-competition systemic use is deemed a risk.
- The current anti-doping policy to control for glucocorticoids is not ideal as it is difficult to distinguish between permitted and prohibited routes of administration. Substance specific urinary reporting concentrations may be more appropriate than a universal reporting limit for all glucocorticoids. The identification of new specific metabolites for each glucocorticoid may also help better discriminate between permitted and prohibited routes of administration.
- Glucocorticoid misuse is less of a concern in sports where use is not beneficial to performance but widely occurs for legitimate therapeutic reasons. Misuse in these sports is likely to be due to inappropriate medical practice. Some international federations have introduced "no needle" policies to improve the governance around the medical use of glucocorticoids and other injectable substances. These medical rules compliment the current anti-doping regulations for controlling glucocorticoid use within sport.

20.6 References

Anti-Doping Denmark (2015) Report on Doping in Danish Cycling 1998–2015 Available at: http://www.doping.nl/media/kb/3493/Report_on_Doping_in_Danish_Cycling%201998-2015_ENGLISH_VERSION.pdf (Accessed 21 July 2017).

Arlettaz, A., Collomp, K., Portier, H. et al. (2006). Effects of acute prednisolone intake during intense submaximal exercise. *International Journal of Sports Medicine* 27: 673–679.

Arlettaz, A., Portier, H., Lecoq, A-M. et al. (2007) Effects of short-term prednisolone intake during submaximal exercise. *Medicine and Science in Sports and Exercise* 39: 1,672–1,678.

Arlettaz, A., Collomp, K., Portier, H. et al. (2008a) Effects of acute prednisolone administration on exercise endurance and metabolism. *British Journal of Sports Medicine* 42: 250–254.

Arlettaz, A., Portier, H., Lecoq, A-M. et al. (2008b). Effects of acute prednisolone intake on substrate utilization during submaximal exercise. *International Journal of Sports Medicine* 29: 21–26.

Barel, M., Perez, O.A., Giozzet, V.A., et al. (2010). Exercise training prevents hyperinsulinemia, muscular glycogen loss and muscle atrophy induced by dexamethasone treatment. *European Journal of Applied Physiology* 108: 999–1007.

Barnes, P.J. (2006) Corticosteroid effects on cell signalling. *European Respiratory Journal* 27: 413–426.

Baume, N., Steel, G., Edwards, T. et al. (2008) No variation of physical performance and perceived exertion after adrenal gland stimulation by synthetic ACTH (Synacthen®) in cyclists. *European Journal of Applied Physiology* 104: 589–600.

Borresen, S.W., Klose, M., Rasmussen, A.K. and Feldt-Rasmussen, U. (2015) Adrenal insufficiency caused by locally applied glucocorticoids: Myth or fact? *Current Medicinal Chemistry* 22: 2,801–2,809.

Brillon, D.J., Zheng, B., Campbell, R.G. and Matthews, D.E. (1995). Effect of cortisol on energy expenditure and amino acid metabolism in humans. *American Journal of Physiology* 268: e501–513.

Brukner, P. and Nicol, A. (2004). Use of oral corticosteroids in sports medicine. *Current Sports Medicine Reports* 3: 181–183.

Buttgereit, F., Burmester, G-R. and Lipworth, B.J. (2005) Optimised glucocorticoid therapy: The sharpening of an old spear. *Lancet* 365: 801–803.

Charmandari, E., Chrousos, G.P., Ichijo, T. et al. (2005) The human glucocorticoid receptor (hGR) β isoforms suppresses the transcriptional activity of hGRα by interfering with formation of active coactivator complexes. *Molecular Endocrinology* 19: 52–64.

Cole, M.A., Murray, A.J., Cochlin, L.E. et al. (2011) A high fat diet increases mitochondrial fatty acid oxidation and uncoupling to decrease efficiency in rat heart. *Basic Research in Cardiology* 106: 447–457.

Collomp, K., Arlettaz, A., Buisson, C. et al. (2016) Glucocorticoid administration in athletes: Performance, metabolism and detection. *Steroids* 115: 193–202.

Collomp, K., Arlettaz, A., Portier, H. et al. (2008) Short-term glucocorticoid intake combined with intense training on performance and hormonal responses. *British Journal of Sports Medicine* 42: 983–988.

Czock, D., Keller, F., Rasche, F.M. and Häussler, U. (2005) Pharmacokinetics and pharmacodynamics of systemically administered glucocorticoids. *Clinical Pharmacokinetics* 44: 61–98.

Davis, J.M. (1995) Central and peripheral factors in fatigue. *Journal of Sports Science* 13: S49–53.

De Oliveira, G.S., Almeida, M.D., Benzon, H.T. and McCarthy, R.J. (2011) Perioperative single dose systemic dexamethasone for postoperative pain. *Anesthesiology* 115: 575–588.

Del Corral, P., Howley, E.T., Hartsell, M. et al. (1998) Metabolic effects of low cortisol during exercise in humans. *Journal of Applied Physiology* 84: 939–947.

Duclos, M. (2010) Glucocorticoids: A doping agent? *Endocrinology Metabolic Clinics North America* 39: 107–126.

Duclos, M., Gatti, C, Bessiere, B. and Mormède, P. (2009) Tonic and phasic effects of corticosterone on food restriction-induced hyperactivity in rats. *Psychoneuroendocrinology* 34: 436–445.

Duclos, M., Guinot, M., Colsy, M. et al. (2007) High risk of adrenal insufficiency after a single articular steroid injection in athletes. *Medicine and Science in Sports and Exercise* 39: 1,036–1,043.

Dvorak, J., Feddermann, N. and Grimm, K. (2006). Glucocorticosteroids in football: Use and misuse. *British Journal of Sports Medicine* 40: i48–i54.

Fardet, L., Petersen, I. and Nazareth, I. (2011). Prevalence of long-term oral glucocorticoid prescriptions in the UK over the past 20 years. *Rheumatology (Oxford)* 50: 1,982–1,990.

Fitch, K. (2016). Glucocorticoids at the Olympic Games: State-of-the-art review. *British Journal of Sports Medicine* 50: 1,267.

Freire, V. and Bureau, N.J. (2016) Injectable corticosteroids: Take precautions and use caution. *Semin: Musculoskeletal Radiology* 20: 401–408.

Gorostiaga, E.M., Czerwinski, S.M. and Hickson, R.C. (1988). Acute glucocorticoid effects on glycogen utilization, O_2 uptake, and endurance. *Journal of Applied Physiology* 64: 1,098–1,106.

Guinot, M., Duclos, M., Idres, N. et al. (2007) Value of basal serum cortisol to detect corticosteroid-induced adrenal insufficiency in elite cyclists. *European Journal of Applied Physiology* 99: 205–216.

Habib, G., Jabbour, A., Artul, S. and Hakim, G. (2014). Intra-articular methylprednisolone acetate injection at the knee joint and the hypothalamic-pituitary-adrenal axis: A randomized controlled study. *Clinical Rheumatology* 33: 99–103.

Härfstrand, A., Fuxe, K., Cintra, A. et al. (1986) Glucocorticoid receptor immunoreactivity in monoaminergic neurons of rat brain. *Proceedings of the National Academy of Science USA* 83: 9,779–9,783.

Harmon, K.G. and Hawley, C. (2003). Physician prescribing patterns of oral corticosteroids for musculoskeletal injuries. *Journal of the American Board Family Practice* 16: 209–212.

Henzen, C., Suter, A., Lerch, E. et al. (2000) Suppression and recovery of adrenal response after short-term, high-dose glucocorticoid treatment. *Lancet* 355: 542–545.

Horber, F.F., Scheidegger, J.R., Grünig, B.E. and Frey, F.J. (1985) Evidence that prednisone-induced myopathy is reversed by physical training. *Journal of Clinical Endocrinology and Metabolism* 61: 83–88.

IOC (2016) Anti-doping rules for the Games of the XXXI Olympiad in Rio de Janeiro in 2016: Needle Policy. Available at: https://stillmed.olympic.org/media/Document%20Library/OlympicOrg/IOC/What-We-Do/Protecting-Clean-Athletes/Fight-against-doping/EN-IOC-Needle-Policy-Rio-2016.pdf (accessed 24 July 2017).

Johnston, P.C., Lansang, M.C., Chatterjee, S. and Kennedy, L. (2015) Intra-articular glucocorticoid injections and their effect on hypothalamic–pituitary–adrenal (HPA)-axis function. *Endocrine* 48: 410–416.

Jollin, L., Thomasson, R., Le Panse, B. et al. (2010) Saliva DHEA and cortisol responses following short-term corticosteroid intake. *European Journal of Clinical Investigation*, 40: 183–186.

Kino, T., Manoli, I., Kelkar, S. et al. (2009) Glucocorticoid receptor (GR) β has intrinsic, GRα-independent transcriptional activity. *Biochemical and Biophysical Research Communications* 381: 671–675.

Le Panse, B., Thomasson, R., Jollin, L. et al. (2009) Short-term glucocorticoid intake improves exercise endurance in healthy recreationally trained women. *European Journal of Applied Physiology* 107: 437–443.

Lewis-Truffin, L.J., Jewell, C.M., Bienstock, R.J. et al. (2007) Human glucocorticoid receptor β binds RU-486 and is transcriptionally active. *Molecular and Cellular Biology* 27: 2,266–2,282.

McMahon, M., Gerich, J. and Rizza, R. (1988) Effects of glucocorticoids on carbohydrate metabolism. *Diabetes/Metabolism Reviews* 4: 17–30.

Marquet, P., Lac, G., Chassain, A.P., Habrioux, G. and Galen F.X. (1999) Dexamethasone in resting and exercising men. I. Effects on bioenergetics, minerals, and related hormones. *Journal of Applied Physiology* 87: 175–182.

Matabosch, X., Pozo, O.J., Perez-Mana, C. et al. (2012) Identification of budesonide metabolites in human urine after oral administration. *Analytical and Bioanalytical Chemistry* 404: 325–340.

Matabosch, X., Pozo, O.J., Perez-Mana, C. et al. (2013a) Discrimination of prohibited oral use from authorized inhaled treatment of budesonide in sports. *Therapeutic Drug Monitoring* 35: 118–128.

Matabosch, X., Pozo, O.J., Monfort, N. et al. (2013b) Urinary profile of methylprednisolone and its metabolites after oral and topical administrations. *Journal of Steroid Biochemistry and Molecular Biology* 138: 214–221.

Matabosch, X., Pozo, O.J., Papaseit, E. et al. (2014b) Detection and characterization of triamcinolone acetonide metabolites in human urine by liquid chromatography/tandem mass spectrometry after intramuscular administration. *Rapid Communication Mass Spectrometry* 28: 1,829–1,839.

Matabosch, X., Pozo, O.J., Monfort, N. et al. (2015a) Detection and characterization of betamethasone metabolites in human urine by LC-MS/MS. *Drug Testing and Analysis* 7: 663–672.

Matabosch, X., Pozo, O.J., Perez-Mana, C. et al. (2015b). Detection and characterization of prednisolone metabolites in human urine by LC-MS/MS. *Journal of Mass Spectrometry* 50: 633–642.

Matabosch, X., Pozo, O.J., Perez-Mana, C. et al. (2015c) Evaluation of the reporting level to detect triamcinolone acetonide misuse in sports. *Journal of Steroid Biochemistry and Molecular Biology* 145: 94–102.

Millar, David (2016) How to get away with doping. *New York Times*, 14 October. Available at: https://www.nytimes.com/2016/10/16/opinion/sunday/how-to-get-away-with-doping.html?mcubz=0 (Accessed 21 July 2017).

Morrison-Nozik, A., Ananda, P., Zhua, H. et al. (2015) Glucocorticoids enhance muscle endurance and ameliorate Duchenne muscular dystrophy through a defined metabolic program. *Proceedings of the National Academy of Sciences*, 112, e6780–e6789.

Murray, A.J., Panagia, M., Hauton, D. et al. (2005) Plasma free fatty acids and peroxisome proliferator-activated receptor α in the control of myocardial uncoupling protein levels. *Diabetes* 54: 3,496–3,502.

Nichols, A.W. (2005) Complications associated with the use of corticosteroids in the treatment of athletic injuries. *Clinical Journal of Sports Medicine* 15: E370.

Oakley, R.H., Sar, M. and Cidlowski, J.A. (1996) The human glucocorticoid receptor beta isoforms. Expression, biochemical properties, and putative function. *Journal of Biological Chemistry* 271: 9,550–9,559.

Oakley, R.H., Webster, J.C., Sar, M. et al. (1997) Expression and subcellular distribution of the β-isoform of the human glucocorticoid receptor. *Endpcrinology* 138: 5,028–5,038.

Petrides, J.S., Gold, P.W., Mueller, G.P. et al. (1997) Marked differences in functioning of the hypothalamic-pituitary-adrenal axis between groups of men. *Journal of Applied Physiology* 82: 1,979–1,988.

Piazza, P.V., Barrot, M., Rougé-Pont, F. et al. (1996a) Suppression of glucocorticoid secretion and antipsychotic drugs have similar effects on the mesolimbic dopaminergic transmission. *Proceedings of the National Academy of Science USA* 93: 15,445–15,450.

Piazza, P.V., Rougé-Pont, F., Deroche, V. et al. (1996b) Glucocorticoids have state-dependent stimulant effects on the mesencephalic dopaminergic transmission. *Proceedings of the National Academy of Science USA* 93: 8,716–8,720.

Pinheiro, C.H., Sousa Filho, W.M., Oliveira Neto, J.D. et al. (2009) Exercise prevents cardiometabolic alterations induced by chronic use of glucocorticoids. *Arquivos Brasileiros de Cardiologia* 93: 392–400.

Plihal, W., Krug, R., Pietrowsky, R. et al. (1996) Corticosteroid receptor mediated effects on mood in humans. *Psychoneuroendocrinology* 21: 515–523.

Pozo, O.J., Marcos, J., Matabosch, X. et al. (2012) Using complementary mass spectrometric approaches for the determination of methylprednisolone metabolites in human urine. *Rapid Communications Mass Spectrometry* 26: 541–553.

Pujols, L., Mullol, J., Roca-Ferrer, J. et al. (2002) Expression of glucocorticoid receptor α- and β-isoforms in human cells and tissues. *American Journal of Physiological Cell Physiology* 283: C1324–C1331.

Qi, D., Pulinilkunnil, T., An, D. et al. (2004) Single-dose dexamethasone induces whole-body insulin resistance and alters both cardiac fatty acid and carbohydrate metabolism. *Diabetes* 53: 1,790–1,797.

Romundstad, L., Breivik, H., Niemi, G. et al. (2004) Methylprednisolone intravenously 1 day after surgery has sustained analgesic and opioid-sparing effects. *Acta Anaesthesiologica Scandinavica* 48: 1,223–1,231.

Roussel, D., Dumas, J-F., Simard, G. et al. (2004) Kinetics and control of oxidative phosphorylation in rat liver mitochondria after dexamethasone treatment. *Biochemical Journal* 382: 491–499.

Ruzzin, J. and Jensen, J. (2005) Contraction activates glucose uptake and glycogen synthase normally in muscles from dexamethasone-treated rats. *American Journal of Physiology and Endocrinological Metabolism* 289: E241–E250.

Sarpolsky, R.M., Romero, M. and Munck, A.U. (2000) How do glucocorticoids influence stress responses? Integrating permissive, suppressive, stimulatory, and preparative actions. *Endocrinology Reviews* 21: 55–89.

Schäcke, H., Döcke, W-D. and Asadullah, K. (2002) Mechanisms involved in the side effects of glucocorticoids. *Pharmacology and Therapeutics* 96: 23–43.

Soetens, E., De Meirleir, K. and Hueting, J.E. (1995) No influence of ACTH on maximal performance. *Psychopharmacology* 118: 260–266.

Son, G.H., Chung, S. and Kim, K. (2011) The adrenal peripheral clock: Glucocorticoid and the circadian timing system. *Frontiers in Neuroendocrinology* 32: 451–465.

Stahn, C., Löwenberg, M., Hommes, D.W. and Buttgereit, F. (2007) Molecular mechanisms of glucocorticoid action and selective glucocorticoid receptor agonists. *Molecular and Cellular Endocrinology* 275: 71–78.

Stavinoha, M.A., RaySpellicy, J.W., Essop, M.F. et al. (2004) Evidence for mitochondrial thioesterase 1 as a peroxisome proliferator-activated receptor-α-regulated gene in cardiac and skeletal muscle. *American Journal of Physiology and Endocrinological Metabolism* 287: E888–E895.

Streck, W.F. and Lockwood, D.H. (1979) Pituitary adrenal recovery following short-term suppression with corticosteroids. *The American Journal of Medicine* 66: 910–914.

Swinburn, C.R., Wakefield, J.M., Newman, S.P. and Jones, P.W. (1988) Evidence of prednisolone induced mood change ("steroid euphoria") in patients with chronic obstructive airways disease. *British Journal of Clinical Pharmacology* 26: 709–713.

The Times (2017) Thomas Dekker: The doping cheat comes clean. Available at: https://www.thetimes.co.uk/article/thomas-dekker-the-doping-cheat-comes-clean-0rqlglps2 (Accessed 21 July 2017).

Thomasson, R., Rieth, N., Jollin, L. et al. (2011) Short-term glucocorticoid intake and metabolic responses during long-lasting exercise. *Hormone Metabolism Research* 43: 216–222.

Tops, M., Van Peer, J.M., Wijers, A.A. and Korf, J. (2006) Acute cortisol administration reduces subjective fatigue in healthy women. *Psychophysiology* 43: 653–656.

Turner, N., Bruce, C.R., Beale, S.M. et al. (2007). Excess lipid availability increases mitochondrial fatty acid oxidative capacity in muscle. *Diabetes*, 56, 2,085–2,092.

UCI (2015) Cycling Regulations: Part 13 Medical Rules. Available at: http://www.uci.ch/mm/Document/News/Rulesandregulation/16/26/69/13-SEC-20150101-E_English.pdf (Accessed 24 July 2017).

Vegiopoulos, A., and Herzig, S. (2007). Glucocorticoids, metabolism and metabolic diseases. *Molecular and Cellular Endocrinology* 275: 43–61.

WADA (2014) Technical Document: TD2014 MRPL (Technical document for minimum required performance levels for detection and identification of non-threshold substances). Available at: https://www.wada-ama.org/en/resources/science-medicine/td2014-mrpl (Accessed 21 July 2017).

WADA (2015) Technical Document: TD2015MRPL (Technical document for minimum required performance levels for detection and identification of non-threshold substances). Available at: https://www.wada-ama.org/en/resources/science-medicine/td2015-mrpl (Accessed 21 July 2017).

WADA (2016) Anti-Doping Testing Figures 2009–2015. Available at: https://www.WADA-ama.org/en/resources/laboratories/anti-doping-testing-figures (Accessed 21 July 2017).

WADA (2017) International Standard: The 2017 Prohibited List. Available at: https://www.WADA-ama.org/en/resources/science-medicine/prohibited-list-documents (Accessed 21 July 2017).

Young, E.A., Abelson, J. and Lightman, L. (2004) Cortisol pulsatility and its role in stress regulation and health. *Frontiers in Neuroendocrinology* 25: 69–76.

Chapter 21

Alcohol

David R. Mottram

21.1 Introduction

Fermented beverages have been used from ancient times. Alcohol continues to feature prominently in contemporary life. With respect to sport, alcohol is closely associated with sponsorship and branding as well as with consumption by players and spectators (Palmer, 2011). Alcohol consumption is part of the social aspects of many sporting events and is claimed to be the most widely used drug among sport participants and athletes (El-Sayed et al., 2005).

21.2 Mode of action of alcohol

Metabolism of alcohol

Ethanol or ethyl alcohol is obtained by the fermentation of sugar. It is non-toxic, except in large and chronic doses, and has been enjoyed as a beverage for many centuries.

Ethyl alcohol is both a drug and a food. Its energy value per unit weight (kcal/g) is seven compared with a value of nine for fat and four for both carbohydrate and protein. The value of alcohol as a food stuff is limited, as it is metabolized mainly in the liver at a fixed rate of about 100mg per kg body weight per hour. For a 70kg individual this amounts to 7g of alcohol hourly. The energy is not available to active skeletal muscle and consequently it is not possible to exercise oneself to sobriety. The diuretic effect of drinking beer makes it less than the ideal agent of rehydration after hard physical training.

Alcohol is a polar substance which is freely miscible in water. It easily penetrates biological membranes and can be absorbed unaltered from the stomach and more quickly from the small intestine. Absorption is quickest if alcohol is drunk on an empty stomach, if gas molecules are present in the drink and if the alcohol content is high. Intense mental concentration, lowered body temperature and physical exercise tend to slow the rate of absorption.

From the gastrointestinal tract alcohol is transported to the liver in the hepatic circulation. The activity of the enzyme alcohol dehydrogenase, present chiefly in the liver, governs the disappearance of alcohol from the body. In the liver, alcohol dehydrogenase converts the alcohol to acetaldehyde; it is then converted to acetic acid or acetate by aldehyde dehydrogenase. About 75 per cent of the alcohol taken up by the blood is released as acetate into the circulation. The acetate is then oxidized to carbon dioxide and water within the Krebs (or citric acid) cycle. An alternative metabolic route for acetate is its activation to acetyl coenzyme A and further reactions to form fatty acids, ketone bodies, amino acids and steroids.

Ethyl alcohol is distributed throughout the body and enters all the body water pools and tissues, including the central nervous system. Initially, alcohol moves rapidly from blood into the tissues.

The metabolism of alcohol in the liver is unaffected by its concentration in the blood. Some alcohol is eliminated in the breath, but this is usually less than 5 per cent of the total amount metabolized. This route is utilized in assessing safe levels for driving, forming the basis for breathalyser tests. Small amounts of alcohol are excreted in urine and also in sweat if exercise is performed whilst drunk. Higher excretion rates through the lungs, urine and sweat are produced at high environmental temperatures and at high blood alcohol levels.

With a single drink the blood alcohol level usually peaks about 45 minutes after ingestion. This is the point where any influence on performance will be most evident.

Action of alcohol on the nervous system

Alcohol has differential effects on the central neurotransmitters, acetylcholine, serotonin, noradrenaline and dopamine.

Activity in the neurones of serotonergic pathways is important for the experience of anxiety; output of corticosteroid hormones from the adrenal cortex increases the activity in these neurones. Alcohol decreases serotonin turnover in the central nervous system therefore may reduce the tension that is felt by the individual in a stressful situation.

Alcohol increases activity in central noradrenergic pathways. This is transient and is followed, some hours later, by a decrease in activity. Catecholaminergic pathways are implicated in the control of mood states, activation of these pathways promoting happy and merry states. The fall in noradrenaline turnover as the blood alcohol concentration drops ties in with the reversal of mood that follows the initial drunken euphoric state. This is exacerbated by large doses of alcohol giving rise to depression.

Alcohol stimulates the brain to release dopamine. Dopamine is regarded as a "pleasure-related" hormone and its release is triggered in the limbic system. Stimulation of sweat glands also affects the limbic system whilst cerebral cortical activity is depressed. Pain sensors are numbed and later the cerebellum is affected, causing difficulty with balance.

Alcohol also affects cerebral energy metabolism by increasing glucose utilization in the brain. As glucose is the main substrate furnishing energy for nerve cells, the result is that the lowered glucose level may induce mental fatigue. This will be reflected in failing cognitive functions and a decline in mental concentration and information processing.

The disruption of acetylcholine synthesis and release means that alcohol acts as a depressant, exerting its effect on the reticular activating system, whose activity represents the level of physiological arousal. It also has a depressant effect on the cortex. Alcohol first affects the reasoning centres in the frontal lobes and sedates inhibitory nerves; at higher levels of blood alcohol, the centres for speech, vision and motor control are affected and eventually awareness is lost. In smaller doses, alcohol inhibits cerebral control mechanisms, freeing the brain from its normal inhibition. This release of inhibition has been blamed for aggressive and violent conduct of individuals behaving out of character when under the influence of alcohol.

Progressive effects of alcohol at different blood alcohol concentrations are summarized in Table 21.1. An important effect of alcohol, not listed, is that it diminishes the ability to process appreciable amounts of information arriving simultaneously from two different sources.

Table 21.1 Demonstrable effects of alcohol at different blood alcohol concentrations

Concentration level (mg/100 ml blood)	Effects
30 (0.03%)	Enhanced sense of well-being; retarded simple reaction time; impaired hand-eye coordination
60 (0.06 %)	Mild loss of social inhibition; impaired judgement
90 (0.09%)	Marked loss of social inhibition; coordination reduced; noticeably "under the influence"
120 (0.12 %)	Apparent clumsiness; loss of physical control; tendency towards extreme responses; definite drunkenness is noted
150 (0.15 %)	Erratic behaviour; slurred speech; staggering gait
180 (0.18 %)	Loss of control of voluntary activity; impaired vision

It is thought that moderate drinking provides a degree of protection against coronary heart disease. In a prospective cohort study over 20 years in Denmark, Pedersen et al. (2008) showed that engaging in physical activity was linked to a 25-30 per cent decrease in risk of death from heart disease; moderate alcohol intake was also linked to a smaller reduction, with the risk of death from heart disease reduced by 17 per cent in men and 24 per cent in women.

21.3 Adverse effects of alcohol

The effects of alcohol on health are usually viewed in terms of chronic alcoholism. Persistent drinking leads to a dependence on alcohol so that it becomes addictive. Most physicians emphasize that alcoholism is a disease or a behavioural disorder rather than a vice and devise therapy accordingly.

The result of excessive drinking is ultimately manifested in liver disease: cirrhosis, a serious hardening and degeneration of liver tissue, is fatal for many heavy drinkers. Cancer is also more likely to develop in a cirrhotic liver. Cancers of the bowel, pharynx, larynx and oesophagus have also been linked to alcohol consumption.

Cardiomyopathy or damage to the heart muscle can result from years of heavy drinking. Other pathological conditions associated with alcohol abuse include generalized skeletal myopathy and pancreatitis. Impairment of brain function also occurs, alcoholic psychoses being a common cause of hospitalization in psychiatric wards. There are potentially fatal consequences of "binge" drinking where excessive amounts of alcohol are drunk in one session.

Alcohol use modulates the immune system and impairs host defence mechanisms. Van der Horst Graat et al. (2007) reported an association between alcohol intake and frequency of respiratory infections in apparently healthy elderly people. Alcohol taken with a meal increases post-prandial lipaemia, an effect that is the opposite of response to exercise.

The suppression of fat oxidation would increase the propensity for weight gain and increased abdominal adiposity (Suter and Schutz, 2008). Alcohol may impair absorption of minerals and vitamins. Vitamin D was deficient in 90 per cent of the men and 76 per cent of the female alcoholics studied by Malik et al. (2009): the link between alcohol consumption and osteoporosis was more evident in the men, raised levels of oestradiol providing a degree of protection for the women. Alcohol decreases resting levels of testosterone and cortisol; it also blunts the cortisol and growth hormone responses to submaximal exercise, factors that could impair performance.

21.4 Alcohol use in sport

Alcohol as an anti-anxiety drug

Amongst athletes, participation in sports brings its own unique form of stress, not only before important contests but also due to frequent participation in competitive events. Though a certain amount of pre-competition anxiety is inevitable, the anxiety response varies enormously between individuals, with some people coping extremely poorly. Many find their own solutions to attenuate anxiety levels, without exogenous aids. Anxiety may adversely affect performance, especially in activities highly demanding of mental concentration and steadiness of limbs. This likely impairment has prompted the use of anti-anxiety drugs.

The psychological reaction to impending sports competition is variously referred to as anxiety, arousal, stress or activation. Anxiety suggests worry or emotional tension, arousal denotes a continuum from sleep to high excitement, stress implies an agent that induces strain in the organism and activation refers to the metabolic state in the "flight or fight" reaction. A moderate level of "anxiety" about the forthcoming activity is desirable to induce the right levels of harnessed motivation for action. The simpler the task the higher is the level of anxiety that can be tolerated before performance efficiency begins to fall.

Over-anxiety has a detrimental effect on the physical and psychomotor elements that comprise sports performance. In such instances anxiety-reducing strategies will have an ergogenic effect. The athlete or mentor may have to choose between mental relaxation techniques or drugs to alleviate anxiety. Where alcohol is used to reduce stress in overanxious individuals, the benefits must be balanced against any adverse effects on physical and neuromotor performance that might be introduced.

Anxiety level depends very much on the nature of the sport as well as on the individual concerned. High anxiety is mostly associated with brief and high-risk activities. Anxiety responses pre-start of competition, as reflected in emotional tachycardia, show motor-racing, ski-jumping and downhill skiing to be top of the list (Reilly, 1997).

In aiming sports, such as archery, a steady limb is needed to provide a firm platform for launching the missile at its target or to keep the weapon still.

Residual effects of alcohol may carry over to the following day, affecting training or subsequent competitive performance. There are also possibilities of tolerance to the drug with chronic use or of drug dependence developing.

Alcohol use in a social sporting context

Heavy drinking is not compatible with serious participation in sport. For the athlete, drinking is usually done only in moderation, an infrequent respite for the ascetic regimens of physical training, though the odd end of season binge may be customary. Nevertheless, drinking is a social convention in many sports where there may be peer-group pressure to take alcohol following training or competition or at club social functions. A study of rugby union players revealed high alcohol consumption, with more than 30 per cent of the athletes binge drinking at least once per week (Sekulic et al., 2014). Those individuals who can tolerate competitive stress still need to relax following competition or at times of a series of important competitions. The same applies to athletes in team sports gathered together in training camps for a sustained period. In these cases drinking alcohol is a frequent method of facilitating relaxation among athletes. The practice is sometimes condoned by the team's management as a means of "bonding" among the players. Indeed, victories are celebrated and defeats accepted by post-event drinking in many sports. In a study with elite Australian athletes, Dunn et al. (2011) found that alcohol was nominated as a drug of concern only by a small proportion of athletes.

The sensible athlete drinks moderately and occasionally, avoiding alcohol for at least 24 hours before competing. Hangovers may persist for a day and disturb concentration in sports involving complex skills.

For a healthy athlete in a good state of training, occasional drinking of alcohol in moderation will have little adverse effect. It is important to emphasize that any such occasional bouts of drinking should be restrained and should follow rather than precede training sessions.

Adverse effects of alcohol in sport and exercise

The deleterious effects of alcohol on the nervous system will have consequences for performance in sports that require fast reactions, complex decision making and highly skilled actions. It will also have an impact on hand–eye coordination, on tracking tasks, such as driving, and on vigilance tasks such as long-distance sailing. An effect on tracking tasks is that control movements lose their normal smoothness and precision and become more abrupt or jerky. At high doses of alcohol, meaningful sport becomes impractical or even dangerous.

Alcohol intoxication may adversely affect a sportsperson's dietary choices by displacing carbohydrate from the diet at a time when restoration of glycogen stores should be a priority (Maughan, 2006).

Impairment in carbohydrate synthesis post-exercise would delay the restoration of muscle glycogen stores and adversely affect endurance performance. Burke et al. (2003) showed that alcohol delayed glycogen re-synthesis the day following strenuous exercise but not when carbohydrate intake was high. Acute alcohol consumption, post-exercise, may negatively alter normal immunoendocrine function, blood flow and protein synthesis so that recovery from skeletal muscle injury may be impaired (Barnes, 2014).

Alcohol decreases peripheral vascular resistance. This response is because of the vasodilatory effect of alcohol on the peripheral blood vessels, which would increase heat loss from the surface of the skin and cause a drop in body temperature. This consequence would be dangerous if alcohol were taken in conjunction with exercise in cold conditions. Sampling whisky on the ski slopes may bring an immediate feeling of warmth but its disturbance of normal thermoregulation may put the recreational skier at risk of hypothermia. Frost-bitten mountaineers especially should avoid drinking alcohol as the peripheral vasodilation it induces would cause the body temperature to fall further. In hot conditions, alcohol is also inadvisable as it acts as a diuretic and would exacerbate problems of dehydration.

A review by Pesta et al. (2013) concluded that alcohol is a uniformly ergolytic agent that has significant detrimental effects on exercise performance and that use of alcohol during competitive activity should be minimized for athlete safety and so as to maximize athletic performance.

Alcohol and sports accidents

Peak effects on motor performance following administration of alcohol are typically observed 45-60min later but impairment is evident for up to three hours after dosing (Kelly et al., 1993). This could render the drinker susceptible to accidents if alcohol is imbibed after sports competitions before driving the journey home. Even at blood alcohol concentrations within the legal limit (about 0.03%), accident risk is increased when driving after sleep restricted to four hours the previous night (Vakulin et al., 2007) or after a prolonged period (18-21 hours) awake (Howard et al., 2007).

Alcohol can compound the hangover effects of some sleeping tablets and is likely to disturb complex skills more than simpler motor tasks performed on the morning of the next day (Kunsman et al., 1992). Attention and reaction time tasks were impaired by concentrations of temazepam and ethanol in combinations which alone did not cause decrements in performance. Subjects tend to be unaware of their reduced performance capabilities when taking these drugs in combination, a factor likely to increase injury risk. Of 402 victims of ski accidents, 20 per cent were positive for alcohol, 8.5 per cent had taken benzodiazepines and 2.5 per cent were positive for both drugs. There is also a diurnal variation in the effects of alcohol as drinking at lunch time has a more detrimental effect on psychomotor performance than alcohol taken in the evening (Horne and Gibbons, 1991). Consequently recreational skiers place themselves at increased risk of injury by drinking at lunch time rather than solely après ski.

A review by El-Sayed et al. (2005) concluded that alcohol is the most frequently used drug among athletes and that it is directly linked to the rate of injury sustained in sport events. In addition, alcohol appears to evoke detrimental effects on exercise performance capacity.

Alcohol in sport: commercial sponsorship

Apart from the specific issue of alcohol use by athletes, there is a much wider association between alcohol and sport. Palmer (2011) provides a detailed review of these wider issues, which include the commercial aspects of sponsorship and advertising in sport by manufacturers of alcoholic drinks. The social practices of spectators with associated issues of crime, violence and health are also addressed.

A UK study showed that students who play sport and who personally receive alcohol sponsorship or whose club or team receives alcohol industry sponsorship appear to have more problematic drinking behaviour than sports students who receive no sponsorship (O'Brien et al., 2014). It is interesting to note that the Fédération Internationale de Football Association (FIFA) asked Brazil to suspend a national ban on the sales of alcohol beverage in soccer stadiums during the 2014 Soccer World Cup (Caetano et al., 2012).

A study on alcohol consumption in community football clubs in Australia suggested that there were high levels of risky alcohol consumption by members leading to alcohol-related harm in the community (Rowland et al., 2015). A related study indicated that implementing a multi-strategy intervention policy to improve alcohol management practices in community sports clubs was successful (Kingsland et al., 2015).

A 2016 systematic review, assessing the evidence on the relationship between alcohol, sport's sponsorship and alcohol consumption, found that all the seven studies investigated indicated that exposure to alcohol sport sponsorship is associated with increased levels of consumption and risky drinking amongst school children and sportspeople (Brown, 2016).

21.5 Alcohol and the WADA Prohibited List

Alcohol was first included on the International Olympic Committee (IOC) Prohibited List in 1988 as part of a group of drugs referred to as "Classes of Drugs Subject to Certain Restrictions". In 2003, following the establishment of the World Anti-Doping Agency (WADA), the joint IOC/WADA Prohibited List re-defined the group of drugs that included alcohol as "Classes of Prohibited Substances in Certain Sports". This Prohibited List stated that, where the rules of the governing body so provide, tests will be conducted for ethanol. This rather loose protocol was strengthened the following year when the first WADA Prohibited List came into force on 1 January 2004. Alcohol was then classified under "Substances Prohibited in Particular Sports" with the International Federations who had requested alcohol to be prohibited being clearly identified. This classification has continued to the current, 2017 Prohibited List.

In which sports is alcohol prohibited?

In 2004, there were 14 sports in which alcohol was prohibited. There were variable threshold levels (between 0.02g/L and 0.50g/L) of alcohol being specified by some sport federations, while others instituted a complete ban. As a result of the continued annual review by International Federations, by 2017 the number of sports in which alcohol was prohibited had reduced to four and a standard threshold level of 0.10g/L established (Table 21.2).

The 2017 list of sports in which alcohol was prohibited included sports in which participation under the influence of alcohol could have serious consequences not just for the athlete but also for fellow competitors and spectators.

PREVALENCE OF ADVERSE ANALYTICAL FINDINGS FOR ALCOHOL

Although alcohol is undoubtedly used by many athletes in a social context, WADA prohibits its use in particular sports only within competition. Consequently, there have been few cases of adverse analytical findings involving alcohol from WADA accredited laboratories (Table 21.3).

Table 21.2 Particular sports in which alcohol was prohibited, according to the WADA Prohibited List (2017)

Alcohol (ethanol) is prohibited in-competition only, in the following sports. Detection will be conducted by analysis of breath and/or blood. The doping violation threshold is equivalent to a blood alcohol concentration of 0.10g/L.

• Air sports (FAI)	• Automobile (FIA)
• Archery (WA)	• Powerboating (UIM)

Table 21.3 WADA statistics for the annual number of adverse analytical findings for alcohol

Year	Number of cases
2003 to 2008	0
2009	5
2010	9
2011	5
2012	5
2013	8
2014	0
2015	0

21.6 Summary

- Alcohol is the most abused drug within society and athletes are not immune to the social conventions of using alcohol to relax, socialize and reduce stress.
- Alcohol is used as an ergogenic aid in a limited number of sports but its use in social contexts is pervasive.
- The acute and chronic effects of alcohol have potentially serious implications for the health of athletes who use it and for fellow competitors.

21.7 References

Barnes, M.J. (2014) Alcohol: Impact on sports performance and recovery in male athletes. *Sports Medicine* 44: 909–919.

Brown, K. (2016) Association between alcohol sports sponsorship and consumption: A systematic review. *Alcohol and Alcoholism* 51(6): 747–755.

Burke, L.M., Collier, G.R., Broad, E.M. et al. (2003). Effect of alcohol intake on muscle glycogen storage after prolonged exercise. *Journal of Applied Physiology* 95: 983–990.

Caetano, R., Pinsky, I. and Laranjeira, R. (2012) Should soccer and alcohol mix? Alcohol sales during the 2014 World Soccer Cup games in Brazil. *Addiction* 107: 1,722–1,723.

Dunn, M., Thomas, J.O., Swift, W. et al. (2011) Recreational substance use among elite Australian athletes. *Drug and Alcohol Review* 30: 63–68.

El-Sayed, M.S., Ali, N. and Ali, Z.E. (2005) Interaction between alcohol and exercise. *Sports Medicine* 35(3): 257–269.

Horne, J.A. and Gibbons, H. (1991). Effects on vigilance performance and sleepiness of alcohol given in the early afternoon (post lunch) vs. early evening. *Ergonomics* 34: 67–77.

Howard, M.E., Jackson, M.L., Kennedy, G.A. et al. (2007). The interaction effects of extended wakefulness and low-dose alcohol on simulated driving and vigilance. *Sleep* 30: 1,334–1,340.

Kelly, T. H., Fultin., R. W., Emurian, C. S. et al. (1993) Performance based testing for drugs of abuse: Dose and time profiles of marijuana, amphetamine, alcohol and diazepam. *Journal of Analytical Toxicology* 17: 264–272.

Kingsland, M, Wolfenden, L., Tindall, J. et al. (2015) Improving the implementation of responsible alcohol management practices by community sporting clubs: A randomised controlled trial. *Drug and Alcohol Review* 34: 447–457.

Kunsman, G. W., Manno, J. B., Przekop, M.A. et al. (1992). The effects of temazepam and ethanol on human psychomotor performance. *European Journal of Clinical Pharmacology* 43: 603–611.

Malik, P., Gasser, R.W., Kemmler, G. et al. (2009). Low bone mineral density and impaired bone metabolism in young adolescent patients without cirrhosis: A cross-sectional study. *Alcoholism: Clinical Experimental Research* 33(2): 375–381.

Maughan, R.J. (2006). Alcohol and football. *Journal of Sports Science* 24: 741–748.

O'Brien, K.S. Ferris, J., Greenlees, I. et al. (2014) Alcohol industry sponsorship and hazardous drinking in UK university students who play sport. *Addiction* 109: 1,647–1,654.

Palmer, C. (2011) Key themes and research agendas in the sport-alcohol nexus. *Journal of Sport and Social Issues* 35: 168–185.

Pedersen, J.O., Heitmann, B.L., Schnoir, P. et al. (2008). The combined influence of leisure-time physical activity and weekly alcohol intake on fatal ischaemic heart disease and all-cause mortality. *European Heart Journal* 29: 204–212.

Pesta, D.H., Angadi, S.S., Burtscher, M. and Roberts, C.K. (2013) The effects of caffeine, nicotine, ethanol and tetrahydrocannabinol on exercise performance. *Nutrition and Metabolism* 10: 71–86.

Reilly, T. (1997). Alcohol: Its influence in sport and exercise. In T. Reilly and M. Orme (eds) *The Clinical Pharmacology of Sport and Exercise*. Elsevier, Amsterdam, 281–290.

Rowland, B., Tindall, J., Wolfenden, L. et al. (2015) Alcohol management practices in community football clubs: Association with risky drinking at the clubs and overall hazardous alcohol consumption. *Drug and Alcohol Review* 34: 438–446.

Sekulic, D., Bjelanovic, L., Pehar, M. et al. (2014) Substance use and misuse and potential doping behaviour in rugby union players. *Research in Sports Medicine* 22: 226–239.

Suter, P.M. and Schutz, P. (2008) The effect of exercise, alcohol or both combined on health and physical performance. *International Journal of Obesity (London)* 32(Suppl. 6): 548–552.

Vakulin, A., Baulk, S.D., Catcheside, P.G. et al. (2007). Effect of moderate sleep deprivation and low-dose alcohol on driving simulator performance and perception in young men. *Sleep* 30: 1,327–1,333.

Van der Horst Graat, J.M., Terpstra, J.S., Kok, F.J. et al. (2007). Alcohol, smoking and physical activity related to respiratory infections in elderly people. *Journal of Nutrition Health and Aging* 11: 80–85.

Chapter 22

Beta blockers

David R. Mottram

22.1 Introduction

Beta blockers are drugs that are used to treat a wide variety of clinical conditions, primarily associated with the cardiovascular system. Pharmacological properties of beta blockers, such as alleviating anxiety and reducing hand tremor, are used by some athletes in order to improve performance. Beta blockers are only prohibited in particular sports, where these properties may be advantageous.

22.2 What are beta blockers?

The first beta blockers were synthesised by the pharmaceutical industry in 1958. They have since become one of the most frequently prescribed classes of drugs providing therapeutic support for a wide range of clinical conditions, principally associated with the cardiovascular system.

Mode of action of beta blockers

Beta blockers antagonise beta receptors, one of the subclasses of adrenoreceptors through which nordadrenaline (norepinephrine) and adrenaline (epinephrine) produce their effects in the body in both the central nervous system (CNS), where they act as neurotransmitters and in the periphery, where noradrenaline is a neurotransmitter in the sympathetic nervous system and adrenaline is a hormone, released from the adrenal medulla during times of stress.

Adrenoceptors are sub-classified into alpha (α) and beta (β). The β-adrenoceptors are further sub-classified into at least three types of receptor β_1, β_2, and β_3. These receptors are found in a variety of tissues and organs of the body, the principal ones being shown in Table 22.1. This table also shows the pharmacological effects that occur when beta blockers occupy these receptors. Clearly, the effects of beta blockers are wide ranging.

The pharmaceutical industry has developed beta blockers that act selectively on particular sub-classes of β-adrenoceptors, in an attempt to target their therapeutic action more precisely and to reduce unwanted side effects. Table 22.2 lists some of the more common beta blockers, indicating their respective selectivity for beta receptor subclasses.

In addition to receptor selectivity, there are a number of other characteristics that distinguish one beta blocker from another. Some beta blockers, such as oxprenolol, pindolol, acebutolol and celiprolol, possess intrinsic sympathomimetic activity (ISA), or partial agonist activity, which represents the capacity of these beta blockers to stimulate as well as

Table 22.1 The main tissues and organs of the body (other than the brain) that contain
β-adrenoceptors and the pharmacological effects produced by beta blockers

Organ	Receptor type	Principal effects of beta blockers
Heart	β_1	Decrease rate and force of beating
Arteries	β_2	Constriction
Veins	β_2	Constriction
Respiratory tract	β_2	Bronchoconstriction
Gastrointestinal tract	β_2	Increase motility
Bladder	β_2	Contraction of the bladder wall
Kidney	β_1	Inhibition of renin secretion
Skeletal muscle	β_2	Reduction in tremor
		Reduction of glycogenolysis
Liver	β_2	Reduction of glycogenolysis
Fat tissue	β_3	Reduction of lipolysis

Table 22.2 Beta blockers and their receptor selectivity

Non-selective beta blockers

Alprenolol
Bunolol
Carteolol
Levobunolol
Metipranolol
Nadolol
Oxprenolol
Pindolol
Propranolol
Sotalol
Timolol

Selective beta blockers (cardioselective for $\beta 1$-adrenoceptors)

Acebutolol
Atenolol
Betaxolol
Bisoprolol
Celiprolol
Esmolol
Metoprolol
Nebivolol

Combined alpha/beta blockers

Carvedilol
Labetalol

block adrenergic receptors. They tend to produce less slowing of the heart (bradycardia)
than other beta blockers and may also reduce coldness of extremities, a common side effect
of beta blockers (Head, 1999).

Beta blockers have variable degrees of solubility between lipid and water phases. Atenolol,
celiprolol, nadolol and sotalol are the most water soluble. This property restricts their ability to cross the blood brain barrier, and therefore decreases centrally mediated side effects
(Turner, 1983).

22.3 Clinical uses of beta blockers

The main clinical uses for beta blockers are shown in Table 22.3.

Many of these uses relate to the effects of beta blockers on the cardiovascular system. Blocking the β_1-adrenoceptors in the heart reduces cardiac rate and force of beating, an effect of benefit in the treatment of patients with angina pectoris. This condition is characterised by severe chest pain due to insufficient oxygen reaching cardiac muscle, during exertion, in patients with compromised cardiac arteries. Beta blockers reduce heart rate thereby delaying the onset of an anginal attack and improving exercise tolerance. Blockade of β_1-adrenoceptors in the heart is important in the management of some types of cardiac dysrhythmias, particularly supraventricular tachycardias. Bisoprolol and carvedilol are particularly useful in stable heart failure. Beta blockers are used to reduce blood pressure in hypertension. They achieve this antihypertensive effect through reduction in heart rate, alteration of baroreceptor reflex sensitivity, depression of renin secretion and possibly central effects, particularly with those beta blockers that can easily cross the blood-brain barrier.

Beta blockers have been shown to be effective in preventing secondary heart attacks in patients who have experienced a myocardial infarction, although for some patients with co-morbidities such as uncontrolled heart failure, bradyarrhythmias or obstructive airways disease, beta blockers are contraindicated.

Phaeochromocytoma is a benign cancer of the adrenal medulla, leading to increased release of the hormone, adrenaline. Beta blockers, in combination with alpha blockers are used to block the systemic effects of this over production of adrenaline.

Migraine is a condition that is treated prophylactically by beta blockers through effects on blood vessels. Not all migraine sufferers respond to beta blockers and more effective treatment regimes are available.

Glaucoma, a condition characterised by increased intra-ocular pressure in the eye, is treated by beta blockers. Although their mode of action is not fully understood, beta blockers are one of the first-line classes of drugs for this condition.

Beta blockers are used in the management of anxiety. The most widely used class of drugs to treat anxiety, the benzodiazepines, treat the psychological symptoms of anxiety, such as worry, tension and fear, mediated through central nervous system. Beta blockers, on the other hand, treat the symptoms of anxiety mediated through the peripheral autonomic nervous system. They decrease heart rate by blocking β_1-adrenoceptors, thereby reducing palpitations, and reduce hand tremor mediated through β_2-adrenoceptors in

Table 22.3 The main clinical conditions for which beta blockers are used

Cardiovascular
  Hypertension
  Angina pectoris
  Cardiac dysrhythmias
  Heart failure
  Prevention of secondary myocardial infarction

Other uses
  Phaeochromocytoma (benign cancer of the adrenal medulla)
  Migraine
  Glaucoma
  Anxiety
  Essential tremor

skeletal muscle (Bowman and Anden, 1981). This, in turn, may prevent the onset of worry and fear.

Essential tremor is a condition characterised by an involuntary rhythmic shaking of a part of the body, most commonly the arms, hands and head. Beta blockers, by blocking the β_2-adrenoceptors in skeletal muscle, can reduce the severity of tremor, particularly in the hands.

Side effects of beta blockers

Common side effects associated with beta blockers are fatigue, due to reduced cardiac output and reduced muscle perfusion in exercise, coldness in the extremities (hands and feet) due to peripheral vasoconstriction and sleep disturbances (Cruickshank, 1981). Those beta blockers with associated ISA are less likely to produce cold extremities whilst those which are water-soluble tend not to cross the blood-brain-barrier and are therefore less likely to produce sleep disturbances such as nightmares, insomnia and occasionally depression.

Beta blockers are contraindicated in asthmatic patients because they block the β_2-adrenoceptors in the respiratory tract, leading to bronchoconstriction with associated airways resistance. This effect is less pronounced in those beta blockers that have selectivity for β_1-adrenoceptors (see Table 22.2) but it should be noted that at higher doses, these beta blockers lose their cardioselectivity.

Hypoglycaemia is associated with beta blocker use. Glucose release in response to adrenaline is important to diabetic patients and to other patients prone to hypoglycaemic attacks. Hypoglycaemia triggers symptoms to warn patients of the urgent need for carbohydrate. Beta blockers reduce these symptoms, therefore beta blockers are contraindicated in patients with poorly controlled diabetes.

22.4 History of beta blockers in sport

Beta blockers are of potential benefit in sports where hand tremor and high anxiety play a role.

Beta blockers were, for many years, first line drugs for the treatment of a number of cardiovascular diseases such as angina and hypertension. Under this pretext, a number of high ranking professional snooker players tested positive for beta blockers at the 1987 World Professional Snooker Championships, as had occurred a few years earlier by competitors in shooting events in the 1984 Olympic Games in Los Angeles (Reilly, 2005). The argument that beta blockers were indispensable drugs for these conditions was, however, unsustainable as other, equally effective first line drugs were available to treat the cardiovascular conditions in question.

At the 1984 Games, the IOC Medical Commission, aware that some athletes were taking beta blockers to improve performance in shooting events, demanded a medical certificate to justify their use. These "Medical Certificates" were submitted by 18 athletes (Fitch, 2012).

Beta blockers were added to the IOC Prohibited List in 1985, as one of the major classes of prohibited substances. It was clear that the pharmacological effects of beta blockers would have an adverse, rather than enhancing, effect on performance in most sports. This led the IOC Medical Commission to test for beta blockers only in high-risk sports where beta blockers may be used for their anti-anxiety effect or in sports where hand steadiness was important. This policy was adopted at the Summer and Winter Olympic Games from 1988 to 1993 (Reilly, 2005). Thereafter the IOC re-classified beta blockers from Section I, Doping

Classes, to Section II, Class of Drugs Subject to Certain Restrictions, where they were only prohibited in specified sports. This policy continued when WADA took over responsibility for the Prohibited List in 2004 and beta blockers were classed as Classes of Prohibited Substances in Certain Sports. Current (2017) WADA regulations are shown in Table 22.4.

Case studies relating to beta blockers

There have been relatively few cases involving beta blockers.

Box 22.1   Kim Jong-Su (2008)

During the 2008 Beijing Olympic Games, the North Korean shooter, Kim Jong-Su was stripped of two medals and was expelled from the Games when he tested positive for the beta blocker, propranolol (Wendt, 2009).

22.5 The action and use of beta blockers in sport

Use of beta blockers in sport

Stress and anxiety are common responses to competitive sport. Therapeutically, benzodiazepines are widely used as tranquillisers and anti-anxiety drugs. They exert their effect in the CNS through inhibition of the release of a number of neurotransmitters, most notably serotonin (Reilly, 2005). However, beta blockers are usually preferred as anti-anxiety agents in sport as they produce their effects peripherally rather than centrally and do not possess the addictive properties of benzodiazepines. Their peripheral anti-anxiety effects are principally associated with blockade of β_1-adrenoceptors in the heart where they reduce stress-induced tachycardia and by the reduction of limb tremor through blockade of β_2-adrenoceptors in skeletal muscle. With respect to the reduction in tremor, a study on the effect of oxprenolol on pistol shooting found a significant improvement in shooting scores but only in slow-firing events (Antal and Good, 1980).

In 1986, Kruse et al. showed that there was a clear (13.4 per cent) improvement in the performance of pistol shooters using metoprolol compared with placebo control. The most skilled marksmen showed the greatest improvement. No correlation was found between shooting improvement and cardiovascular variables, such as heart rate and blood pressure, leading the authors to conclude that the improvement was caused by an effect of metoprolol on hand tremor.

One particular sport has been associated with high levels of anxiety that has led to a specific term to describe the phenomenon, the "Yips" in golf (Smith et al., 2003). It has been defined as a motor phenomenon of involuntary movements affecting golfers and is associated with high stress levels performance anxiety. The physical symptoms of the yips are tremor, jerks or freezing of the hands and forearms, particularly associated with putting strokes. For this reason, some golfers have used alcohol and/or beta blockers to alleviate the symptoms. In 2009, WADA added golf to the list of sports in which beta blockers are prohibited within competition, at the request of the International Golf Federation. In the same year, Doug Barron became the first golfer to test positive for beta blockers, although he argued that he took beta blockers and testosterone for legitimate medical needs (Chamblee, 2012).

Beta blockers are also prohibited in sports requiring motor vehicle control (Shrivastav et al., 2010). These authors describe the various analytical methods available for the detection of beta blockers in plasma and urine. More recent analytical techniques for detecting beta blockers have been described by Santos et al. (2015).

Adverse effects of beta blockers in sport

Beta blockers produce metabolic effects including a decrease in the rate of glycogenolysis in skeletal muscle. This may have implications for performance at sub-maximal levels. Similarly, in sustained exercise, the inhibition of glycogenolysis in liver will affect performance by reducing blood glucose levels (Reilly, 2005). These effects on glycogenolysis are mediated through blockade of β_2-adrenoceptors and are more evident with non-selective beta blockers such as propranolol. Prolonged exercise may be adversely affected by the inhibition of lipolysis that is produced by beta blockers. The availability of free fatty acids is reduced thereby causing an earlier onset of fatigue. A thorough description of the metabolic effects of beta blockers in exercise can be found in a review paper by Head (1999).

A study by Rusko et al. (1980) examined the effect of beta blockers on short-term high-intensity exercise. A series of anaerobic tasks were performed by subjects comparing the beta blocker, oxprenolol, with placebo control. Oxprenolol reduced power output on a cycle ergometer with a concomitant reduction in heart rate and peak blood lactate. The drug had no effect on isometric strength of leg extension, stair running or vertical jumping. In a study on alpine skiers, it was reported that short-term maximal muscle power, recorded during a 30-second submaximal cycling test, was reduced by beta blockers (Karlsson et al., 1983). Beta blockers have been shown to reduce maximal oxygen uptake (VO_{2max}) (Head, 1999).

In prescribing medication for hypertensive patients who participate in sport, Derman (2008) recommended caution in the use of beta blockers as they are not the most efficacious class of antihypertensives and their effects on exercise are detrimental to competition.

22.6 Beta blockers and the WADA Prohibited List

WADA regulations with respect to beta blockers

The 2017 WADA Prohibited List classes beta blockers under "substances prohibited in particular sports" (Table 22.4).

For most of these sports, beta blockers are prohibited in-competition only. However, in the sports of Archery and Shooting, beta blockers are also prohibited out-of-competition. The list of sports reflects the potential benefit of beta blockers in producing anti-anxiety and anti-tremor effects.

Prevalence of adverse findings for beta blockers

Annual statistics from WADA accredited laboratories show that there are few adverse analytical findings (AAFs) for beta blockers (Table 22.5).

The sports in which beta blockers were identified are shown in Figure 22.1.

Table 22.4 2017 WADA regulations for beta blockers

Beta-blockers are prohibited in-competition only, in the following sports, and also prohibited out-of-competition where indicated.

- Archery (WA)*
- Automobile (FIA)
- Billiards (all disciplines) (WCBS)
- Darts (WDF)
- Golf (IGF)
- Shooting (ISSF, IPC)*
- Skiing/snowboarding (FIS) in ski jumping, freestyle aerials/halfpipe and snowboard halfpipe/big air
- Underwater sports (CMAS) in constant-weight apnoea with or without fins, dynamic apnoea with and without fins, free immersion apnoea, jump blue apnoea, spearfishing, static apnoea, target shooting, and variable weight apnoea.

*Also prohibited out-of-competition

Reports of AAFs include findings that underwent the Therapeutic Use Exemption (TUE) approval process. However, in general, beta blockers are not used as first-line therapy in athletes because of adverse effects on exercise (Oliveira et al., 2010).

It should be noted that beta blockers are first-line drugs in the treatment of the eye condition, glaucoma. Ophthalmologists need to be aware of the need for a Therapeutic Use Exemption certificate for athletes receiving eye drops containing beta blockers, particularly within competition, as reported by Nicholson et al. (2012) at the time of the London 2012 Olympic and Paralympic Games.

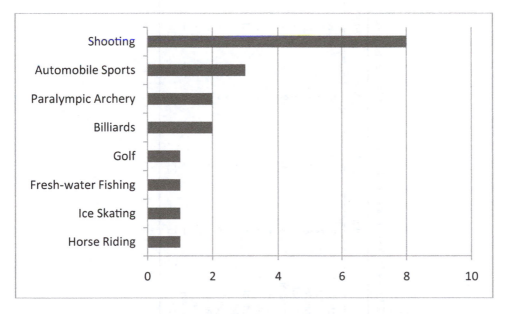

Figure 22.1 Sports in which beta blockers were identified through WADA test results, for 2015

Table 22.5 WADA statistics for the number of adverse analytical findings for beta blockers (2006–2015)

	2006	2007	2008	2009	2010	2011	2012	2013	2014	2015
Atenolol	9	3	6	8	4	4	2	3	6	–
Bisoprolol	2	6	5	7	6	5	–	7	5	7
Metoprolol	6	6	4	10	4	4	5	5	3	6
Acebutolol	–	–	2	–	2	–	–	–	–	–
Propranolol	6	8	9	11	10	4	–	8	7	3
Carteolol	–	1	–	–	–	–	–	1	–	–
Sotalol	–	–	–	1	1	–	–	–	–	–
Carvedilol	3	2	1	–	–	–	–	–	–	–
Timolol	2	1	–	–	–	–	–	–	1	–
Betaxolol	–	–	3	–	–	–	–	–	–	–
Labetalol	–	–	1	–	–	2	2	–	–	–
Nadolol	–	–	–	–	2	–	–	–	–	1
Celiprolol	–	–	–	–	–	1	–	1	–	–
Total	28	27	31	38	30	21	13	25	25	19

22.7 Summary

- Beta blockers are used widely to treat medical conditions, particularly associated with the cardiovascular system.
- There have been few cases of misuse of beta blockers in sport.
- For most sports, the adverse effects of beta blockers outweigh any potential performance enhancing effect.
- WADA regulations restrict the use of beta blockers in particular sports, where reduction of hand tremor and high levels of anxiety may be beneficial.

22.8 References

Antal, L.C. and Good, C.S. (1980) Effects of oxprenolol on pistol shooting under stress. *Practitioner* 224: 755–760.

Bowman, W. and Anden, N. (1981) Effects of adrenergic activators and inhibitors on the skeletal muscles. In L. Szekeres (ed.) *Adrenergic activators and inhibitors*. Berlin, Springer, 47–128.

Chamblee, B. (2012) Keeping it clean. *Golf Magazine* 54(11): 120.

Cruickshank, J.M. (1981) β-blockers, bradycardia and adverse effects. *Acta Therapeutica* 7: 309–321.

Derman, W. (2008) Antihypertensive medications and exercise. *International SportsMed Journal* 9(1): 32–38.

Fitch, K. (2012) Proscribed drugs at the Olympic Games: Permitted use and misuse (doping) by athletes. *Clinical Medicine* 12(3): 257–260.

Head, A. (1999) Exercise metabolism and β-blocker therapy. *Sports Medicine* 27(2): 81–96.

Karlsson, J., Kjessel, T. and Kaiser, P. (1983) Alpine skiing and acute beta-blockade. *International Journal of Sports Medicine* 4(3): 190–193.

Kruse, P., Ladefoged, J., Nielsen, U. et al. (1986) Beta-blockade used in precision sports: Effect on pistol shooting performance. *Journal of Applied Physiology* 61(2): 417–420.

Nicholson, R.G.H., Thomas, G.P.L., Potter, M.J. et al. (2012) London 2012: Prescribing for athletes in ophthalmology. *Eye* 26(8): 1,036–1,038.

Oliveira, L.P.J. and Lawless, C.E. (2010) Hypertension update and cardiovascular risk reduction in physically active individuals and athletes. *Physician and Sportsmedicine* 38(1): 11–20.

Reilly, T.R. (2005) Alcohol, antianxiety drugs and sport. In D.R. Mottram (ed.) *Drugs in Sport*, 4th edition. London, Routledge, 258–287.

Rusko, H., Kantola, H., Luhtanen, R. et al. (1980) Effect of beta-blockade on performances requiring force, velocity, coordination and/or anaerobic metabolism. *Journal of Sports Medicine and Physical Fitness* 20: 139–144.

Santos, M.G., Tavares, I.M.C., Boralli, V.B. and Figueiredo, E.C. (2015) Direct doping analysis of beta blocker drugs from urinary samples by online molecular imprinted solid-phase extraction coupled with liquid chromatography/mass spectrometry. *Analyst* 140(8): 2,696–2,703.

Shrivastav, P.S., Buha, S.M., Shailesh, M. et al. (2010) Detection and quantitation of beta blockers in plasma and urine. *Bioanalysis* 2(2): 263–276.

Smith, A.M., Adler, C.H., Crews, D. et al. (2003) The "Yips" in golf: A continuum between a focal dystonia and choking. *Sports Medicine* 33(1): 13–31.

Turner, P. (1983) β-blockade and the human central nervous system. *Drugs* 25(Suppl 2): 262–273.

Wendt, J.T. (2009) Reflections on Beijing. *Entertainments and Sports Lawyer* 26(4): 10–18.

Substances and methods permitted in sport

Chapter 23

Non-steroidal anti-inflammatory drugs

Nick Wojek

23.1 Introduction

Musculoskeletal and joint injuries are frequently encountered in sport and lead to time lost from training and competition. In most instances, these types of injuries are minor but they can account for numerous days of inactivity and ultimately lead to losses in performance. The pressure to perform or make selection for a team may tempt athletes to continue training or competing with such injuries. The challenge faced in sports medicine is to find interventions that hasten an athlete's return to activity without compromising tissue repair.

One common intervention used in the management of acute or chronic musculoskeletal injuries is the use of non-steroidal anti-inflammatory drugs (NSAIDs). They are used to control pain and to limit the amount and duration of inflammation. There is a general acceptance by athletes that exercise and pain coexist which has led to the widespread use of NSAIDs within sport at all levels. Although the use of NSAIDs has become a widely-accepted treatment of minor musculoskeletal injuries in sport, there is a growing view that NSAIDs have only modest results in the management of such injuries and that some athletes use NSAIDs without a clear clinical need.

This chapter will describe how NSAIDs work, explore their effectiveness, and investigate their prevalence of use amongst athletes. Finally, some ethical considerations about the use of NSAIDs within sport will be presented.

23.2 What are NSAIDs?

NSAIDs possess analgesic, anti-inflammatory, antipyretic and antithrombotic properties (Joint Formulary Committee, 2017a). They exert their effects by inhibiting cyclo-oxygenase (COX) enzyme activity which is involved in the synthesis of prostaglandins from arachidonic acid (Figure 23.1). NSAID inhibition of COX enzyme activity causes a decrease in the formation of prostaglandins which in turn diminishes the inflammatory response. Prostaglandins are mediators of the inflammatory process as they initiate vasodilation, increase capillary permeability, and attract inflammatory cells to areas of cell damage leading to pain and inflammation (Smith et al., 1991; Mitchell et al., 1995). They also have important cardiovascular, renal and gastrointestinal (GI) regulatory functions (Warden, 2009).

NSAIDs are categorised by their selectivity for inhibiting the activity of the two isoforms of COX; COX-1 and COX-2. COX-1 is the constitutive form which is expressed in a variety of cells including endothelial, gastric mucosal, blood platelet and kidney cells. COX-2 is inducible and becomes over expressed in cases of inflammation such as when rheumatoid

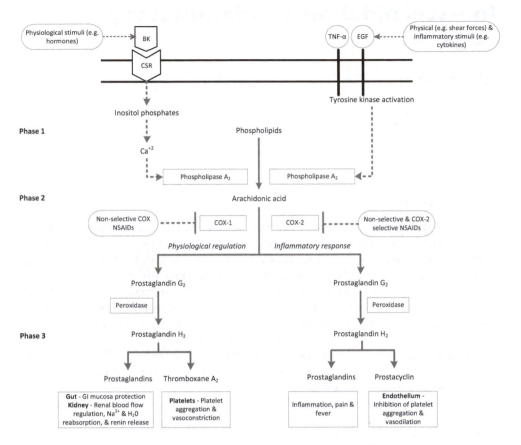

Figure 23.1 Biosynthesis of prostaglandins and the mode of action of NSAIDs

arthritis occurs or following skeletal muscle damage. Non-selective NSAIDs inhibit both COX-1 and COX-2 activity to some degree whereas selective COX-2 inhibitors predominately inhibit COX-2 enzyme activity (Figure 23.1).

23.3 Clinical uses and efficacy

NSAIDs are administered by oral, topical, intramuscular, and less commonly by intravenous routes. They are routinely used to relieve pain following operative procedures and when associated with fever, headaches, migraines, and dysmenorrhea (Day and Graham, 2013). Low-dose aspirin, unlike other NSAIDs, is prescribed to individuals at high risk of having a heart attack or stroke as it has specific anti-platelet effects that reduce the likelihood of these cardiovascular events from occurring (Joint Formulary Committee, 2017b). NSAIDs are also useful as adjunctive medication in the treatment of rheumatic conditions such as rheumatoid arthritis, osteoarthritis, gout and lupus. There are over 20 NSAIDs available for clinical use in the UK, some of which are available for general purchase (Table 23.1).

In sport, NSAIDs are used to treat a wide range of acute musculoskeletal injuries such as ligament sprains, ligament and muscle-tendon strains, muscle contusions and muscle

Table 23.1   Examples of selective and non-selective COX inhibitors available in the UK (data obtained
from the following medicine databases: Medicines.org.uk and MHRA.gov.uk, 2017)

Type	Non-proprietary name	Proprietary name
Non-selective NSAIDs (only available as POM)	Aceclofenac	Preservex™
	Acemetacin	Emflex™
	Dexibuprofen	Seractil™
	Dexketoprofen	Keral™
	Etodolac	Eccoxolac™, Etopan™, Lodine™
	Indometacin	Indocid™, Indolar™
	Ketorolac	Acular™, Toradol™
	Ketoprofen	Axorid™, Larafen™, Oruvail™, Powergel™, Tiloket™, Valket™
	Mefenamic acid	Ponstan™
	Nabumetone	Reliflex™
	Piroxicam	Feldene™
	Tenoxicam	Mobiflex™
	Tiaprofenic acid	Surgam™
	Tolfenamic acid	Clotam™
Non-selective NSAIDs (available as GSL, P, or POM)	Aspirin (GSL, P, POM)	Anadin™, Asasantin™, Atransipar™, Beechams™, Codis™, Danamep™, Disprin™, Migramax™, Molita™, Nu-Seals™, Radian™, Resprin™
	Diclofenac (P, POM)	Adacium™, Arthrotec™, Dicloflex™, Diclomax™, Econac™, Fenactol™, Masidemen™, Motifene™, Rheumatac™, Rhumalgan™, Solaraze™, Volsaid™, Voltarol™
	Flurbiprofen (P, POM)	Froben™, Ocufen™, Strefen™
	Ibuprofen (GSL, P, POM)	Anadin™, Brufen™, Calprofen™, Cuprofen™, Feminax™, Fenbid™, Fenpaed™, Flarin™, Hedex™, Ibuderm™, Ibugel™, Ibuleve™, Ibumousse™, Ibuspray™, Lemsip™, Nurofen™, Nuromol™, Pedea™, Phorpain™, Radian B™, RobiCold™, Soleve™, Solpadeine™, Sudafed™
	Naproxen (P, POM)	Feminax™, Naprosyn™, Stirlescent™, Vimovo™
Selective COX-2 inhibitors (only available as POM)	Celecoxib	Celebrex™
	Etoricoxib	Arcoxia™
	Parecoxib	Dynastat™

POM – prescription only medicine; P – pharmacy; GSL – general sales list

soreness (Alkmekinders, 1999; Paoloni et al., 2009). They are also used in painful chronic musculoskeletal conditions such as osteoarthritis, tenosynovitis, inflammatory bursitis and soft tissue injuries involving nerve impingement (Alkmekinders, 1999; Paoloni et al., 2009). These acute and chronic injuries provoke an inflammatory response that results in pain, stiffness, swelling and consequently a loss of function. Athletes require analgesic drugs to inhibit the pain component of the injury. However, as these injuries are also normally associated with an inflammatory element, the logical choice is to use a NSAID instead of an analgesic to counter both components together. The inflammatory process at times can also be excessive and cause oedema, resulting in anoxia and further cell death (Paoloni et al., 2009). In these instances, NSAIDs may be beneficial by acting to restrict the amount of inflammation and oedema that appears.

Inflammation is an important step in the healing process of injury as it facilitates the removal of cellular debris and damaged tissue which allows healing to begin. There is increasing evidence, albeit mainly from animal studies, that NSAIDs have a deleterious effect on long-term tissue regeneration as a result of preventing inflammation. Indeed, long-term tendon (Marsolais et al., 2003; Cohen et al., 2006), ligament (Elder et al., 2001; Warden et al., 2006) and muscle (Thorsson et al., 1998; Shen et al., 2005) healing has been found to be impaired in animal models with acute injury. Regular use may also impair bone healing following fracture due to the inhibition of COX-2 (Simon and O'Connor, 2007; Geusens et al., 2013).

Knowledge of the effect of NSAID use on tissue healing in humans is largely unknown. Whilst animal data may have limited translation to the clinical setting, the clinical implications of animal models infers that in humans prolonged use will likely enhance injury susceptibility, impair mechanical strength and delay injury repair. There is also a potential concern that prolonged use of NSAIDs may impair the adaptive response to exercise by impairing protein metabolism (Trappe et al., 2002) and satellite cell activity (Mackey et al., 2007). Many athletes are thought to take NSAIDs prophylactically, which may be contraindicative to the aim of resistance training, although this has yet to be proven (Warden, 2009). In contrast, short-term use of NSAIDs does not seem to have a detrimental effect on post-exercise protein synthesis in humans despite a detrimental effect in animal models (Schoenfield, 2012; Morelli et al., 2017).

NSAID use is controversial in the treatment of injuries where inflammation is not the primary feature (Magra and Maffulli, 2006; Paoloni et al., 2009). In chronic tendinopathies, NSAIDs are used with the primary goal to relieve pain, which may lead to further damage if individuals ignore the early symptoms of the injury due to pain masking (Magra and Maffulli, 2006). In such scenarios, use of a NSAID over paracetamol (acetaminophen) is questionable since inflammation is not present and paracetamol has an analgesic action comparable to NSAIDs, but with fewer potential side effects (Woo et al., 2005; Dalton and Schweinie, 2006). Furthermore, evidence-based working groups on pain management recommend using paracetamol as first line treatment in chronic musculoskeletal pain management (Schnitzer, 2006; Paoloni et al., 2009).

23.4 Adverse effects

NSAIDs are not without their adverse effects, especially when administered at high doses or for a prolonged period. The use of non-selective NSAIDs can lead to gastrointestinal (GI) adverse effects, including dyspepsia, haemorrhage, intestinal bleeding, intestinal cramps, peptic ulceration, and perforation (Wolfe et al., 1999; Michels et al., 2012). These adverse effects occur due to the direct toxic effects of NSAIDs on the gastroduodenal mucosa and their indirect effects whereby they decrease the synthesis of prostaglandins that normally protect the gastroduodenal mucosa from hydrochloric acid damage (Schoen and Vender, 1989; Wolfe et al., 1999).

Recently, selective COX-2 inhibitors have been introduced to clinical practice with the aim of inhibiting the formation of inflammatory prostaglandins without inhibiting COX-1 activity. A lower incidence of adverse GI effects has been observed with the use of selective COX-2 inhibitors compared to traditional non-selective NSAIDs (Deeks et al., 2002; Takemoto et al., 2008). However, COX-2 inhibitors have also been associated with cardiovascular events as they disturb the prostacyclin-thromboxane balance, thereby increasing the risk of the development of pro-thrombotic states (Burnier, 2005; Warden, 2005; Grosser et al., 2017). The adverse cardiovascular effect profile of rofecoxib has even led this COX-2 inhibitor to be withdrawn from the market (Burnier, 2005; Day and Graham, 2013). It is unknown whether this is an isolated drug effect or a class-specific problem.

NSAIDs are known to have adverse effects on kidney function. Acute renal changes during exercise are thought to be regulated predominantly via COX-2 inhibition as selective COX-2 inhibitors and non-selective NSAIDs both induce significant inhibition of free water clearance (Baker et al., 2005). The occurrence of renal dysfunction in the form of hyponatremia has been observed during endurance (Walker et al., 1994; Baker et al., 2005) and ultra-endurance exercise (Wharam et al., 2006; Page et al., 2007; Lipman et al., 2017) in athletes consuming either selective or non-selective NSAIDs. Furthermore, a combination of NSAID use and dehydration during ultra-endurance races may exacerbate renal injury (Lipman et al., 2017).

Changes in renal function as a result of prolonged use of NSAIDs may also lead to renal failure. In 2007, Croatian footballer Ivan Klasnić suffered kidney failure, which he associated with the prolonged use of NSAIDs to recover from injury (McGrath, 2012).

Topical NSAIDs in the form of creams, gels, sprays and patches may limit some of these adverse effects. Topical preparations are appealing to use as plasma levels remain low reducing the likelihood of adverse effects, and these preparations show good penetration of the drug through the skin to the underlying tissues (Singh and Roberts, 1994). Clinical trials generally demonstrate that topical NSAIDs are slightly more effective than topical placebo preparations when used to relieve musculoskeletal pain and are without the associated side effects of systemic NSAIDs (Massey et al., 2010).

23.5 Prevalence of use and ethical issues of NSAID use within sport

Reports identifying the frequent use of NSAIDs by athletes are well documented. Approximately one in four athletes drug tested at the Sydney 2000 Olympic Games declared the use of a NSAID with use occurring within three days of Doping Control (Corrigan and Kazlauskas, 2003). The estimated frequency of NSAID use decreased at the Athens 2004 Olympic Games to one in ten athletes drug tested, although NSAIDs were still the most declared type of medication (Tsitsimpikou et al., 2009). High incidences of NSAID use were also reported at the XV Pan-American Games (Da Silva, 2011). In addition to multi-sport events, just over half of all male and female football players at some point during each of the last four FIFA World Cups (2002–2014) have been prescribed with a NSAID (Tscholl and Dvorak, 2012; Tscholl et al., 2015; Vaso et al., 2015).

Although these reports indicate that NSAIDs are the most commonly used class of medication by athletes, prevalence of use seems to differ depending on the type of sport. Elite Finnish athletes competing in speed and power sports were found to be more frequent users of NSAIDs than athletes in endurance or motor skill based sports (Alaranta et al., 2006).

Similarly, international-level athletes competing in power and sprint disciplines in track and field athletics declared using more NSAIDs than middle- and long-distance runners (Tscholl et al., 2010). Team sports (e.g. football, handball, volleyball) and sports involving the extensive use of upper and lower limbs (e.g. baseball, fencing, gymnastics, rowing, softball, tennis) appear to have the highest incidence of NSAID use even above power and speed based sports according to data gathered from the 1996 and 2000 Canadian Olympic teams (Huang et al., 2006), and medication declarations monitored over a four-year period from Doping Control forms analysed by the Ghent WADA-accredited laboratory (van Thuyne and Delbeke, 2008).

The above reports do not explore the reasons why NSAIDs are the most frequently used type of medication amongst athletes. In a comparison study, it was estimated that athletes use approximately four-fold more NSAIDs than age-matched controls from the general population (Alaranta et al., 2006). Such higher usage rates are likely to be primarily reflective of the greater occurrence of musculoskeletal injuries because of the physical demands of sport over normal daily activities, and common disorders encountered such as fever, headaches, and migraines. The specific injury profile (i.e. the rate of acute or chronic injuries) and the physical demands of a sport are also likely to account for some of the observed differences between the types of sports in which higher rates of use are observed.

There is also the potential for the overuse of NSAIDs within the athlete population. Athletes have relatively unrestricted access to these drugs as many can be purchased over the counter or via the internet, and the class of drug itself is not regulated by the World Anti-Doping Agency (WADA, 2017). It has become apparent that some athletes use at least two different preparations concurrently (Corrigan and Kazlauskas, 2003; Tscholl et al., 2008; Tsitsimpikou et al., 2009), which increases the risk of experiencing side effects. In other cases, use has been found to occur on a prophylaxis basis in an attempt to prevent the onset of pain associated with muscle contusions and the delayed-onset of muscle soreness (Warner et al., 2002; Tscholl et al., 2008; Gorski et al., 2011). Use may even form part of an athlete's pre-competition routine or superstition rather than due to an actual therapeutic need (Warden, 2009).

Worryingly, it appears that athletes have a very limited knowledge and awareness regarding the effects of NSAIDs, their indications for use, and possible side effects (Gorski et al., 2011; Küster et al., 2013). More effort is required to educate athletes about the efficacy of use and adverse effects of NSAIDs in order to address the growing concerns about usage rates and the incidence of adverse effects within sport at all levels (Warden, 2009; Matava, 2016).

23.6 Summary

- NSAIDs possess analgesic, anti-inflammatory, antipyretic and antithrombotic properties as they inhibit COX activity, which prevents the production of prostaglandins.
- COX-1 and COX-2 are responsible for the production of different prostaglandins. Non-selective NSAIDs inhibit both COX-1 and COX-2 activity to some degree whereas selective COX-2 inhibitors predominately inhibit COX-2 enzyme activity.
- NSAIDs are widely used in sports medicine to treat acute and chronic musculoskeletal injuries to reduce pain and inflammation and allow the early return of an athlete to activity.
- The potential beneficial effect of NSAIDs in the early phase of injury when inflammatory signs and symptoms are present is not maintained in the long-term and may even delay the repair process if use becomes prolonged.

- The use of NSAIDs in the treatment of fractures, muscle strains and chronic tendinopathies is controversial. In these clinical scenarios, paracetamol appears to be a more suitable first line treatment option as it has a similar analgesic efficacy to NSAIDs and has a lower side-effect profile.
- NSAID-induced inhibition of prostaglandin formation can lead to adverse GI, renal and cardiovascular effects if NSAIDs are used for prolonged periods of time, at high doses or concurrently with multiple NSAIDs.
- NSAIDs are not prohibited in sport and are readily available over the counter.
- NSAIDs appear to be overused by athletes. More effort is required to educate athletes about the efficacy of NSAID use and their side effects in order to address concerns about usage rates and the incidence of adverse effects within sport at all levels.

23.7 References

Alaranta, A., Alaranta, H., Heliövaara, M. et al. (2006) Ample use of physician-prescribed medications in Finnish elite athletes. *International Journal of Sports Medicine* 27: 919–925.

Almekinders, L.C. (1999) Anti-inflammatory treatment of muscular injuries in sport: An update of recent studies. *Sports Medicine* 28: 383–388.

Baker, J., Cotter, J.D., Gerrard, D.F. et al. (2005) Effects of indomethacin and celecoxib on renal function in athletes. *Medical Science in Sports Exercise* 37: 12–17.

Burnier, M. (2005) The safety of rofecoxib. *Expert Opinion on Drug Safety* 4: 491–499.

Cohen, D.B., Kawamura, S., Ehteshami, J.R. and Rodeo, S.A. (2006) Indomethacin and celecoxib impair rotator cuff tendon-to-bone healing. *American Journal of Sports Medicine* 34: 362–369.

Corrigan, B. and Kazlauskas, R. (2003) Medication use in athletes selected for doping control at the Sydney Olympics. *Clinical Journal of Sports Medicine* 13: 33–40.

Dalton, J.D. and Schweinie, J.E. (2006) Randomized controlled noninferiority trial to compare extended release acetaminophen and ibuprofen for the treatment of ankle sprains. *Annals of Emergency Medicine* 48: 615–623.

Da Silva, E.R., De Rose, E.H., Ribeiro, J.P. et al. (2011) Non-steroidal anti-inflammatory use in the XV Pan-American Games (2007). *British Journal of Sports Medicine* 45: 91–94.

Day, R.O. and Graham, G.G. (2013) Republished research: Non-steroidal anti-inflammatory drugs (NSAIDs). *British Journal of Sports Medicine* 47: 1,127.

Deeks, J.J., Smith, L.A. and Bradley, M.D. (2002) Efficacy, tolerability, and upper gastrointestinal safety of celecoxib for treatment of osteoarthritis and rheumatoid arthritis: Systematic review of randomised controlled trials. *British Medical Journal* 325: 619.

Elder, C.L., Dahners, L.E. and Weinhold, P.S. (2001) A cyclooxygenase-2 inhibitor impairs ligament healing in the rat. *American Journal of Sports Medicine* 29: 801–805.

Geusens, P., Emans, P.J., de Jong, J.J. and van den Bergh, J. (2013) NSAIDs and fracture healing. *Current Opinion in Rheumatology* 25: 524–531.

Gorski, T., Cadore, E.L., Pinto, S.S. et al. (2011) Use of NSAIDs in triathletes: Prevalence, level of awareness and reasons for use. *British Journal of Sports Medicine* 45: 85–90.

Grosser, T., Ricciotti, E. and FitzGerald, G.A. (2017) The cardiovascular pharmacology of nonsteroidal anti-inflammatory drugs. *Trends in Pharmacological Sciences* 38: 733–748.

Huang, S-H., Johnson, K. and Pipe, A.L. (2006) The use of dietary supplements and medications by Canadian Athletes at the Atlanta and Sydney Olympic Games. *Clinical Journal of Sports Medicine* 16: 27–33.

Joint Formulary Committee (2017a) Non-steroidal anti-inflammatory drugs. *British National Formulary*. London, BMJ Group and Pharmaceutical Press. Available at: https://bnf.nice.org.uk/treatment-summary/non-steroidal-anti-inflammatory-drugs.html (Accessed on 30 July 2017).

Joint Formulary Committee (2017b) Aspirin: Indications and doses. Available at: https://bnf.nice.org.uk/drug/aspirin.html#indicationsAndDoses (Accessed on 30 July 2017).

Küster, M., Renner, B., Oppel, P. et al. (2013) Consumption of analgesics before a marathon and the incidence of cardiovascular, gastrointestinal and renal problems: A cohort study. *British Medical Journal Open* 3(4), e002090.

Lipman, G.S., Shea, K., Christensen, M. et al. (2017) Ibuprofen versus placebo effect on acute kidney injury in ultramarathons: A randomised controlled trial. *Emergency Medical Journal*. Available at http://emj.bmj.com/content/early/2017/06/28/emermed-2016-206353 (Accessed 30 July 2017).

McGrath, M. (2012) Fifa alarmed at widespread "abuse" of painkillers. Available at: http://www.bbc.co.uk/news/science-environment-18064904 (Accessed on 30 July 2017).

Mackey, A.L., Kjaer, M., Dandanell, S. et al. (2007) The influence of anti-inflammatory medication on exercise-induced myogenic precursor cell responses in humans. *Journal of Applied Physiology* 103: 425–431.

Magra, M. and Maffulli, N. (2006) Nonsteroidal antiinflammatory drugs in tendinopathy: Friend or foe. *Clinical Journal of Sports Medicine* 16: 1–3.

Marsolais, D., Côté, C.H. and Frenetta, J. (2003) Nonsteroidal anti-inflammatory drug reduces neutrophil and macrophage accumulation but does not improve tendon regeneration. *Laboratory Investigations* 83: 991–999.

Massey, T., Derry, S., Moore, R.A. and McQuay, H.J. (2010) Topical NSAIDs for acute pain in adults. *Cochrane Database Systematic Review* 6: 1–99.

Matava, M.J. (2016) Ethical considerations for analgesic use in sports medicine. *Clinical Journal of Sports Medicine* 35: 227–243.

Medicines.org.uk (2017) *Summary of Product Characteristics (SPC) Search: Electronic Medicines Compendium (eMC)*. Available at: http://www.medicines.org.uk/emc/ (Accessed on 30 July 2017).

MHRA.gov.uk (2017) *Medicines Information: SPC and PILs*. Available at: http://www.mhra.gov.uk/spc-pil/?subsName (Accessed on 30 July 2017).

Michels, S.L., Collins, J., Reynolds, M.W. et al. (2012) Over-the-counter ibuprofen and risk of gastrointestinal bleeding complications: A systematic literature review. *Current Medical Research and Opinion* 28: 89–99.

Mitchell, J.A., Larkin, S. and Williams, T.J. (1995) Cyclooxygenase-2: Regulation and relevance in inflammation. *Biochemical Pharmacology* 50: 1,535–1,542.

Morelli, K.M., Brown, L.B. and Warren, G.L. (2017) Effect of NSAIDs on recovery from acute skeletal muscle injury: A systematic review and meta-analysis. *The American Journal of Sports Medicine*. Available at: https://www.ncbi.nlm.nih.gov/pubmed/28355084 (Accessed 30 July 2017).

Page, A.J., Reid, S.A., Speedy, D.B. et al. (2007) Exercise-associated hyponatremia, renal function, and nonsteroidal antiinflammatory drug use in an ultraendurance mountain run. *Clinical Journal of Sports Medicine* 17: 43–48.

Paoloni, J.A., Milne, C., Orchard, J. and Hamilton, B. (2009) Non-steroidal anti-inflammatory drugs in sports medicine: guidelines for practical but sensible use. *British Journal of Sports Medicine* 43: 863–865.

Schnitzer, T.J. (2006) Update on guidelines for the treatment of chronic musculoskeletal pain. *Clinical Rheumatology* 25: S22–S29.

Schoen, R.T. and Vender, R.J. (1989) Mechanisms of nonsteroidal anti-inflammatory drug-induced gastric damage. *American Journal of Medicine* 86: 449–458.

Schoenfeld, B.J. (2012) The use of nonsteroidal anti-inflammatory drugs for exercise-induced muscle damage: Implications for skeletal muscle development. *Sports Medicine* 2: 1,017–1,028.

Shen, W., Li, Y., Tang, Y., Cummins, J. and Huard, J. (2005) NS-398, a cyclooxygenase-2-specific inhibitor, delays skeletal muscle healing by decreasing regeneration and promoting fibrosis. *American Journal of Pathology* 167: 1,105–1,117.

Simon, A.M. and O'Connor, J.P. (2007) Dose and time-dependent effects of cyclooxygenase-2 inhibition on fracture-healing. *Journal of Bone and Joint Surgery of America* 89: 500–511.

Singh, P. and Roberts, M.S. (1994) Skin permeability and local tissue concentrations of nonsteroidal anti-inflammatory drugs after topical application. *Journal of Pharmacology and Experimental Therapy* 268: 144–151.

Smith, W.L., Marnett, L.J. and DeWitt, D.L. (1991) Prostaglandin and thromboxane biosynthesis. *Pharmacological Therapy* 49: 153–179.

Takemoto, J.K., Reynolds, J.K., Remsberg, C.M. et al. (2008) Clinical pharmacokinetic and pharmacodynamic profile of etoricoxib. *Clinical Pharmacokinetics* 47: 703–720.

Thorsson, O., Rantanen, J., Hurme, T. and Kalimo, H. (1998) Effects of nonsteroidal antiinflammatory medication on satellite cell proliferation during muscle regeneration. *American Journal of Sports Medicine* 26: 172–176.

Trappe, T.A., White, F., Lambert, C.P., Cesar, D., Hellerstein, M. and Evans, W.J. (2002) Effect of ibuprofen and acetaminophen on postexercise muscle protein synthesis. *American Journal of Physiology and Endocrinological Metabolism* 282: e551–e556.

Tscholl, P.M., Alonso, J.M., Dollé, G., Junge, A. and Dvorak, J. (2010) The use of drugs and nutritional supplements in top-level track and field athletes. *American Journal of Sports Medicine* 38: 133–140.

Tscholl, P.M. and Dvorak, J. (2012) Abuse of medication during international football competition in 2010: Lesson not learned. *British Journal of Sports Medicine* 46: 1,140–1,141.

Tscholl, P.M., Junge, A. and Dvorak, J. (2008) The use of medication and nutritional supplements during FIFA World Cups 2002 and 2006. *British Journal of Sports Medicine* 42: 725–730.

Tscholl, P.M., Vaso, M., Weber, A. and Dvorak, J. (2015) High prevalence of medication use in profressional football tournaments including the World Cups between 2002 and 2014: A narrative review with a focus on NSAIDs. *British Journal of Sports Medicine* 49: 580–582.

Tsitsimpikou, C., Tsiokanos, A., Tsarouhas, K. et al. (2009) Medication use by athletes at the Athens 2004 Summer Olympic Games. *Clinical Journal of Sports Medicine* 19: 33–38.

van Thuyne, W. and Delbeke, F.T. (2008) Declared use of medication in sports. *Clinical Journal of Sports Medicine* 18: 143–147.

Vaso, M., Weber, A., Tscholl, P.M. et al. (2015) Use and abuse of medication during 2014 FIFA World Cup Brazil: A retrospective survey. *BMJ Open* 5. Available at: http://bmjopen.bmj.com/content/5/9/e007608 (Accessed on 30 July 2017).

WADA (2017) International Standard: The 2017 Prohibited List. Available at: https://www.wada-ama.org/en/resources/science-medicine/prohibited-list-documents (Accessed on 21 July 2017).

Walker, R.J., Fawcett, J.P., Flannery, E.M. and Gerrard, D.F. (1994) Indomethacin potentiates exercise-induced reduction in renal hemodynamics in athletes. *Medical Science in Sports Exercise* 26: 1,302–1,306.

Warden, S.J. (2005) Cyclooxygenase-2 inhibitors (COXIBs): Beneficial or detrimental for athletes with acute musculoskeletal injuries? *Sports Medicine* 35: 271–283.

Warden, S.J., Avin, K.G., Beck, E.M. et al. (2006) Low-intensity pulsed ultrasound accelerates and a nonsteroidal anti-inflammatory drug delays knee ligament healing. *American Journal of Sports Medicine* 34: 1,094–1,102.

Warden, S.J. (2009) Prophylactic misuse and recommended use of non-steroidal antiinflammatory drugs by athletes. *British Journal of Sports Medicine* 43: 548–549.

Warner, D.C., Schnepf, G., Barrett, M.S. et al. (2002) Prevalence, attitudes, and behaviors related to the use of nonsteroidal anti-inflammatory drugs (NSAIDs) in student athletes. *Journal of Adolescent Health* 30: 150–153.

Wharam, P.C., Speedy, D.B., Noakes, T.D. et al. (2006). NSAID use increases the risk of developing hyponatremia during an Ironman triathlon. *Medical Science in Sports Exercise* 38: 618–622.

Wolfe, M.M., Lichtenstein, D.R. and Singh, G. (1999) Gastrointestinal toxicity of nonsteroidal anti-inflammatory drugs. *New England Journal of Medicine* 340: 1,888–1,899.

Woo, W.W., Man, S.Y., Lam, P.K. and Rainer, T.H. (2005) Randomized double-blind trial comparing oral paracetamol and oral nonsteroidal antiinflammatory drugs for treating pain after musculoskeletal injury. *Annals of Emergency Medicine* 46: 352–361.

Chapter 24

Sports supplements and herbal preparations

Neil Chester

24.1 Introduction

It is beyond the remit of a book entitled *Drugs in Sport* to review, in detail, all supplements that might be used by athletes for the purpose of enhancing performance and maintaining health. Indeed many supplements that are pharmacological in nature are covered elsewhere in this book. Other, countless supplements that are available to the athlete and not prohibited in sport are reviewed extensively in other texts. The author directs interested readers to the reviews on nutritional supplements in the *British Journal of Sports Medicine* (Volumes 43 to 47) for further information relating to specific supplements.

Meanwhile the use of products labelled as sports supplements does bring with it a number of important challenges from an anti-doping perspective. Indeed inadvertent doping is a real and serious problem for athletes, their entourage and anti-doping organisations alike. The regulation of the sports supplements industry is not as comprehensive as that surrounding the pharmaceutical industry and therefore in recent years many issues have come to light as a consequence of the contamination, adulteration and mislabelling of supplements. In addition the use of herbal supplements where the active ingredients are often unclear or unknown may put an athlete at risk of contravening anti-doping rules.

Whilst strict liability remains WADA's guiding principle, both the significance and risk of inadvertent doping cannot be underestimated. Indeed a positive test can have a huge impact on an athlete's career. Therefore a major challenge remains in terms of limiting the chances of an anti-doping rule violation (ADRV) occurring as a consequence of supplement use.

This chapter will examine the use of supplements in sport and discuss the challenges to athletes, their support staff and anti-doping organisations in allowing legitimate use, yet preventing indiscriminate use and ensuring the World Anti-Doping Program is both credible and operational.

24.2 What are sports supplements?

Sports supplements may encompass a wide range of dietary interventions that might be used to maintain health and promote exercise performance. Supplements may be characterised into three broad categories, including:

1   Medication such as over-the-counter (OTC) products used to alleviate symptoms or treat an illness or long-term condition;

2   Health-related products including micronutrients that may supplement the diet with nutrients that may be required due to the demands of the sport or due to a poor diet; and
3   Ergogenic aids, that is, products designed to enhance sports performance.

Clearly, ergogenic aids is a particularly broad category and may encompass many of the performance and image-enhancing drugs (PIED) outlined throughout this book. However, it also includes numerous supplements that are generally accepted in sport due to their availability in a regular diet (possibly in smaller amounts) or their presence naturally in the body.

Whilst ergogenic aids, particularly those not typically classified as PIEDs, will be the focus of this chapter, it is clear that this category of dietary supplements is positioned in a 'grey area' from an anti-doping perspective. There has been considerable debate surrounding ergogenic aids, particularly when a new product reaches the marketplace, in terms of its safety and legitimacy as a 'legal' ergogenic aid. What constitutes a permitted ergogenic aid and what differentiates it from a prohibited, performance-enhancing substance is particularly important, albeit difficult, to determine.

24.3 Why do athletes use supplements?

An athlete may consider using a wide range of supplements according to their particular health status, training status and the demands of their particular sport. The following factors might be considered potential reasons for supplement use:

1   To substitute for a poor quality diet;
2   To provide additional nutrients to support the demands of training and competition;
3   To help alleviate illness or injury or aid in its recovery;
4   To facilitate recovery from training and competition;
5   To provide ergogenic advantage during training or competition; or
6   To support a diet that is compromised by a busy schedule or travel (e.g. overseas competition or training).

Supplements play an important part in effective sports nutrition. Good nutrition is often compromised by the constraints of everyday living and heavy training and competition schedules. An informed and well-considered supplement plan can therefore ensure that the diet maintains its balance of macro- and micro-nutrients and that these are consumed in the required amounts in a timely manner, thus ensuring optimal health, exercise performance and recovery.

A major focus of many athletes' sports supplement regimes are centred on direct improvement in performance, which might involve consumption prior to, or even during a competition or training session. These supplements will be specific to the demands of the exercise, in terms of the intensity and duration of effort and the nature of the activity, and as to whether it incorporates significant skill-based elements and decision-making. In combination with an event-specific regime typically comes a post-event, recovery supplement plan, whose target is to enhance recovery and adaptation from a competition or training session.

In addition to the seemingly rational justification for supplement use, athletes may simply consider their use because competitors or training partners are using them or in response to enticing marketing by sports nutrition companies or media reports. Also, the drive to be successful will typically result in athletes turning to a variety of supplements, on the understanding that they will offer the improvement required to succeed. In addition, within professional sport the demands to succeed are also shared amongst an athlete's support staff. Therefore, additional pressure to use supplements is placed on athletes by their entourage and possibly by sports supplement companies who may sponsor athletes or sports teams.

24.4 The prevalence of supplement use

It is clear from a sales perspective that sports supplements have grown in popularity over recent years. Indeed, a recent consumer research report stated that UK consumers spent £66 million on sports nutrition products (food and drink) in 2015, which amounted to a rise of 27 per cent since 2013 (Mintel, 2016). The report also stated that 42 per cent of those between 16 and 24 years had used sports nutrition products in the previous three months (three months prior to May 2016). The growth in sales of sports supplements is evidenced by their widespread availability throughout mainstream retail outlets, including supermarkets as well as the internet. It is clear that sports supplement use, once the domain of the competitive athlete, is now widespread across recreational athletes and sedentary individuals alike.

Whilst drug use in sport is practised in a covert manner, unsurprisingly there is less reticence in terms of discussing supplement use amongst athletes. Numerous studies have attempted to provide an accurate estimation of supplement use amongst athletes with varied success. Figures on the scope and extent of supplement use vary widely. It has been suggested that between 40 and 100 per cent of athletes use supplements, often as multiple regimes and at higher than normal doses (Baume et al., 2007).

At the Sydney Olympics in 2000, Corrigan and Kazlauskas (2003) recorded the declarations of supplement use by the 2,758 athletes who were drug tested at the Games. At least 17 different classes of supplements were reported, the most frequently cited being multivitamins (n = 1,116), Vitamin C (n = 810), creatine (n = 316) and amino acids (n = 190). At the Athens Olympics in 2004, Tsitsimpikou et al. (2009) again used athlete declarations during doping control tests to examine medication and supplement use. Just over 75 per cent of athletes declared use of medication and supplements with food supplements the most common (45% of respondents), followed by vitamins (43%) and proteins/amino acids (14%).

A study by Tscholl et al. (2008) examined the use of medication and supplement use amongst players at the FIFA World Cup in 2002 and 2006. Supplement use by players prior to each match was recorded from reports by each team physician. Of all supplements, 43 per cent were categorised as medication whilst 57 per cent were nutritional supplements. Again the most common nutritional supplements were vitamins (41 per cent) followed by minerals (21 per cent) and amino acids (11 per cent).

Sundgot-Borgen et al. (2003) investigated the use of selected supplements within Norwegian elite athletes compared with a control group that comprised of a random sample from the general population. A similar percentage of female athletes (54 per cent) and female controls (52 per cent) reported using supplements, whilst more male athletes (51 per cent) used supplements when compared to male controls (32 per cent). In the athlete group, the main supplements used were minerals (males 26 per cent; females 42 per cent), amino acids (males 12 per cent; females 3 per cent) and creatine (males 12 per cent; females 3 per cent).

Nieper (2005) found that 62 per cent of UK junior international track and field athletes were using supplements, with an average of 2.4 products per athlete and that males used ergogenic aids more often than females. Multivitamins and minerals were the most popular products used. Whilst 25 per cent reported using supplements for ergogenic purposes, the main reasons for their use were for health (45 per cent) and to enhance the immune system (40 per cent).

Erdman et al. (2006) surveyed Canadian high-performance athletes and found that 88 percent reported using dietary supplements during the previous six months, with an average of 3.08 supplements per user. Sport drinks (22 per cent), sport bars (14 per cent), multivitamins and minerals (14 per cent), protein supplements (9 per cent) and Vitamin C (6 per cent) were the most frequently reported supplements used. Protein supplements were significantly more likely to be used by athletes at the highest performance level.

A recent unpublished report examined elite rugby league players in England (n = 166) and found that 95 per cent of players reported supplement use (Woolfenden, 2017). The reasons for the use of supplements included recovery (90 per cent of respondents), to build muscle (86 per cent) and for energy (40 per cent). A significant proportion of players (16 per cent) also reported fat loss as a reason for their supplement use.

A recent systematic review by Knapik et al. (2016) concluded that whilst there was variability in the estimates of prevalence of supplement use amongst athletes, elite athletes tended to use more supplements than non-elite athletes. In addition, supplement use was found to be similar between males and females although whilst the use of iron was most prevalent in females, the use of protein, creatine and vitamin D was preferred by males.

24.5 The risks associated with supplement use

As mentioned above, the sports supplement market is particularly buoyant and is currently experiencing rapid growth. Manufacturers are capitalising on the perceived need by many individuals to supplement their diet for the demands of exercise training and competition. Whilst many products are deemed to be rather innocuous, the safety associated with high doses and their long-term use is often unknown.

Clearly, regulations exist concerning the manufacture and sale of both pharmaceuticals and dietary supplements to protect the consumer. However, unlike the pharmaceutical industry, manufacturers of dietary supplements are not required to test their products or the ingredients in clinical trials to prove their safety or efficacy before marketing (Clarkson, 1996). They are also not subject to the same independent, scientific scrutiny as that for regulated medicines (Herbert, 1999; Maughan, 2005). Whilst dietary supplements may be removed from the market and production may cease in response to safety concerns the regulatory bodies must typically provide proof of such concerns.

In addition to the concerns associated with long-term use and relatively high doses of particular supplements, there has also been concern regarding their use as a gateway to the future use of illicit performance enhancers. Several researchers have attempted to elucidate the relationship between supplement use and possible use of prohibited substances in the future (Backhouse et al., 2013; Hildebrandt et al., 2012). Understandably this link remains under debate but it does pose the question, whether by advocating or encouraging ergogenic aids we are normalising their use and blurring the boundary between acceptable supplementation and doping.

Whilst evidence shows that the minority of athletes use prohibited substances to enhance sport performance (see Chapter 3) there is clear evidence of widespread supplement use. Debate in terms of the legitimacy and the ethics surrounding the use of particular sports supplements remains; however, the ambitious, yet responsible athlete will use whatever is deemed to be acceptable and ensure prohibited PIEDs are avoided. Nevertheless, whilst this course of action might have been acceptable in the past, the significant risks associated with supplement use have become clear over the last decade. Indeed, there have been numerous ADRVs attributed to the use of seemingly innocuous sports supplements, and research studies have revealed the real issue of supplement contamination and potential adulteration.

Indeed, whilst sport supplements manufacturers exploit the innate competitiveness of those participating in sport, some products can fall into a 'grey area' in relation to doping and contravening the 'spirit of sport'. Many products may contain additional active ingredients either from herbal extracts or as synthetically synthesised pharmaceuticals. It is therefore essential that athletes and their support personnel are fully aware of the ingredients contained in any supplements used, to ensure that they limit the chances of falling foul of the anti-doping regulations. The World Anti-Doping Agency (WADA) upholds a strict liability policy whereby athletes are responsible for any prohibited substance found in their blood or urine. Ignorance or negligence is not considered an acceptable defence for an ADRV. Indeed, determining whether an individual bears no fault or negligence is particularly difficult to establish.

As part of this chapter several herbal supplements are reviewed to highlight the link between what might be deemed natural, safe supplements and potentially hazardous doping agents (Section 24.6). The major concern with herbal supplements is that there are no assurances in terms of their content (and the exact quantity) of active ingredients. Also, many herbs have been found to contain high quantities of heavy metals (e.g. mercury and lead) as a consequence of the level of soil contamination in countries where the herbs are grown, such as China (Mueller and Hingst, 2013).

Athletes are also asked to be vigilant and keep their drinks bottles with them at all times to avoid the possibility of sabotage by fellow competitors. Secure storage of supplements should also be considered to limit the possibility of cross contamination and sabotage. Whilst evidence to support this practice is lacking, it would seem plausible that sabotage might be a possible option for an extremely motivated athlete where pressure to out-perform their competitor(s) is critical.

Contamination

Many sports supplements have been found to be affected by contamination due to sub-optimal manufacturing and quality control procedures. Inadvertent contamination may occur through contamination of the raw materials used or cross-contamination during the manufacturing process. Clearly, safety is a major issue when the label and packaging does not reflect the contents of a particular product. Since the regulations set out for the manufacture of dietary supplements rely on the compliance of the manufacturer and are not under the strict constraints of the production of pharmaceuticals there is an opportunity for quality control standards to fall significantly below those of pharmaceutical-grade operations.

Research carried out over the last ten years and more has demonstrated how real the problem of supplement contamination actually is. Between 10 and 25 per cent of products tested were found to be contaminated (Baume et al., 2007). Many of these contaminants are liable to result in an adverse analytical finding during drug testing. Two sources of contamination have been proposed (Burke, 2004):

1   Cross-contamination due to poor manufacturing practice; and
2   Undeclared additions of active ingredients to supplements in order to increase their efficacy.

Whilst the first source would appear to be true contamination that could be alleviated through improved manufacturing procedures, the second source would seem to describe adulteration of sports supplements.

The main contaminants in supplements have been shown to be stimulants, such as ephedrine, anabolic androgenic steroids (AAS) and their precursors, often referred to as prohormones (Baume et al., 2007). Prohormones are available as sports supplements and aggressively marketed as having enormous potential to increase muscle growth and strength (Geyer et al., 2008). The most common are the precursors of testosterone and nandrolone including, 4-androstenedione, 4-androstenediol, 5-androstenediol (precursors of testosterone) 19-norandrostenedione and 19-norandrostenediol (precursors of nortestosterone) as well as dehydroepiandrosterone (DHEA) (Yonamine et al., 2004).

An international study found that from a total of 634 products purchased from shops and the internet a significant proportion (almost 15 per cent) of supplements contained AAS and related substances (including prohormones) not declared on their packaging. Also, the extent of contaminated supplements varied between countries, with the Netherlands (25.8 per cent), Austria (22.7 per cent), UK (18.8 per cent) and USA (18.8 per cent) all reporting higher contamination than the average (Geyer et al., 2004).

A similar study was conducted on 103 dietary supplements purchased from the internet (Baume et al., 2006). The products were screened for the presence of stimulants, AAS and their precursors and metabolites. Results showed that approximately one in five supplements were contaminated with substances not declared on the label, all of which would have resulted in an adverse analytical finding if an athlete had used these products prior to undergoing a drugs test.

A more recent study by Russell et al. (2013) performed a prohibited drugs screen on 114 products obtained from the largest sports supplement companies in Europe. Supplements were chosen randomly and included a wide range of products, none of which were part of a routine drug screen programme. Results found that 10 per cent of products were contaminated with prohibited substances including AAS and stimulants with a total of 20 prohibited substances identified. Despite the increased awareness of contamination issues, relating to sports supplements, this research highlights that the problem remains a real issue.

A review by Outram and Stewart (2015) examined the number of ADRVs that could be attributed to inadvertent doping following supplement use. Outram and Stewart (2015) examined the cases of athletes from the USA, Australia and the UK who had tested positive for a prohibited substance over an eight- or nine-year period and had subsequently been judged to be an ADRV. Of all ADRVs within the designated period up to and including 2013, between 6.4 and 8.8 per cent were attributed to supplement use. The authors however provide a caveat, stating that their findings offer only an indication of the ADRVs attributed to supplements since the evidence available cannot categorically confirm such a link.

Indeed, athletes should be aware that WADA-accredited laboratories can detect prohibited substances and their metabolites at much lower concentrations (parts per billion; $\mu g.L^{-1}$) than the levels detectable by the majority of supplement manufacturers (parts per million; $mg.L^{-1}$) (Mottram, 2011). In reality, this means that supplement companies may abide by manufacturing guidelines from a general health and safety perspective and yet still be at risk of producing supplements that might put an athlete at risk of a positive drugs test.

The contamination of sports supplements is not only an issue with regards to prohibited substances but also concerning the purity of products and the cleanliness of the manufacturing process. Indeed, in addition to prohibited substances, contaminants including broken glass and animal faeces have been discovered (Maughan et al., 2011).

Adulteration, counterfeiting and mislabelling

In light of the differences in how pharmaceuticals and dietary supplements are regulated there is sufficient scope for unscrupulous supplement manufactures to take advantage of the lag between regulation and potential enforcement. As mentioned previously, there may be a more sinister motive behind the presence of a prohibited substance in a sports supplement. Adulteration of sports supplements during the manufacturing process may provide enhanced ergogenic properties to otherwise innocuous products through the addition of a prohibited substance. Also, substitution of one active ingredient for another (i.e. counterfeiting) is not uncommon in the manufacture of products from the illicit market (Graham et al., 2009).

Mislabelling is another major issue associated with the adulteration of products. Research has shown that not only do products sometimes contain substances not stated on the label but also that they might contain substances in different quantities (Van Thuyne et al., 2006). Recent reports have determined the presence of a variety of adulterants in dietary supplements (Cohen et al., 2014b; 2015). Indeed, those supplements that appear to be most at risk of adulteration are those targeted at weight loss, muscle growth and pre-workout formulas. Most worrying is the continued presence of adulterants in products that have been recalled for safety reasons (Cohen et al., 2014a). According to Olivier (2015), whilst awareness of contamination of supplements has increased, scrupulous manufacturers have looked to minimise the risk through improved practice; however, adulteration remains a significant problem that can only be addressed through heighted regulation.

Accuracy and quality of information and advice concerning sports supplements

Heavy advertising through magazines and the internet has allowed athletes unrestricted access to a wide range of supplements (Baume et al., 2007). Manufacturers may make exaggerated claims regarding the ergogenic properties of their products (Beltz and Doering, 1993). Such claims are rarely substantiated by sound scientific data in peer-reviewed journals (Nieman and Pedersen, 1999).

Athletes often self-prescribe supplements but may seek advice from a variety of sources. Coaches were found to be the main advisors on supplement use for male (58 per cent) and female (52 per cent) elite Norwegian athletes (Sundgot-Borgen et al., 2003). Erdman et al. (2007) also reported that athletes found coaches a valuable source of advice in terms of supplement use (41 per cent of respondents); however, family and friends (52.7 per cent) and team mates (44 per cent) were considered most valuable. In a survey by Nieper (2005), 72 per cent of respondents claimed to have access to a sports dietician but tended to underutilise this resource. Subjects indicated that coaches (65 per cent) had the greatest influence on their supplement use, with doctors (25 per cent) and sports dieticians (30 per cent) being less important. Recent data from elite rugby league highlighted strength and conditioning coaches were particularly influential and were often assigned roles relating to nutritional supplementation despite no formal qualifications in sports nutrition (Woolfenden, 2017).

Considering the specific dangers that have been highlighted with respect to the indiscriminate use of sports supplements from both an anti-doping and health and safety perspective there is a need to ensure that accurate information is readily available. Greater enforcement of the regulations in place that limit sports supplements companies making unrealistic claims is required. Advertising should also be sensitive to a potential young market to ensure that children are not unduly influenced by the marketing of sports supplements. Considering their influence it is also necessary to educate not only athletes but their entourage, in the safe use of supplements.

24.6 Herbal supplementation

Plants are an essential source of nutrients and phytochemicals which are central to the diet but also help in maintaining health and treating illness and disease. Although the term herbal relates to an extract from an herbaceous plant (i.e. a plant without a consistent woody stem) it is typically used collectively to describe any plant source which might be used in cooking or for its medicinal properties. Herbals (or botanicals) have been used in traditional medicine for thousands of years and form the basis of many modern medicines. Whilst mass produced synthetic pharmaceuticals are the mainstay of modern medicine, traditional herbal medicines remain central to medical care in the developing world (Wachtel-Galor and Benzie, 2011). Herbals used as medicines (e.g. traditional Chinese medicine) are classified as such and their use and manufacture is regulated in a way that is similar to pharmaceuticals in the European Union and the USA. Herbal medicines therefore require authorisation prior to being released to the market in the European Union (Miroddi et al., 2013). In the USA this process is rather more stringent involving testing to establish both the safety and efficacy of any herbal medicinal products (Miroddi et al., 2013). Herbals may however be included in or form the basis of dietary supplements and therefore regulated in much the same way as food. The determining factor in terms of their classification and thus their regulation is generally dependent on their purpose of use and their marketing.

Herbs may contain many active ingredients and the exact quantities and contents are seldom labelled. Whilst herbal products contain active ingredients they are often classified as food supplements rather than medicinal products. Classified as food they undergo less stringent quality control procedures prior to their sale. Most herbal supplements have not been subject to extensive scientific scrutiny and rigorous clinical trials. This poses a significant problem in terms of the safety of herbal supplement use. The major risks of taking herbal supplements include the purity of the ingredients and the possibility of contamination, and possible interactions between the ingredients and between other supplements or indeed drugs that maybe consumed simultaneously. Athletes should therefore exercise extreme caution when contemplating the use of natural/herbal supplements.

Whilst it is beyond the scope of this book to provide a comprehensive review of the countless herbal supplements available it is pertinent to highlight two distinct groups of herbs that athletes may contemplate using. Many supplements aimed at the weight loss market contain herbal ingredients that are natural sources of stimulants related to ephedrine and caffeine. Also, a recent area of growth in the sports supplements industry is the development of the pre-workout supplement. These supplements are aimed at those individuals who might require a boost by way of a stimulant to enhance performance during a training session. Another area of growth in the supplements market is in products designed to enhance muscle bulk. Whilst there are many examples of supplements which contain prohormones in an attempt to enhance testosterone levels and subsequent muscle gains (see Chapter 9), there are also several herbs that are termed 'natural testosterone boosters' that have reputed benefits in promoting muscle growth.

Natural testosterone boosters

Supplements promoted as testosterone boosters typically contain prohormones, however natural testosterone boosters include several herbs that allegedly increase circulating testosterone via other mechanisms. Clearly, enhanced testosterone levels offer the potential for increased muscle bulk and function.

Tribulus terrestris

Tribulus terrestris (TT) is one of the most commonly used natural testosterone boosters and is promoted as a supplement to produce gains in lean muscle mass and strength. These gains are claimed to occur in response to increased luteinising hormone and subsequent increases in testosterone. Whilst the mechanisms by which TT might exert its effects have not been elucidated it is believed to be in response to steroidal saponins contained in the herb (Ganzera et al., 2001).

Despite its widespread use there has been limited research into its reputed ergogenic effects. Studies that have examined supplementation have failed to report any significant effects in terms of gains in lean body mass and muscular strength (Antonio et al., 2000; Poprzecki et al., 2005; Rogerson et al., 2007). Whilst anti-doping organisations would actively discourage the use of TT due to the many claims made surrounding its efficacy, Rogerson and colleagues (2007) investigated whether through the use of the supplement an individual might increase their testosterone/epitestosterone (T:E) ratio and thus lead to the possible failure of a drugs test. However, the T:E ratio was not altered following five weeks of supplementation with TT. A recent systematic review by Qureshi et al. (2014) concluded that evidence was insufficient to support the notion that supplementation with TT has a significant effect on increasing circulating testosterone levels in humans.

Eurycoma longfolia Jack

Eurycoma longifolia Jack (EL) is a popular herb in the countries of South East Asia and is commonly known as Tongkat Ali in Malaysia (Chen et al., 2012). In Asian countries it is used for its reputed health benefits pertaining to a wide range of conditions (Chen et al., 2012). It is, however, its potential effect on sexual function and anabolic effect on skeletal muscle that has created recent interest in terms of its use as an ergogenic aid. Although there are no studies that have examined the prevalence of its use it is now starting to infiltrate the sports supplement market in the West. The mechanisms behind the reputed efficacy of EL have not been elucidated, however the phytochemical, eurycomanone (contained in EL), a quassinoid is deemed to provide testosterone boosting properties (Low et al., 2013). It has been reported that eurycomanone is able to enhance testosterone levels in an animal model by aromatase inhibition in Leydig cells, thus reducing the conversion of testosterone to estradiol (Low et al., 2013). However, Chen et al. (2014) found that six weeks of supplementation with EL (400mg.day^{-1}) did not raise urinary T:E ratio in male recreational athletes.

Recent studies have also examined the potential of EL as an ergogenic aid in terms of increasing muscle mass and improving exercise performance. Preliminary data has been provided by Hamzah and Yusuf (2003) which revealed improvements in muscle strength and muscle size following five weeks of supplementation with EL (150mg.day^{-1}) in combination with resistance training. Similarly George et al. (2013) reported improvements in muscle strength following EL supplementation (300mg.day^{-1}) without resistance training. Research is required to further examine the effects of EL on exercise performance and provide information on potential mechanisms in humans, to address concerns from an anti-doping perspective.

Herbal stimulants

There are a large number of products available for weight reduction, combating drowsiness, relieving fatigue and enhancing sports performance all containing a variety of herbal stimulants. Many herbal stimulants contain caffeine and related methylxanthines of which the most common are coffee and tea. A full review of caffeine is provided in Chapter 25. Herbal stimulants may also contain natural sources of ephedrine and related sympathomimetic amines (Chapter 17).

Guarana

Guarana is a South American plant whose seeds contain caffeine (2.5 to 5 per cent) and theophylline and theobromine in small amounts, together with large amounts of tannins (Carlini, 2003). Guarana is widely available as a constituent of numerous OTC supplements designed to suppress appetite, relieve tiredness and enhance sports performance. The effects of guarana are mediated largely through its active ingredients caffeine and theophylline via adenosine receptor antagonism, described in more detail in Chapter 25. There has been limited research into the efficacy of guarana supplementation in humans. Research examining the effects of herbal supplements containing guarana and Ma Huang has shown significant fat reduction and weight loss in humans (Boozer et al., 2001). Research using animal models has shown that guarana reduced fatigue in forced swimming in mice and increased memory in rats (Espinola, 1997). Supplementation of doses of caffeine equivalent to that contained in the guarana extract did not show any improvement in performance. It has been suggested that additional phytochemicals, other than methylxanthines, such as tannins contained in guarana may be responsible for the improvements in performance observed (Espinola, 1997).

Ephedra sinica/Ma Huang

Ma Huang is the name in Chinese medicine given to the plant species *Ephedra sinica*. *Ephedra sinica* is a natural source of ephedrine, pseudoephedrine, norephedrine (phenylpropanolamine) and norpseudoephedrine (cathine). *Ephedra sinica* is typically an ingredient in weight-loss preparations as a consequence of ephedrine's thermogenic and anorectic properties. Ma Huang typically contains up to 24mg of ephedrine and related sympathomimetics per unit dose (Bucci, 2000). Limited research has examined the use of Ma Huang as an ergogenic aid and whilst it is likely that it offers the same ergogenic benefits as its isolated constituents further work is necessary to elucidate the effects of consuming combined sympathomimetics in herbal form.

Citrus aurantium

Weight loss products often marketed as 'ephedra free' typically contain *Citrus aurantium* (Seville orange or bitter orange extract) as a substitute for ephedra. The peel of bitter orange is known as Zhi Shi in traditional Chinese medicine and is used in the treatment of gastrointestinal complaints such as indigestion and constipation. The principal active ingredients of Citrus aurantium include the sympathomimetics synephrine (~6 per cent) and octopamine (Haller et al., 2005).

Synephrine acts at the α_1-adrenergic receptors leading to vasoconstriction and increased blood pressure (Bui et al., 2006). Evidence from animal models suggests that octopamine activates lipolysis via the β_3-adreneroreceptors of adipocytes thus accounting for *Citrus aurantium*'s purported thermogenic effect in humans (Carpene et al., 1999). However, β_3-adrenoreceptor agonists are less active in human adipocytes (Fugh-Berman and Myers, 2004) and therefore it is likely that any positive effect on weight loss may be attributed to the effects on appetite suppression. However, 'ephedra-free' weight loss products not only contain *Citrus aurantium* but also other herbs such as guarana and green tea, all rich in methylxanthines. It is this combination of sympathomimetics and methylxanthines which is thought to produce marked effects in weight loss.

Whilst 'ephedra-free' products are deemed to be safer than their ephedra counterparts there has been limited research examining their safety. It is possible that the combined effects of synephrine and caffeine may be similar to the reported effects from ephedrine and caffeine including hypertension, myocardial infarction and stroke. Haller et al. (2005) demonstrated significant cardiovascular stimulation following the administration of a supplement containing synephrine, octopamine and caffeine. However no effect on blood pressure was found following administration of a supplement containing only synephrine (46.9mg). Bui et al. (2006) has shown increases in heart rate and systolic and diastolic blood pressure in young, healthy adults following a single 900mg dose of a *Citrus aurantium* (6 per cent synephrine) supplement. It is also ironic that the term 'ephedra free' is used to highlight the fact that the supplement does not contain ephedrine, which is prohibited substance and yet *Citrus aurantium* is a source of octopamine (albeit in small amounts), which is also a prohibited substance (WADA, 2016a).

Other herbal supplements

In addition to herbals that are centred on their reputed stimulant or testosterone boosting effects there are many others that are used widely for other potential ergogenic effects. These effects are often wide ranging and lacking in substantive supporting scientific evidence. Examples of such herbal supplements include ginseng and *Rhodiola rosea*.

Ginseng

Ginseng has been used for centuries in traditional Chinese medicine and is a particularly common herbal supplements used for its purported health and performance-enhancing properties. Whilst Korean ginseng (*Panax ginseng*), also known as Chinese or Asian ginseng, is most commonly used as an ergogenic aid there are other species, namely American (*Panax quinquefolius*) and Siberian (*Eleutherrococcus senticosis*) ginseng. The main active ingredients in Korean ginseng are ginsenocides, which are believed to have wide-ranging benefits particularly relating to resistance of fatigue, possibly by modulating the hypothalamic-pituitary-adrenal cortex axis and alleviation of the catabolic effects of cortisol (Williams, 2006). Nevertheless, despite the widespread use as an ergogenic aid there is limited good quality research to support its reputed performance-enhancing properties (Bach et al., 2016).

Rhodiola rosea

Rhodiola rosea (RR) is an herbaceous plant found in the Arctic and mountainous regions in Europe and Asia. It has been used for a variety of reasons and has gained particular interest as a sports supplement due to its reputed benefits in alleviating fatigue. A systematic review by Ishaque et al. (2012) concluded that whilst RR supplementation might have a positive effect on physical and psychological performance there is a lack of well-conducted research studies to elucidate its efficacy. A recent study has examined the use of RR as an immuno-protective agent following a competitive marathon (Ahmed et al., 2015). It was suggested that RR supplementation might reduce virus replication following prolonged, vigorous exercise thus going someway to counteracting the typical immuno-suppression experienced following heavy exercise. However, no anti-bacterial activity was observed in this study. Research is needed to further elucidate the potential benefits of RR and mechanisms of action.

24.7 Anti-doping violations involving the use of sports supplements

It is not uncommon for any athlete who tests positive for a prohibited substance to claim that it was an inadvertent offence and likely to be due to supplement contamination, adulteration or sabotage. Whilst several of the claims that reach the headlines appear implausible there are many which may be considered true. Despite such claims there are few athletes that avoid sanctions due to the principle of 'strict liability'.

Nandrolone

Around the turn of the century there were a number of high profile cases involving athletes who had tested positive for the AAS nandrolone. In most cases athletes claimed that they had ingested the steroid in a contaminated nutritional supplement, an assertion which was considered plausible (Ayotte, 1999).

The tennis player Greg Rusedski tested positive for nandrolone in July 2003, claiming it was a result of taking contaminated electrolyte supplement pills that the Associated of Tennis Professionals (ATP) had been giving out to tennis players through its trainers. A number of other tennis players similarly tested positive for nandrolone between September 2002 and May 2003. Many of these players were below the cut-off level that was in place for testing purposes and were therefore not sanctioned. However, Rusedski and another six players were above the cut-off level but were exonerated by the ATP. The ATP Anti-Doping Tribunal acknowledged that it could not prosecute a case when it had created the situation itself by the action of its trainers distributing contaminated supplements.

Subsequently, the ATP commissioned an anti-doping expert to investigate the source of the nandrolone but found no trace of nandrolone in around 500 pills tested. His conclusion was ambiguous: 'While the circumstantial evidence points to nandrolone-related contamination of the electrolyte-replacement products as the source . . . there is insufficient evidence to prove that the electrolytes were the cause of the test results. Similarly there is not sufficient evidence to prove they were not the cause' (Mottram, 2011).

Methylhexaneamine

The numerous doping cases involving methylhexanamine over recent years have clearly high-lighted the serious issues around the supplement industry from an anti-doping and health and safety perspective. The significant number of adverse analytical findings (AAF) involving methylhexaneamine have been a particular concern. Indeed according to the 2012 WADA Anti-Doping testing figures, 46 per cent of AAFs involving stimulants were attributed to meth-ylhexaneamine which accounted for 320 occurrences worldwide (WADA, 2013). In 2015, WADA Anti-Doping testing figures indicated a drop in AAFs involving methylhexaneamine (see Table 17.1; WADA, 2016b) with 11 per cent (n = 56) of all those attributed to stimulants (n = 528). Nevertheless, this still accounts for a significant proportion of AAFs.

Methylhexaneamine (2-amino-4-methylhexane; 1,3-dimethylamylamine; DMAA) was first manufactured synthetically by the pharmaceutical company Eli Lily and marketed as a vasoconstrictor under the name Forthane (Zhang et al., 2012). Despite its removal as a pharmaceutical in 1970, DMAA has recently been reintroduced as a constituent of numer-ous sports supplements promoted as 'fat-burners' and 'pre-workout' aids (Mueller and Hingst, 2013). The growth in this sector of the sports supplements market, demonstrated by the increased use of DMAA-containing products, coincided with its addition as a non-specified stimulant to the WADA Prohibited List in 2010. Subsequently there has been a plethora of AAFs attributed to DMAA contained in such products.

What is particularly interesting in the case of DMAA is that its presence in sports sup-plements was disguised as a natural herb ingredient on the label of these products. Indeed, each of these products made reference to an ingredient known as geranium stem, geranium oil extract or geranamine. Reference to a natural herb ingredient allowed manufacturers to market their products as a dietary supplement despite them containing a pharmacological active ingredient. Whilst reference material quoted a research study that claimed the ingre-dient was a natural constituent of geranium oil this finding has been disputed by Lisi et al. (2011) and Zhang et al. (2012). Indeed recent work examining geranium oil has concluded that DMAA is not an active constituent (Zhang et al., 2012) and that products that are labelled with geranium oil but contain DMAA have been adulterated (Lisi et al., 2011).

Despite the numerous doping cases involving DMAA the most disturbing aspect of these sports supplements are the reports of several fatalities attributed to their use. Indeed, the tragic case of Claire Squires highlights the huge health risk that sports supplements pose. As a recreational athlete, Claire Squires' death due to acute cardiac failure in the 2012 London Marathon was attributed to extreme exertion and the use of a DMAA-containing supple-ment (Hill, 2013). In 2012 the Medicines and Healthcare products Regulatory Agency (MHRA) classified all DMAA-containing products as medicines due to concerns regarding their safety and as such, products containing DMAA require appropriate authorisation to be marketed in the UK (MHRA, 2017). However, despite the removal of many products from the marketplace and increased education, recent positive tests involving DMAA suggest it continues to be a problem in elite sport (WADA, 2016b).

24.8 Safeguarding athletes against inadvertent doping through supplement use

Whilst the dangers surrounding supplement use have been described it is essential to con-sider a proactive approach in terms of limiting the possibility of a positive drugs test and the potential harm caused by the use of a sports supplement.

Are supplements necessary?

Clearly a key question that needs to be considered is whether supplements confer any advantage to the athlete. In a review by Deldicque and Francaux (2008) it was stated that several types of supplements have demonstrated improved sport performance at a higher level than that expected with a well-balanced diet. Nevertheless, the evidence base for the efficacy of many supplements is not robust. Indeed, due to the lucrative nature of the sports supplements industry there are numerous products marketed that do not have strong scientific research to support their use. A suitably qualified sports nutritionist would advocate a healthy diet and would typically recommend the use of whole foods in the first instance to obtain sufficient nutrients before promoting supplement use.

Product testing

Not only is it unrealistic to expect athletes to avoid sport supplements but in doing so it may also put them at a distinct disadvantage when up against their competitors. Indeed, there are several reasons why supplements may be helpful to the athlete (Section 24.3) and whilst that might not include the use of the latest product offered on the internet it is clear that even a somewhat responsible athlete can risk a doping offence through the use of a seemingly ordinary/innocuous supplement. It is for this reason that schemes involving product testing have been developed to safeguard athletes.

In the UK and beyond, numerous manufacturers subscribe to a supplement testing programme known as 'Informed Sport' whereby each batch of a specified product is analysed for the presence of substances contained on the WADA Prohibited List. A negative result provides confidence to both the athlete and the manufacturer that a registered product is safe to use without the repercussions of a doping offence.

The Informed Sport supplement testing programme involves testing of products to ISO 17025 standards. This is an internationally recognised standard for analytical laboratories that ensures that testing is performed to the required high standards and that the limits of detection relating to a contaminant is in line with WADA-accredited laboratory testing.

In addition the programme includes an assessment of each stage involved in the manufacture of a product from the source of raw materials to packaging and storage of products. Analysis of raw materials for possible contaminants is an important stage in terms of ensuring the safety of a product. Only when all analytical tests (including batch testing) report negative results, can companies use the 'Informed Sport' logo to market their products. Misuse of the logo is nevertheless an issue – highlighting the need to check specific batch numbers with those products that have been tested and are highlighted by the scheme.

There are also inherent limitations with such a testing programme. Indeed, a 100 per cent guarantee that the use of a registered product will not result in a positive drugs test cannot be given. Since WADA do not provide a definitive list of all substances that are prohibited it is not possible to test products for all prohibited substances. Also, by its very nature batch testing cannot be completely reliable since only a very small sample of all products are tested and therefore there is always the likelihood of products 'slipping through the net'. Whilst Informed Sport is a global company, there are similar schemes operating in Germany, the USA, Australia and the Netherlands.

Recommendations for athletes

Current recommendations from anti-doping organisations are that athletes should avoid the use of supplements. Clearly, this recommendation allows WADA to uphold its strict liability policy. A more practical solution is that when supplements are used they should only be those from reputable manufacturers that test their products for the presence of prohibited substances.

Whilst the risk of supplement contamination is genuine, athletes may safeguard themselves against the possibility of a doping offence by taking the following precautions:

- Perform a needs analysis – do you need to supplement your diet?
- Consult a suitably qualified nutritionist and/or the scientific literature to determine the efficacy of a supplement.
- Be wary of products that appear to be too good to be true – manufacturers are likely to be making false claims.
- Exercise caution when considering the use of products that are described as natural and contain herbal ingredients.
- Read the label on all products – consult an anti-doping organisation for advice with respect to the status of any unknown ingredients.
- Only use products from reputable manufacturers that subscribe to a supplement testing programme.
- Be wary of purchasing products from the internet or independent sport supplements shops.
- Keep sight of your personal feeding bottle at all times during training and competition.

Athletes not only risk jeopardising their reputation and career but also their health if they do not ensure a responsible approach to supplement use. Clearly, athletes intent on using supplements need to be vigilant with respect to the validity of the source of their products.

24.9 Summary

Supplement use is particularly common amongst athletes and non-athletes alike. Indeed, the sports nutrition marked has burgeoned with widespread availability of supplements from high street retailers and supermarkets to internet-based retailers. Despite the prevalence of use there is a need for the athlete and their entourage to be aware of the risks that supplements pose from a health and anti-doping perspective. Inadvertent doping as a consequence of supplement contamination and adulteration with prohibited supplements is particularly rife highlighting the need to exercise due diligence and employ clear risk minimisation strategies. The use of supplements from reputable companies that batch test their products for the presence of prohibited substances is an effective strategy to minimise the risk of inadvertent doping attributed to supplement use. Herbal supplements are a particular cause for concern in light of the fact they often contain many active ingredients and are not often fully characterised. Evidence regarding the efficacy of such supplements is also generally lacking.

24.10 References

Ahmed, M., Henson, D.A., Sanderson, M.C. et al. (2015) *Rhodiola rosea* exerts anti-viral activity in athletes following a competitive marathon race. *Frontiers in Nutrition* 2: 24.

Antonio, J., Uelmen, J., Rodriguez, R. and Earnest, C. (2000) The effects of *Tribulus Terrestris* on body composition and exercise performance in resistance-trained males. *International Journal of Sport Nutrition and Exercise Metabolism* 10: 208–215.

Ayotte, C. (1999). Nutritional supplements and doping controls. *New Studies in Athletics* 14: 37–42.

Bach, H.V., Kim, J., Myung, S.K. and Cho, Y.A. (2016) Efficacy of ginseng supplements on fatigue and physical performance: A meta-analysis. *Journal of Korean Medical Science* 31: 1,879–1,886.

Backhouse, S.H., Whitaker, L. and Petroczi, A. (2013) Gateway to doping? Supplement use in the context of preferred competitive situations, doping attitude, beliefs and norms. *Scandinavian Journal of Medicine and Science in Sports* 23: 244–252.

Baume, N., Hellemans, L. and Saugy, M. (2007) Guide to over-the-counter sports supplements for athletes. *International Sports Medicine Journal* 8(1): 2–10.

Baume, N., Mahler, N., Kamber, M. et al. (2006) Research of stimulants and anabolic steroids in dietary supplements. *Scandanavian Journal of Medical Science in Sports* 16: 41–48.

Beltz, S.D. and Doering, P.L. (1993) Efficacy of nutritional supplements used by athletes. *Clinical Pharmacy* 12: 900–908.

Boozer, C.N. Nasser, J.A., Heymsfield, S.B. et al. (2001) An herbal supplement containing Ma Huang-Guarana for weight loss: A randomised, double-blind trial. *International Journal of Obesity* 25: 316–324.

Bucci, L.R. (2000) Selected herbals and human exercise performance. *American Journal of Clinical Nutrition* 72(Suppl): 624S–636S.

Bui, L.T., Nguyen, D.T. and Ambrose, P.J. (2006) Blood pressure and heart rate effects following a single dose of bitter orange. *Annals of Pharmacotherapy* 40: 53–57.

Burke, L.M. (2004) Contamination of supplements: An interview with Professor Ron Maughan. *International Journal of Sport Nutrition and Exercise Metabolism* 14: 493–496.

Carlini, E.A. (2003) Plants and the central nervous system. *Pharmacology and Biochemistry and Behaviour* 75: 501–512.

Carpene, C., Galitzky, J., Fontana, E. et al. (1999) Selective activation of β_3-adrenoceptors by octopamine: Comparative studies in mammalian fat cells. *Naunyn-Schmiedeberg's Archives of Pharmacology* 359: 310–321.

Chen, C.K., Mohamed, W.M., Ooi, F.K. et al. (2014) Supplementation of *Eurycoma longifoliaI Jack* extract for 6 weeks does not affect urinary testosterone: Epitestosterone ratio, liver and renal functions in male recreational athletes. *International Journal of preventative Medicine* 5(6): 728–733.

Chen, C.K., Muhamad, A.S. and Ooi, F.K. (2012) Herbs in exercise and sports. *Journal of Physiological Anthropology* 31(4): 1–7.

Clarkson, P.M. (1996). Nutrition for improved sport performance: Current issues on ergogenic aids. *Sports Medicine* 21: 393–401.

Cohen, P.A., Maller, G., DeSouza, R. and Neal-Kababick, J. (2014a) Presence of banned drugs in dietary supplements following FDA recalls. *Journal of American Medical Association* 312(16): 1,691–1,693.

Cohen, P.A., Travis, J.C. and Venhuis, B.J. (2014b) A methylamphetamine analog (N,α-diethylphenylethylamine) identification in mainstream dietary supplements. *Drug Testing and Analysis* 6(7–8): 805–807.

Cohen, P.A., Travis, J.C. and Venhuis, B.J. (2015) A synthetic stimulant never tested in humans, 1,3-methylbutylamine (DMBA), is identified in multiple dietary supplements. *Drug Testing and Analysis* 7(1): 83–87.

Corrigan, B. and Kaslauskas, R. (2003) Medication use in athletes selected for doping control at the Sydney Olympiad (2000). *Clinical Journal of Sports Medicine* 13: 33–40.

Deldicque, L. and Francaux, M. (2008) Functional food for exercise performance: Fact or foe? *Current Opinions in Clinical Nutrition and Metabolic Care* 11: 774–781.

Erdman, K.A., Fung, T.S. and Reimer, R.A. (2006) Influence of performance level on dietary supplementation in elite Canadian athletes. *Medicine and Science in Sports and Exercise* 38(2): 349–356.

Erdman, K.A., Fung, T.S., Doyle-Baker, P.K. et al. (2007) Dietary supplementation of high performance Canadian athletes by age and gender. *Clinical Journal of Sports Medicine* 17: 458–464.

Espinola, E.B., Dias, R.F., Mattei, R. et al. (1997) Pharmacological activity of Guarana (Paullinia cupana Mart.) in laboratory animals. *Journal of Ethnopharmacology* 55: 223–229.

Fugh-Bernam, A. and Myers, A. (2004) Citrus aurantium, an ingredient of dietary supplements marketed for weight loss: Current status of clinical and basic research. *Experimental Biology and Medicine* 229: 698–704.

Ganzera, M., Bedir, E. and Khan, I.A. (2001) Determination of steroidal saponins in Tribulus terrestis by reversed-phase high performance liquid chromatography and evaporative light scattering detection. *Journal of Pharmaceutical Sciences* 90(11): 1,752–1,758.

George, A., Liske, E., Chen, C.K. and Ismail, S.B. (2013) The Eurycoma longifolia freeze-dried water Extract-Physta® does not change normal ratios of testosterone to epitestosterone in healthy males. *Journal of Sports Medicine and Doping Studies* 3(2): 1–6.

Geyer, H., Parr, M.K., Mareck, U. et al. (2004) Analysis of non-hormonal nutritional supplements for anabolic androgenic steroids: Results of an international study. *International Journal of Sports Medicine* 25: 124–129.

Geyer, H., Parr, M.K., Koehler, K. et al. (2008) Nutritional supplements cross-contaminated and faked with doping substances. *Journal of Mass Spectrometry* 43: 892–902.

Graham, M.R., Ryan, P., Baker, J.S. et al. (2009) Counterfeiting in performance and image-enhancing drugs. *Drug Testing and Analysis* 1: 135–142.

Haller C.A., Benowitz, N.L. and Jacob, P. (2005) Hemodynamic effects of ephedra-free weight-loss supplements in humans. *American Journal of Medicine* 118: 998–1,003.

Hamzah, S. and Yusuf, A. (2003) The ergogenic effects of Tongkat Ali (Eurycoma longifolia): A pilot study. *British Journal of Sports Medicine* 37(Abstract 007): 465–466.

Herbert, D.L. (1999) Recommending or selling nutritional supplements enhances potential legal liability for sports medicine practitioners. *Sports Medicine Alert* 5(11): 91–92.

Hildebrandt, T., Harty, S. and Langenbucher, J.W. (2012) Fitness supplements as a gateway substance for anabolic-androgenic steroid use. *Psychology of Addictive Behaviours* 26(4): 955–962.

Hill, A. (2013) Claire Squires: Amphetamine stimulant had role in runner's fatal heart attack. Available at: https://www.theguardian.com/uk/2013/jan/30/claire-squires-runner-dmaa-fatal (Accessed on 31 July 2017).

Ishaque, S., Shamseer, L., Bukutu, C. and Vohra, S. (2012) *Rhodiola rosea* for physical and mental fatigue: A systematic review. BMC *Complementary and Alternative Medicine* 12: 70.

Knapik, J.J., Steelmann, R.A., Hoedebecke, S.S. et al. (2016) Prevalence of dietary supplement use by athletes: Systematic review and meta-analysis. *Sports Medicine* 46(1): 103–123.

Lisi, A., Hasick, N., Kazlauskas, R. and Goebel, C. (2011) Studies of methylhexaneamine in supplements and geranium oil. *Drug Testing and Analysis* 3(10–11): 873–876.

Low, B.S., Choi, S-B., Abdul Wahab, H. et al. (2013) Eurycomanone, the major quassinoid in *Eurycoma longifolia* root extract increases spermatogenesis by inhibiting the activity of phosphodiesterase and aromatase in steroidogenesis. *Journal of Ethnopharmacology* 149: 201–207.

Maughan, R.J. (2005) Contamination of dietary supplements and positive drug tests in sport. *Journal of Sports Sciences* 23(9): 883–889.

Maughan, R.J., Greenhaff, P.L. and Hespel, P. (2011) Dietary supplements for athletes: Emerging trends and recurring themes. *Journal of Sport Sciences* 29(S1): S57–S66.

MHRA (2017) MHRA warns athletes to avoid potentially dangerous DMAA. Available at: https://www.gov.uk/government/news/mhra-warns-athletes-to-avoid-potentially-dangerous-dmaa (Accessed 31 July 2017).

Mintel (2016) Sports nutrition bulks up: UK market sales rise by 27% in two years as one in four Brits use the products. Available at: http://www.mintel.com/press-centre/social-and-lifestyle/sports-nutrition-bulks-up-uk-market-sales-rise-by-27-in-two-years-as-one-in-four-brits-use-the-products (Accessed 30 July 2017).

Miroddi, M., Mannucci, C., Mancari, F. et al. (2013) Research and development for botanical products in medicinals and food supplements market. *Evidence Based Complementary and Alternative Medicine* 2013: 1–6.

Mottram, D.R. (2011) Supplement use in sport. In D.R. (ed.) *Drugs in Sport*, 5th edition. London, Routledge.

Mueller, K. and Hingst, J. (2013) *The Athlete's Guide to Sports Supplements*. Champaign, IL, Human Kinetics.

Nieman, D.C. and Pedersen, B.K. (1999). Exercise and immune function: Recent developments. *Sports Medicine* 27: 73–80.

Nieper, A. (2005) Nutritional supplement practices in UK junior national track and field athletes. *British Journal of Sports Medicine* 39: 645–649.

Olivier, R. (2015) Dietary supplements and sport: Stronger regulation needed! *Planta Medica* 81, Congress Abstract.

Outram, S. and Stewart, B. (2015) Doping through supplement use: A review of the available empirical data. *International Journal of Sports Nutrition and Exercise Metabolism* 25(1): 54–59.

Poprzecki, S., Zebrowska, A., Cholewa, J. et al. (2005) Ergogenic effects of *Tribulus Terrestris* supplementation in men. *Journal of Human Kinetics* 13: 41–50.

Qureshi, A., Naughton, D.P. and Petroczi, A. (2014) A systematic review on the herbal extract *Tribulus Terrestis* and the roots of its putative aphrodisiac and performance enhancing effect. *Journal of Dietary Supplements* 11(1): 64–79.

Rogerson, S., Riches, C., Jennings, C. et al. (2007) The effect of five weeks of *Tribulus Terrestris* supplementation on muscle strength and body composition on muscle strength and body composition during preseason training in elite rugby league players. *Journal of Strength and Conditioning Research* 21(2): 348–353.

Russell, C., Hall, D. and Brown, P. (2013). *HFL Sport Science European Supplement Contamination Survey*. Fordham, Cambridgeshire, HFL Sport Science.

Sundgot-Borgen, J., Berglund, B. and Torstveit, M.K. (2003) Nutritional supplements in Norwegian elite athletes: Impact of international ranking and advisors. *Scandanavian Journal of Medical Science in Sports* 13: 138–144.

Tscholl, P.M., Junge, A. and Dvorak, J. (2008) The use of medication and nutritional supplements during FIFA World Cups™ 2002 and 2006. *British Journal of Sports Medicine* 42(9): 725–730.

Tsitsimpikou, C., Tsiokanos, A., Tsarouhas, K. et al. (2009) Medication use by athletes at the Athens 2004 Summer Olympic Games. *Clinical Journal of Sports Medicine* 19(1): 33–38.

Van Thuyne, W., Van Eenoo, P. and Delbeke, F.T. (2006) Nutritional supplements: prevalence of use and contamination with doping agents. *Nutrition Research Reviews* 19: 147–158.

Wachtel-Galor, S. and Benzie, I.F.F. (2011) Herbal medicine: An introduction to its history, usage, regulation, current trends and research needs. In S. Wachtel-Galor and I.F.F. Benzie (eds) *Herbal Medicine: Biomolecular and Clinical Aspects*, 2nd edition. London, CRC Press.

WADA (2013) 2012 Anti-Doping Testing Figures Report. Available at: https://www.wada-ama.org/sites/default/files/resources/files/WADA-2012-Anti-Doping-Testing-Figures-Report-EN.pdf (Accessed on 31 July 2017).

WADA (2016a) The 2017 Prohibited List International standard. Available at: https://www.wada-ama.org/sites/default/files/resources/files/2016-09-29_-_wada_prohibited_list_2017_eng_final.pdf (Accessed on 31 July 2017).

WADA (2016b) 2015 Anti-Doping Testing Figures: Laboratory Report. Available at: https://www.wada-ama.org/sites/default/files/resources/files/2015_wada_anti-doping_testing_figures_report_0.pdf (Accessed on 25 July 2017).

Williams, M. (2006) Dietary supplements and sports performance: Herbals. *Journal of the International Society of Sports Nutrition* 3(1): 1–6.

Woolfenden, A. (2017) Supplement use in professional rugby league. Unpublished MPhil thesis. Liverpool John Moores University, Liverpool, UK.

Yonamine, M., Garcia, P.R. and de Moraes Moreau, R.L. (2004). Non-intentional doping in sports. *Sports Medicine* 34(1): 697–704.

Chapter 25

Caffeine

Neil Chester

25.1 Introduction

Caffeine is a phytochemical found in a wide variety of plant species distributed throughout the world, the most notable sources being coffee, tea and cocoa. Since it is a constituent of a large number of commonly available beverages and foodstuffs (Table 25.1) and its use is generally unregulated and accepted throughout the world, caffeine is believed to be one of the most widely used drugs. It is also a key constituent in numerous over-the-counter (OTC) medications for pain relief and the relief of upper respiratory tract conditions including the common cold and influenza.

Table 25.1 Caffeine content of selected beverages and OTC products

Beverage/OTC product	Caffeine content (mg)
Coffee	
Brewed	163
Espresso	77
Instant	57
De-caffeinated (brewed)	6
De-caffeinated (instant)	3
Tea	
Black	42
Green	25
De-caffeinated (black)	5
Soft drinks	
Coca Cola (355ml)	34
Pepsi Max (355ml)	69
Dr Pepper (355ml)	41
Energy drinks	
Red Bull (250ml)	80
Relentless (500ml)	160
Lucozade Energy (360ml)	46
Caffeinated gum	
Healthspan Elite Kick Start Gum	100/piece*
Military Energy Gum	100/piece
OTC cold and flu medication	
Benylin Cold and Flu Max Strength	25/capsule**
Beechams Powders	50/sachet**
Lemsip Max Cold and Flu	25/capsule**

OTC pain relief medication
    Anadin Extra   45/tablet**
    Solpadine Plus   40/tablet**
    Panadol Extra   65/tablet**
OTC products for the relief of tiredness
    Pro-Plus   50/tablet

Average caffeine levels according to caffeineinformer.com

*Caffeine levels according to manufactures

**Caffeine levels according to the Electronic Medicines Compendium (eMC; www.medicines.org.uk/emc/)

Caffeine has great appeal as an ergogenic aid with extensive scientific research supporting its performance-enhancing properties over a wide range of sporting activities. It is commonly employed, by many individuals for its psychotropic properties, to increase wakefulness, alertness and concentration. Although caffeine is used widely as a performance-enhancing drug there remains conjecture regarding the exact mechanisms supporting its use.

Caffeine was removed from the WADA Prohibited List in 2004 for a number of reasons, including its widespread consumption together with limited side effects at low to moderate doses as well as the fact that it remains extremely difficult, if not impossible, to differentiate via a drugs test, between habitual consumption and that for the purpose of enhancing performance. Although not prohibited, caffeine has been part of the WADA Monitoring Program since its inception. Evidence gathered from this programme would potentially support or oppose the reintroduction of caffeine to the Prohibited List.

Within society as a whole, there appears to have been a general increase in the consumption of caffeine over recent years, not least as a consequence of the growth in the café culture and an expansion of the caffeinated drinks market targeted at the young. In sport, the use of caffeine as an ergogenic aid appears to have increased too, following its removal from the Prohibited List. Although there is a general acceptance of caffeine use in society there appears to be almost an unwillingness to accept or appreciate its negative side-effects and the ethical implications of its use as an ergogenic aid in organised sport.

25.2 Pharmacology

Chemically caffeine is classified as a methylxanthine closely related to two other naturally occurring methylated xanthines namely, theophylline and theobromine (Figure 25.1). Caffeine (1,3,7-trimethylxanthine) is a tri-methylated xanthine whilst theophylline and theobromine are di-methylated xanthines. Pharmacologically, theophylline is considered the most potent of the naturally occurring methylxanthines with theobromine, a constituent of cocoa, the least (Undem and Lichtenstein, 2001).

Following oral ingestion, it is rapidly absorbed via the gastrointestinal tract and reaches peak plasma concentrations between 30 and 60 minutes (Sawynok and Yaksh, 1993). Due to its lipophilic properties, it is widely distributed around the body easily crossing the blood-brain barrier and placenta. The half life of caffeine in healthy individuals is approximately four hours (Lelo et al., 1986a) and it is metabolised extensively through demethylation into paraxanthine (80 per cent), theobromine (11 per cent) and theophylline (4 per cent) by chytochrome P450 enzymes in the liver (Lelo et al., 1986b).

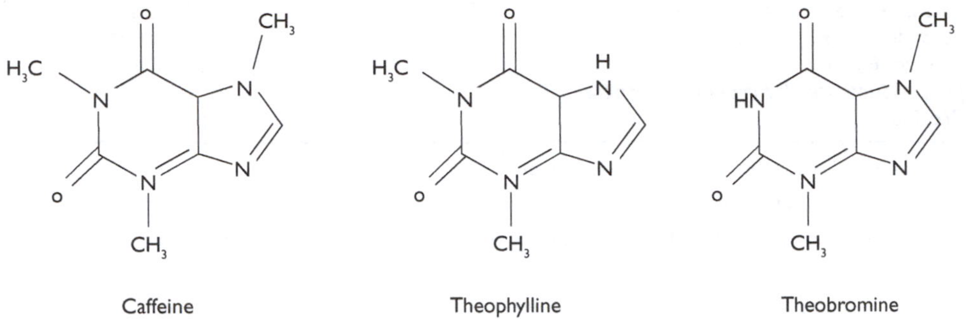

Caffeine   Theophylline   Theobromine

Figure 25.1 Chemical structure of naturally occurring methylxanthines

Caffeinated chewing gum is a recent addition to the marketplace and offers an advantage over traditional methods of caffeine administration/consumption in terms of the speed of absorption. Whilst bioavailability is similar to other methods, chewing gum allows rapid absorption into the circulation via the buccal mucosa (Kamimori et al., 2002) thus bypassing first pass metabolism and limiting the risk of gastrointestinal side effects (Paton et al., 2010).

25.3 Mechanisms of action

Whilst it is accepted that caffeine has marked pharmacological, physiological and performance-enhancing effects there remain some conjecture regarding the exact mechanisms involved. However, the principal mechanism by which caffeine exerts its effects is believed to be as an adenosine receptor antagonist. It is the only mechanism that is believed to occur at caffeine concentrations in the magnitude of those experienced following typical caffeine consumption (Fredholm, 1995).

Adenosine is a ubiquitous molecule essential in physiological function. It is a modulator of various physiological processes both in the CNS and in the peripheral tissues via adenosine receptors. Adenosine receptors are located in most tissues including the brain, heart, smooth muscle, adipocytes and skeletal muscle. The effects of adenosine are therefore widespread. Adenosine receptors, located on the cell membrane and coupled to G-proteins, can be divided into four sub-types, A_1, A_{2A}, A_{2B} and A_3. Stimulation of A_1 receptors typically initiates inhibitory responses through a reduction in cyclic AMP and stimulation of potassium channels. Inhibition of calcium flux is also believed to occur following A_1 receptor activation (Shimada and Suzuki, 2000). Activation also inhibits noradrenergic, dopaminergic, serotonergic and acetylcholinergic neurotransmission. The A_{2A} receptors are linked to dopaminergic neurons and stimulation of these receptors appears to be involved in the inhibition of dopaminergic neurotransmission. The A_{2B} receptors are believed to be low affinity receptors serving a modulating role whilst A_3 receptors are believed to be sparsely distributed in the CNS (Graham, 1997).

Caffeine, which is similar in structure to adenosine, has the most affinity to the A_1 and A_{2A} receptors and its ability to cross the blood–brain barrier means that it readily affects the CNS. Since adenosine has largely an inhibitory effect, caffeine, as an adenosine receptor antagonist, therefore has a stimulatory effect. The complex nature of caffeine's actions relates to the abundance of adenosine receptors and the fact that it is able to operate via the receptors in both a direct or indirect manner.

Despite the importance of adenosine receptor antagonism in characterising the effects of caffeine other related mechanisms are believed to play a role. Inhibition of cyclic nucleotide phosphodiesterase that leads to increased cyclic AMP and increased sensitivity of calcium translocation are both considered key mechanisms.

Caffeine's ability to inhibit cyclic nucleotide phosphodiesterase enzymes is significant since it results in increased intracellular levels of cyclic AMP and cyclic GMP. These molecules act as secondary messengers enabling signal-response pathways to be enhanced. Cyclic AMP is involved in the signal-response pathway that activates inactive hormone-sensitive lipase and stimulates lipolysis in adipose tissue. Increased sympathetic nervous system activity also results in enhanced intracellular cyclic AMP levels leading to increased lipolysis. These mechanisms fit neatly with the positive effects of caffeine associated with endurance exercise performance and the proposed glycogen sparing hypothesis. However, such mechanisms are not considered to account primarily for enhanced endurance following caffeine consumption. Indeed research has found improvements without significant increases in circulating adrenaline and free fatty acids and reduction in the respiratory exchange ratio (RER) (Graham and Spriet, 1991 and 1995).

The ability of caffeine to effect calcium translocation in the muscle may contribute directly to performance enhancement during physical exercise. Increases in intracellular calcium have been observed with caffeine. Caffeine seems to interfere with excitation-contraction coupling. Caffeine activates the release of calcium from the sarcoplasmic reticulum which binds with troponin and activates the myofilaments leading to contraction. Whilst this has been demonstrated *in vitro*, using high caffeine doses, the ability to show similar effects using doses comparable with those taken by humans has proved difficult (Tarnopolsky, 2008).

Since the ability to combat fatigue may relate directly to maintenance of electrolyte homeostasis caffeine may have direct impact as a consequence of its reported effect on potassium levels. Lindinger et al. (1993) reported that plasma potassium increased to a lesser extent during exercise following caffeine administration. The significance of this finding is that fatigue is associated with suppression in resting membrane potential and therefore less motor unit activation and force production. This may occur as a result of loss of potassium from the myocyte, thus increasing plasma potassium levels or less release of calcium from the sarcoplasmic reticulum. The lower plasma potassium levels observed following caffeine administration may be as a consequence of increased plasma clearance or a lower efflux from the active muscle. It has been hypothesised that caffeine works directly or indirectly via adrenaline to stimulate muscle sodium/potassium ATPase and subsequent potassium uptake (Lindinger et al., 1993 and 1996).

25.4 Performance-enhancing properties

As an ergogenic aid caffeine is used extensively across many sports in an attempt to increase alertness and perception, mask the symptoms of fatigue, spare energy substrates and increase muscle force production and endurance. Whilst these effects following caffeine administration have not been demonstrated unequivocally there is widespread support amongst the athletic and scientific community alike.

The effects of caffeine administration on performance show a great inter-individual variation. Individuals who display limited ergogenic effects following caffeine ingestion are often termed non-responders. The factors that are likely to contribute to this variation may relate to the source of caffeine ingestion, the dose and timing of ingestion and individual characteristics relating to caffeine habituation and metabolism. The effects of caffeine have been shown to be most prominent amongst those that do not consume caffeine on a regular basis as opposed to habitual consumers (Bell and McLellan, 2002).

Whilst there is no evidence to support a dose-response relationship in terms of caffeine and performance there appears to be an optimum dose above which adverse side effects may prevail and potentially be detrimental to performance. Positive improvements in performance have been shown following relatively low doses of caffeine (i.e. 2.1mg.kg BW^{-1}) (Kovacs et al., 1998). Responses of low dose caffeine to exercise performance are associated with central effects including increased vigilance, alertness and mood (Spriet, 2014). However, the optimum dose for performance enhancement is believed to be between 3 and 6mg.kg BW^{-1} (Spriet, 2002). Higher doses of caffeine (i.e. 9mg.kg BW^{-1}) have shown no further improvements in performance (Graham and Spriet, 1991; Pasman et al. 1995).

To aid sports performance caffeine is typically ingested one hour before competition. However, whilst caffeine is rapidly absorbed, it is metabolised relatively slowly and remains at high concentrations in the circulation for several hours. There is a suggestion that its metabolic action (i.e. peak FFA levels) may peak at three hours post exercise and therefore may incur the greatest effect on endurance exercise performance (Nehlig and Debry, 1994). However, since caffeine-induced lipolysis is not deemed to be a central mechanism in improved endurance exercise such a proposal is unlikely to significantly influence performance.

Interestingly, although coffee is considered the most widespread source of caffeine, its use as an ergogenic aid has been questioned. Whilst pure caffeine ingestion enhanced endurance performance, Graham et al. (1998) found no effect following caffeine ingestion in the form of coffee. It is suggested that some constituents of coffee may interfere with caffeine and its ergogenic properties (Graham, 2001). Nevertheless, other studies have refuted this claim and have demonstrated ergogenic effects following caffeine ingestion as a constituent of coffee (Wiles et al., 1992; Hodgson et al., 2013). In practice an issue in administering caffeine through coffee relates to the difficulty in standardising the dose of caffeine consumed.

There has been limited research into the effects of other methylxanthines on sports performance. Theophylline is considered to be the most potent of the naturally occurring methylxanthines. However, Morton et al. (1989) found no effects on VO$_{2max}$, muscular performance (strength, power and endurance) and psychomotor performance following 10 to 13mg.kg BW^{-1}.day^{-1} administration of theophylline over a four-day period. Conversely, Greer et al. (2000) examined the effects of both caffeine and theophylline and found both enhanced endurance cycling performance.

Most research has tended to focus on the impact of acute caffeine supplementation on competitive events. Whilst there is a clear rationale for assessing the ergogenic effects of caffeine during competition it may be pertinent to examine the effects of caffeine supplementation during a training regimen. It is realistic to speculate that the use of caffeine as a training aid would have a significant impact on subsequent competitive performance. Nevertheless, it would be important to consider that the habitual use of caffeine in training may attenuate the response of caffeine during competition (Beaumont et al., 2017).

Endurance exercise

Research by Costill et al. (1978) demonstrated significant increases in endurance cycling performance following moderate doses of caffeine. This research paved the way for the huge interest in caffeine as a performance-enhancing substance in endurance exercise. It was proposed that caffeine promoted free fatty acid (FFA) mobilisation through increased catecholamine release. Glycogen sparing was believed to occur as a consequence of greater FFA utilisation by the exercising muscles due to increased availability of circulating FFA. It is now understood that this is not the sole mechanism nor is it the most important. In most instances, exercise performance is not limited by muscle glycogen. Whilst caffeine is clearly able to affect muscle fuel supply, this mechanism does not account for the many ergogenic effects experienced during endurance and short-term exercise alike.

Nonetheless, the ergogenic effects of caffeine on endurance performance would appear to be unquestionable. Caffeine ingestion (3 to 13mg.kg BW^{-1}) has been shown to improve time to exhaustion using exercise protocols at 80 to 85 per cent VO$_{2max}$ (Graham and Spriet, 1995; Pasman et al., 1995). Similarly, in more ecologically valid time trial protocols endurance performance lasting between 30 and 60min has shown improvements following doses of caffeine between 3 and 6mg.kg BW^{-1} (Kovacs et al., 1998; Bridge and Jones, 2006; Laurence et al., 2012). Performance of short-term endurance exercise has also shown improvements following caffeine ingestion. In rowing caffeine ingestion (6 or 9mg.kg BW^{-1}) has significantly enhanced 2000m time trial performance (Anderson et al., 2000; Bruce et al., 2000). In swimming, 1500m time trial performance was enhanced following caffeine ingestion (6mg.kg BW^{-1}) (MacIntosh and Wright, 1995).

Anaerobic exercise

Whilst the effects of caffeine on endurance exercise have been widely documented there has been relatively less attention placed upon the effects of caffeine supplementation on short-term, high intensity exercise. The studies that have been conducted are not conclusive in their support for caffeine as an aid to anaerobic exercise performance.

Very few studies have examined the effects of caffeine on sport-specific sprinting performance. Collomp et al. (1992) assessed whether caffeine ingestion (250mg) had any impact on 100m freestyle swimming. In trained swimmers, swimming velocity significantly increased under caffeine conditions. As part of a protocol to simulate rugby union, Stuart et al. (2005) examined the effects of caffeine (6mg.kg BW^{-1}) on 20 and 30m sprints and found improvements in mean performance.

Maximal accumulated oxygen deficit (MAOD), an indirect measure of anaerobic capacity has been employed to examine the effects of caffeine on anaerobic performance (Doherty, 1998; Bell et al., 2001). Doherty (1998) found that caffeine ingestion (5mg.kg BW^{-1}) improved time to exhaustion in a running protocol by 14 per cent whilst Bell et al. (2001) reported significant improvements in both time to exhaustion and MAOD using a cycling protocol under caffeine conditions (5mg.kg BW^{-1}).

The Wingate test has also been used to assess potential improvements in anaerobic performance in response to caffeine supplementation (Collomp et al., 1991; Kang et al., 1998; Beck et al., 2006; Greer et al., 2006). However, only Kang et al. (1998) demonstrated enhanced performance. Following caffeine doses of 2.5 and 5mg.kg BW^{-1} significant improvements were reported in total, peak and mean power during a 30s Wingate test.

It has been speculated that if caffeine's effects are mediated by the CNS then any effects in competition may be masked by the heightened arousal experienced in competition (Davis and Green, 2009). It is clear that further research is required to establish the ergogenic value of caffeine on anaerobic performance.

Resistance exercise

In light of the reputed effects of caffeine on contractile properties of muscle and on central mechanisms such as motivation it would seem extremely feasible that caffeine would have a positive impact upon resistance exercise. Despite several studies examining the ergogenic properties of caffeine on such exercise there appears to be no conclusive evidence to support its use.

Commonly used methods to assess muscular strength include the determination of one repetition maximum (1 RM), isokinetic peak torque or force produced during an isometric maximal voluntary contraction (MVC). Beck et al. (2006) reported a significant increase in bench-press 1 RM but no increase in leg-press 1 RM following ingestion of a caffeine-containing supplement (201mg). Astorino et al. (2008) however found no increase in bench or leg press 1 RM following caffeine ingestion (6mg.kg BW^{-1}). In a study by Bond et al. (1986) the effects of caffeine ingestion (5mg.kg BW^{-1}) on isokinetic knee flexor and extensor strength were examined. There were no significant differences in peak torque across a range of speeds (30°, 150° and 300°.s^{-1}) between caffeine and placebo trials. In elite athletes Jacobson et al. (1992) however reported greater peak torque for knee flexors at speeds of 30°.s^{-1}, 150°.s^{-1} and 300°.s^{-1} and for knee extensors at speeds of 30°.s^{-1} and 300°.s^{-1} following caffeine consumption (7mg.kg BW^{-1}). Similarly, a recent study by Duncan et al. (2014) demonstrated a significant effect of caffeine ingestion (6mg.kg BW^{-1}) over placebo on peak torque during isokinetic knee extension exercise across three speeds (30°.s^{-1}, 150°.s^{-1} and 300°.s^{-1}) with an augmented effect with increases in angular velocity. Kalmar and Cafarelli (1999) reported a significant increase in MVC following caffeine administration (6mg.kg BW^{-1}), whilst Tarnopolsky and Cupido (2000) found no ergogenic value of caffeine in relation to MVC.

Several studies have examined muscular endurance using repetitions of exercises at a percentage of 1 RM until volitional fatigue. Beck et al. (2006) found no significant effect of caffeine on bench and leg-press exercises (80 per cent 1 RM) to failure. Using a similar protocol (60% 1 RM until failure), Astorino et al. (2008) reported non-significant increases in muscular endurance following caffeine ingestion in the order of 11 and 12 per cent for bench and leg-press exercises, respectively. Muscular endurance has been assessed in other studies through sustained isometric contractions. Caffeine has shown positive effects on isometric knee extensions (50 per cent MVC) in doses of 6mg.kg BW^{-1} (Kalmar and Cafarelli, 1999; Plaskett and Cafarelli, 2001; Meyers and Cafarelli, 2005).

Intermittent exercise

Team games such as football and rugby are characterised by aerobic exercise interspersed with repeated, intermittent bouts of high intensity anaerobic exercise. The ability to assess physiological performance has proved extremely difficult within these sports. Of those researchers that have attempted to assess intermittent exercise few have been successful in recreating the demands of a game. The Yo-Yo intermittent recovery test developed by

Bangsbo et al. (2008) was devised to simulate the activity pattern of sports such as football. Applying this test to an intervention study involving caffeine supplementation (6mg.kg BW^{-1}) showed an enhancement in fatigue resistance over placebo (Mohr et al., 2011). Schneiker et al. (2006) examined the effect of caffeine supplementation (6mg.kg BW^{-1}) on a repeated sprint protocol consisting of two, 36 min halves (18 × 4s sprints and 2min active recovery between each sprint). Performance, with respect to total amount of sprint work and mean power output was enhanced under caffeine conditions. However, Paton et al. (2001) investigated the effects of caffeine ingestion (6mg.kg BW^{-1}) on a repeated 20m sprint protocol (10 × 20m sprint with 10s recovery following each sprint) and found no effect on performance or fatigue.

The difficulty in assessing physiological performance has led many researchers to focus on physiological function or skill performance. Stuart et al. (2005) examined the effects of caffeine (6mg.kg BW^{-1}) on a battery of tests chosen to simulate the physical and skill demands of a rugby union match. Whilst improvements in most tests were evident, performance of tackle speed and reduction in fatigue in 30m sprint speed were performance measures that had been particularly enhanced by caffeine supplementation. Foskett et al. (2009) demonstrated improvements in passing accuracy and jump performance amongst football players participating in a simulated soccer-specific activity following caffeine ingestion (6mg.kg BW^{-1}). Del Coso et al. (2013) used global positioning system technology to determine the effects of caffeine (3mg.kg BW^{-1}) on rugby league performance. Simulated match performance was enhanced as indicated by total distance covered, distance covered at greater than 20km.h^{-1} and number of sprints performed. Such research highlights clearly the multi-faceted effects of caffeine and its ability to enhance not only physiological performance but also cognitive function and psychomotor performance.

Cognitive function

Caffeine is used extensively by the wider population to increase alertness in a variety of situations such as conditions of sleep deprivation, at night time, the post-lunch dip and during periods of long working hours such as studying or prolonged driving. There is a large body of evidence to support the use of caffeine as a cognitive performance enhancer especially in conditions of low arousal. It has been shown to increase cognitive function such as alertness and mood state (Penetar et al., 1993) as well as vigilance, learning and memory (Lieberman et al., 2002) under conditions of sleep deprivation.

Effects on mood and motor performance are believed to be related to caffeine's affinity to A_{2A} receptors and stimulation of dopaminergic neurotransmission. The positive effect of caffeine on mood has been demonstrated via reports of lower anxiety and increased contentedness, self-confidence and motivation following ingestion (Lieberman et al., 1987).

Decreased reaction time typically demonstrates improved selective attention and efficient information processing. The positive effect of caffeine on cognitive performance tasks has been demonstrated with reaction time (Smit and Rogers, 2000) and choice reaction time (van Duinen et al., 2005).

Whilst much of the research has centred on enhancement of generic behavioural characteristics following caffeine ingestion they are clearly transferable to sport. However, it may be difficult to assess the effects on more complex tasks within a sporting context since the heightened state of arousal that is typical of competition may mask any effects likely by caffeine ingestion.

25.5 Caffeine combinations

The co-administration of nutritional and pharmacological substances to enhance performance is common. Combinations of caffeine with additional supplements including carbohydrate and sympathomimetic amines may further enhance sports performance.

Whilst ingestion of carbohydrate supplements during exercise is common amongst endurance athletes, the introduction of caffeine as an ingredient in such supplements (i.e. sports drinks, gels) is relatively new and has no doubt increased following caffeine's removal from the WADA Prohibited List. A study examining the ingestion of a sports drink (carbohydrate-electrolyte solution) with added caffeine (2.1, 3.2 and 4.5mg.kg BW^{-1}) during a 1h cycling time trial led to an improvement in performance (Kovacs et al., 1998). Similarly, Cox et al. (2002) reported improved time trial performance following 2h steady state cycling amongst subjects that co-ingested carbohydrate and caffeine during exercise in the form of Coca-Cola (3 × ~1.5mg.kg BW^{-1}). Caffeine in low doses (~1.5 to 3mg.kg BW^{-1}) ingested with carbohydrate during exercise would therefore appear to have ergogenic benefits.

In work by Pederson et al. (2008) the co-ingestion of carbohydrate with high doses of caffeine (8mg.kg BW^{-1}) after exhaustive exercise resulted in significantly greater muscle glycogen resynthesis during the 4h post exercise when compared with carbohydrate ingestion alone. According to Pederson et al. (2008) the rate of glycogen resynthesis (~60mmol.kg $dw^{-1}.h^{-1}$) was deemed to be the highest that has been observed in humans under physiological conditions. Whilst further research is required, caffeine may play a key role in nutritional strategies designed to promote optimal recovery.

Caffeine in combination with sympathomimetic amines is often employed in weight reduction therapy. Caffeine and ephedrine is a particularly common combination used for its thermogenic and anorectic properties. Boozer et al. (2001) have found significant weight reduction in obese individuals following supplementation with natural sources of caffeine and ephedrine (Guarana and Ma Huang). Indeed, several products marketed as herbal weight loss supplements typically contain caffeine from Guarana, a plant from South America whose seeds contain caffeine, theophylline and theobromine (Espinola et al., 1997). These products also contain natural sources of sympathomimetics such as ephedrine and synephrine in the form of Ma Huang and *Citrus aurantium*, respectively. Both caffeine and ephedrine are also commonly combined with acetylsalicylic acid (aspirin) for its weight reduction properties (Astrup and Toubro, 1993). Whilst the mechanisms behind the weight reducing effects of such drug combinations is not clearly understood, both caffeine and aspirin are believed to work synergistically with the thermogenic effects of ephedrine (Dulloo, 1993).

In addition to weight loss, research in recent years has supported the use of caffeine in combination with ephedrine or pseudoephedrine directly as a performance-enhancing aid (Bell et al., 1998 and 2002; Weatherby and Rogerson, 2002). Bell et al. (1998) demonstrated a significant improvement in time to exhaustion using a cycling protocol (85 per cent VO_{2max}), following caffeine (5mg.kg BW^{-1}) and ephedrine (1mg.kg BW^{-1}) supplementation over placebo and supplementation of caffeine alone. Ephedrine (0.8mg.kg BW^{-1}) and caffeine (4mg. kg BW^{-1}) in combination have also shown improvements in a 10 km run time trial whilst wearing fighting order weighing approximately 11kg (Bell et al., 2002). There is limited support for the combination of caffeine with pseudoephedrine; nevertheless Weatherby and Rogerson (2002) reported an improvement in short-duration, supramaximal cycling exercise following the supplementation of 300mg of caffeine with 120mg of pseudoephedrine. Whilst the combination of caffeine with ephedrines appears to boast performance-enhancing properties there is clearly scope for further research to elucidate the performance-enhancing mechanisms.

25.6 Therapeutic actions

The inclusion of methylxanthines in many over-the-counter medications is as a bronchodilator or an analgesic adjuvant. Theophylline is largely incorporated into cold and flu preparation due to its role as a bronchodilator whilst caffeine is typically incorporated into pain relief medication as an adjuvant to aspirin or acetaminophen (Paracetamol). Evidence suggests that when combining a peripheral acting analgesic such as acetaminophen with caffeine that the pain relief is typical of that experienced when combined with a centrally acting analgesic (Laska et al., 1984). The significance of this is that the side-effects of taking a centrally acting analgesic can be avoided and it precludes the need to take high doses of aspirin and paracetamol. Research has suggested that these effects are mediated by central amplification of cholinergic neurotransmission (Ghelardini et al., 1997). However, the mechanisms behind these properties of caffeine are not clearly understood. Indeed, some studies have questioned the analgesic adjuvant properties of caffeine (Zhang and Li Wan Po, 1996 and 1997).

25.7 Adverse side effects

Plasma caffeine concentrations above $15\mu g.ml^{-1}$ can result in toxic symptoms such as tachycardia, arrhythmia and tremor whilst concentrations greater than $80\mu g.ml^{-1}$ are considered fatal (Riesselmann et al., 1999). Despite the widespread availability and consumption of products containing caffeine there are relatively few reports of caffeine intoxication nevertheless in a recent review by Banerjee et al. (2014) eight adult cases of fatal intoxication within a ten year period (1999 to 2009) are highlighted within the state of Maryland. All cases were solely or in part, attributed to caffeine intoxication via prescription or over-the-counter medication. Whilst no deaths were attributed to over consumption of caffeine containing foods in the Maryland report a recent case in the UK involved the death of a 40-year-old man following the consumption of 12 caffeinated sweets believed to amount to almost one gram of caffeine (Bradley, 2013). Cirrhosis of the liver was believed to have been a confounding factor in the man's death since this would result in reduced metabolism of caffeine and thus lead to an accumulation in the circulation.

The safety of caffeine consumption in relation to the cardiovascular system has long been a contentious issue. Dietary caffeine intake has been linked with cardiovascular mortality and morbidity (James, 2004). Rosenberg et al. (1988) suggested that consumption of caffeinated coffee increased the risk of myocardial infarction. Also, research has shown a positive relationship between coffee consumption and elevations in systolic blood pressure (Jee et al., 1999). However, there is a considerable body of evidence which opposes these conclusions. A large prospective study by Grobbee et al. (1990) found no association with coffee consumption and increased risk of coronary heart disease or stroke. Indeed, low to moderate caffeine consumption in the form of coffee may even have cardio-protective effects attributed to the antioxidants present in coffee (Cornelis and El-Sohemy, 2007).

The most noticeable side-effects are those pertaining to the CNS. Whilst caffeine is ingested for its positive effects on cognitive function excessive doses may cause numerous side effects. Insomnia, headache, nervousness, restlessness, tremors and irritability are examples of side-effects following high dose administration of caffeine. Chronic consumption of caffeine can lead to dependence and tolerance as the body up-regulates the number of adenosine receptors. Withdrawal symptoms are frequently experienced upon abrupt cessation of its consumption. According to Reeves et al. (1997) acute caffeine withdrawal can cause distress and symptoms of nausea, nervousness, tachycardia, arrhythmia and insomnia. Interestingly the symptoms experienced during withdrawal are similar to those following excessive caffeine consumption. Silverman et al. (1992) demonstrated that withdrawal symptoms, including a drop in mood, increased anxiety, fatigue and headache, can also be experienced in low to moderate caffeine consumers. Indeed, Evans and Griffiths (1999) confirmed that withdrawal and physical dependence can occur at low doses and following a short period of exposure (i.e. three consecutive days).

Frequent urination is a commonly stated symptom of caffeine ingestion. Excessive fluid loss through urination may result in diuresis and a reduction in plasma volume. However, such concerns would appear to be unfounded. Whilst mild diuresis was demonstrated following administration of caffeinated drinks there was no significant changes in urine and plasma osmolarity, sweat rate or plasma volume (Wemple et al., 1997). In a recent meta-analysis, Zhang et al. (2015) concluded that although caffeine ingestion caused a minor diuretic effect this was negated when ingestion was combined with exercise. This is thought to be because of reduced renal plasma flow and glomerular filtration rate as a consequence of increased sympathoadrenal activity.

Groups that are believed to be particularly sensitive to caffeine include pregnant women, infants and children. Caffeine consumption is deemed to be particularly problematic due to the extended half-life of caffeine within pregnant women and infants and the high doses of caffeine, in relation to body weight, that are consumed by children. The half-life of caffeine is extended during pregnancy by approximately two-fold in comparison with non-pregnant women (Knutti et al., 1981). The significance of this is that it extends the time at which caffeine can exert its effects and increases the potential for toxicity. Caffeine also freely crosses the placenta and passes into breast milk (Undem and Lichtenstein, 2001). Indeed further evidence has linked caffeine consumption in pregnant women with low birth weight (Care Study Group, 2008).

Caffeine is often mistakenly associated with poor iron absorption. Whilst the consumption of tea and coffee has been shown to negatively affect dietary iron absorption (Morck et al., 1983; Hurrell et al., 1999) this has not been attributed to caffeine intake. Tea and coffee contain polyphenols that can bind to iron, making it difficult to absorb. A recommendation to avoid such beverages at meal times is particularly important for people at risk of iron deficiency.

The widespread availability of caffeine in high doses in a variety of forms poses risk from a health perspective. Caffeinated sweets, gum and drinks are particularly open to misuse or overconsumption leading to significant side-effects. A particular issue is the availability of caffeine as an anhydrous powder purchased in containers as sports supplements. The containers typically include a small measuring utensil to enable the addition of appropriate and safe amounts of caffeine to beverages. Nevertheless, the risk of ingesting caffeine in amounts, way in excess of the recommended dose is particularly high (Eichner, 2014).

25.8 Caffeine use and WADA regulations

In 1984 caffeine was included in the IOC Prohibited List and a urinary concentration threshold of $15\mu g.ml^{-1}$ was set in an attempt to combat inadvertent positive drug tests following 'normal/acceptable' caffeine intake. In 1985 this threshold was reduced to $12\mu g.ml^{-1}$ and caffeine remained on the List until 2004. In 2004 WADA produced its first Prohibited List and specific stimulants such as caffeine, pseudoephedrine and phenylephrine were removed and included on the Monitoring Program.

The purpose of the Monitoring Program was to examine specific substances with the aim of identifying potential misuse (WADA, 2015). This data may be used as evidence to support the reintroduction of substances back to the Prohibited List (WADA, 2003). As a consequence the consumption of caffeine was allowed in sport without restriction. However, the motivation behind the removal of caffeine from the Prohibited List remains unclear. According to the Prohibited List committee there was concern with regards to whether caffeine levels in the urine were a good determinant of misuse due to the high degree of individual variability in urine caffeine levels (WADA, 2003). It would appear that the premise behind the Monitoring Program is to avoid the frustration and adverse publicity caused by an inadvertent positive drug test caused by legitimate use of therapeutic OTC medication or acceptable social consumption of caffeine. This would suggest that whilst caffeine has been removed from the Prohibited List, WADA is not advocating its use as a performance-enhancing supplement. Unfortunately, this message has not been clearly voiced.

Undoubtedly, with the advent of the Monitoring Program there was the potential for caffeine use to increase markedly within sport. However, laboratory data does not support this (Van Thuyne and Delbeke, 2006). Analysis of urinary caffeine levels before and after the removal of caffeine from the List showed the overall percentage of 'positive' samples remained the same. Surprisingly, overall urinary caffeine concentrations actually dropped post-2004. Following the examination of samples in relation to sport, only cycling showed an increase in 'positive' samples. Likewise, Del Coso et al. (2011) in their examination of 20,686 doping control urine samples between 2004 and 2008 found only 0.6 per cent exceeding the former urinary threshold, with endurance sports demonstrating the highest use. With a view to examining the motives of caffeine use pre- and post-2004 Chester and Wojek (2008) surveyed 480 track and field athletes and cyclists. It was revealed that use of caffeine for performance enhancing purposes was high, especially amongst the elite and that this had increased post-2004. Further work assessing the impact of the changes to the Prohibited List in 2004 was carried out by Desbrow and Leveritt (2006). Almost 90 per cent of competitors questioned at the 2005 Ironman Triathlon World Championships intended to use caffeine prior to or during the competition.

The sports supplements market, whilst considered a niche market, has attempted to profit from the re-classification of caffeine in elite sport. Caffeine has been added to numerous products in an attempt to increase their efficacy as an ergogenic supplement. Evidence of the use of caffeinated energy gels, bars and powders in addition to more traditional sources of caffeine (i.e. coffee, energy drinks and pharmaceutical preparations) amongst track and field athletes and cyclists has been shown by Chester and Wojek (2008).

Central to the caffeinated sports supplements market is the caffeinated energy drinks market. This market has grown exponentially in recent years with UK consumption believed to have more than doubled between the years 2006 and 2012 (British Soft Drinks Association, 2013). In 2016 the energy drinks market in the UK was worth two billion pounds, an increase of almost eight per cent in two years (British Soft Drinks Association, 2016). The primary consumers are thought to be those under 35 years of age and predominantly male.

An investigation into the consumption of caffeinated energy drinks amongst college students from the United States found that 51 per cent of participants regularly consumed on average one energy drink per month (Malinauskas et al., 2007). The reasons put forward for their consumption was to increase alertness following insufficient sleep (67 per cent), increase energy (65 per cent) and to consume with alcohol for social reasons (54 per cent). Side-effects were regularly reported, such as headaches (22 per cent) and heart palpitations (19 per cent). Energy drinks accounted for six per cent of total caffeine intake by children and adolescents in the US in the period 2009 to 2010 (Branum et al., 2014).

There is concern regarding the excessive use of caffeinated energy drinks and this has been compounded by reports of several deaths throughout Europe linked with such misuse (Dhar et al., 2005). The sale of high-caffeine energy drinks is banned in a number of countries such as France and Denmark, which have imposed a statutory limit of $150\mu g.ml^{-1}$ of caffeine in soft drinks (Finnegan, 2003). James (2012) argues that widespread regulation should be considered involving the following measures: improved labelling of products with high caffeine content, restrictions placed on advertising of such products, taxation of high caffeine-containing products and age restrictions on their sale.

Clearly only a small proportion of the caffeinated energy drinks market relates to their use in sport. Nevertheless, the expansion in the caffeinated energy drinks market coupled with a 10.4 per cent growth in sales from coffee retail outlets in the UK between 2015 and 2016 to over 3.4 billion pounds (Mintel, 2017) would suggest a significant increase in the consumption of caffeine across the general population. Undoubtedly, a rise in caffeine consumption throughout society is likely to impact on both the social use and ergogenic use of caffeine by those participating in sport.

25.9 Summary

Caffeine is arguably the most widely used performance-enhancing drug in the world due to its wide ranging effects and its appeal to athletes across a broad spectrum of sports. Despite caffeine's clear performance-enhancing properties it still provokes great interest amongst the scientific community. Whilst significant improvements in numerous sporting activities has been shown following moderate dosing with caffeine there remains some conjecture with respect to the mechanisms behind these effects. Although the use or consumption of caffeine is generally accepted, if not embraced, within most cultures of the world it still commands attention from health authorities. With recent growth in coffee sales and the exponential growth in the caffeinated energy drinks market particular attention has been placed on caffeine consumption amongst children. Particular concern relates to the aggressive marketing techniques of such drinks companies and their effect on consumption amongst children. From a sporting perspective it may be difficult to reconcile the anti-doping message whilst caffeine, an established performance-enhancing drug, is condoned and even actively promoted within many sporting bodies.

25.10 References

Anderson, M.E., Bruce, C.R., Fraser, S.F. et al. (2000) Improved 2000 meter rowing performance in competitive oarswomen after caffeine ingestion. *International Journal of Sports Nutrition and Exercise Metabolism* 10: 464–475.

Astorino, T.A., Rohmann, R.L. and Firth, K. (2008) Effect of caffeine ingestion on one-repetition maximum muscular strength. *European Journal of Applied Physiology* 102: 127–132.

Astrup, A. and Toubro, S. (1993) Thermogenic, metabolic and cardiovascular responses to ephedrine and caffeine in man. *International Journal of Obesity* 17: S41–S43.

Banerjee, P., Ali, Z., Levine, B. and Fowler, D.R. (2014) Fatal caffeine intoxication: A series of eight cases from 1999 to 2009. *Journal of Forensic Science* 59(3): 865–868.

Bangsbo, J., Laia, F.M. and Krustrup, P. (2008) The Yo-Yo intermittent recovery test: A useful tool for evaluation of physical performance in intermittent sports. *Sports Medicine* 38: 37–51.

Beaumont, R., Cordery, P., Funnell, M. et al. (2017) Chronic ingestion of a low-dose of caffeine induces tolerance to the performance benefits of caffeine. *Journal of Sports Sciences* 35(19): 1,920–1,927.

Beck, T.W., Housh, T.J., Schmidt, R.J. et al. (2006) The acute effects of caffeine-containing supplement on strength, muscle endurance and anaerobic capabilities. *Journal of Strength and Conditioning Research* 20: 506–510.

Bell, D.G., Jacobs, I. and Ellerington, K. (2001) Effect of caffeine and ephedrine on anaerobic exercise performance. *Medicine and Science in Sports and Exercise* 33: 1,399–1,403.

Bell, D.G., Jacobs, I. and Zamecnik, J. (1998) Effects of caffeine, ephedrine and their combination on time to exhaustion during high-intensity exercise. *European Journal of Applied Physiology and Occupational Physiology* 77: 427–433.

Bell, D.G. and McLellan, T.M. (2002) Exercise endurance 1, 3 and 6h after caffeine ingestion in caffeine users and non-users. *Journal of Applied Physiology* 93: 1,227–12,34.

Bell D.G., McLellan T.M. and Sabiston C.M. (2002) Effect of ingesting caffeine and ephedrine on 10-km run performance. *Medicine and Science in Sports and Exercise* 34: 344–349.

Bond, V., Gresham, K., McRae, J. et al. (1986) Caffeine ingestion and isokinetic strength. *British Journal of Sports Medicine* 20: 135–137.

Boozer, C.N. Nasser, J.A., Heymsfield, S.B. et al. (2001) A herbal supplement containing Ma Huang-Guarana for weight loss: A randomised, double-blind trial. *International Journal of Obesity* 25: 316–324.

Bradley, S. (2013) Dad John Jackson died from caffeine overdose after eating sweet shop mints. *Birmingham Mail.* Available at: http://www.birminghammail.co.uk/news/local-news/dad-john-jackson-died-caffeine-6170091 (Accessed on 25 July 2017).

Bridge, C.A. and Jones, M.A. (2006) The effect of caffeine on 8km run performance in a field setting. *Journal of Sport Sciences* 24: 433–439.

British Soft Drinks Association (2013) The 2013 UK Soft Drinks Report. Available at: http://www.britishsoftdrinks.com/write/MediaUploads/Publications/2013UKsoftdrinksreport.pdf (Accessed on 25 July 2017).

British Soft Drinks Association (2016) Leading the way: Annual report 2016. Available at: http://www.britishsoftdrinks.com/write/MediaUploads/Publications/BSDA_Annual_report_2016.pdf (Accessed on 25 July 2017).

Bruce, C.R., Anderson, M.E., Fraser, S.F. et al. (2000) Enhancement of 2000m rowing performance after caffeine ingestion. *Medicine and Science in Sports and Exercise* 32: 1,958–1,963.

Care Study Group (2008) Maternal caffeine intake during pregnancy and risk of fetal growth restriction: A large prospective observational study. *British Medical Journal* 337: a2332.

Chester, N. and Wojek, N. (2008) Caffeine consumption amongst British athletes following changes to the 2004 WADA Prohibited List. *International of Journal Sports Medicine* 29: 524–528.

Collomp, K., Ahmaidi, S., Audran, M. et al. (1991) Effects of caffeine ingestion on performance and anaerobic metabolism during the Wingate test. *International Journal of Sports Medicine* 12: 439–443.

Collomp, K., Ahmaidi, S., Chatard, J.C. et al. (1992) Benefits of caffeine ingestion on sprint performance in trained and untrained swimmers. *European Journal of Applied Physiology* 64: 377–380.

Cornelis, M.C. and El-Sohemy, A. (2007) Coffee, caffeine and coronary heart disease. *Current Opinion in Clinical Nutrition and Metabolic Care* 10: 745–751.

Costill, D.L., Dalsky, G.P., and Fink, W.J. (1978) Effects of caffeine ingestion on metabolism and exercise performance. *Medicine and Science in Sports* 10: 155–158.

Cox, G.R., Desbrow, B., Montgomery, P.G. et al. (2002) Effect of different protocols of caffeine intake on metabolism and endurance performance. *Journal of Applied Physiology* 93: 990–999.

Davis, J.K. and Green, J.M. (2009) Caffeine and anaerobic performance ergogenic value and mechanisms of action. *Sports Medicine* 39: 813–832.

Del Coso, J., Munoz, G. and Munoz-Guerra, J. (2011) Prevalence of caffeine use in elite athletes following its removal from the World Anti-Doping Agency list of banned substances. *Applied Physiology, Nutrition and Metabolism* 36: 555–561.

Del Coso, J., Ramirez, J.A., Munoz, G. et al. (2013) Caffeine-containing energy drink improves physical performance of elite rugby players during a simulated match. *Applied Physiology Nutrition and Metabolism* 38: 368–374.

Desbrow, B. and Leveritt, M. (2006) Awareness and use of caffeine by athletes competing at the 2005 Ironman Triathlon World Championships. *International Journal of Sports Nutrition and Exercise Metabolism* 16: 545–558.

Dhar, R., Stout, C.W., Link, M.S. et al. (2005) Cardiovascular toxicities of performance enhancing substances in sports. *Mayo Clinic Proceedings* 80: 1,307–1,315.

Doherty, M. (1998) The effects of caffeine on the maximal accumulated oxygen deficit and short-term running performance. *International Journal of Sports Nutrition,* 8: 95–104.

Dulloo, A.G. (1993) Ephedrine, xanthines and prostaglandin-inhibitors: Actions and interactions in the stimulation of thermogenesis. *International Journal of Obesity* 17(Suppl): S35–S40.

Duncan, M.J., Thake, C.D. and Downs, P.J. (2014) The effect of caffeine ingestion on torque and muscle activity during resistance exercise men. *Muscle and Nerve* 50(4): 523–527.

Eichner, R.E. (2014) Fatal caffeine overdose and other risks from dietary supplements. *Current Sports Medicine Reports* 13(6): 353–354.

Espinola, E.B., Dias, R.F., Mattei, R. et al. (1997) Pharmacological activity of Guarana (*Paullinia cupana Mart.*) in laboratory animals. *Journal of Ethnopharmacology* 55: 223–229.

Evans, S.M. and Griffiths, R.R. (1999) Caffeine withdrawal: A parametric analysis of caffeine dosing conditions. *Journal of Pharmacology and Experimental Therapeutics* 289: 285–294.

Finnegan, D. (2003) The health effects of stimulant drinks. *Nutrition Bulletin* 28: 147–155.

Foskett, A., Ali, A. and Gant, N. (2009) Caffeine enhance cognitive function and skill during simulated soccer activity. *International Journal of Sports Nutrition and Exercise Metabolism* 19: 410–423.

Fredholm, B.B. (1995) Adenosine, adenosine receptors and the actions of caffeine. *Pharmacology and Toxicology* 76: 93–101.

Ghelardini, C., Galeotti, N. and Bartolini, A. (1997) Caffeine induces central cholinergic analgesia. *Naunyn Schmiedebergs Archives of Pharmacology* 356: 590–595.

Graham, T.E. (1997) The possible actions of methylxanthines on various tissues. In T. Reilly and M. Orme (eds) *Proceedings of the Estelle Foundation Symposium: The Clinical Pharmacology of Sport and Exercise* Vol. 7. Elsevier, Amsterdam, 257–270.

Graham, T.E. (2001) Caffeine and exercise: Metabolism, endurance and performance. *Sports Medicine* 31: 785–807.

Graham, T.E., Hibbert, E. and Sathasivam, P. (1998) Metabolic and exercise endurance effects of coffee and caffeine ingestion. *Journal of Applied Physiology* 85: 883–889.

Graham, T.E., Spriet, L.L. (1991) Performance and metabolic responses to a high caffeine dose during prolonged exercise. *Journal of Applied Physiology* 71: 2,292–2,298.

Graham, T.E., Spriet, L.L. (1995) Metabolic, catecholamine and exercise performance responses to various doses of caffeine. *Journal of Applied Physiology* 78: 867–874.

Greer, F., Friars, D. and Graham, T.E. (2000) Comparison of caffeine and theophylline ingestion: Exercise metabolism and endurance. *Journal of Applied Physiology* 89: 1,837–1,844.

Greer, F., Morales, J. and Coles, M. (2006) Wingate performance and surface EMG frequency variables are not affected by caffeine ingestion. *Applied Physiology Nutrition and Metabolism* 31: 597–603.

Grobbee, D.E., Rimm, E.B., Giovannucci, E. et al. (1990) Coffee, caffeine and cardiovascular disease in men. *New England Journal of Medicine* 324: 991–992.

Hodgson, A.B, Randell, R.K. and Jeukendrup, A.E. (2013) The metabolic and performance effects of caffeine compared to coffee during endurance exercise. *PLoS ONE* 8(4): e59561.

Hurrell, R.F., Reddy, M. and Cooke, J.D. (1999) Inhibition of non-haem iron absorption in man by polypenolic-containing beverages. *British Journal of Nutrition* 81: 289–295.

Jacobson, B.H., Weber, M.D., Claypool, L. et al. (1992) Effects of caffeine on maximal strength and power in elite male athletes. *British Journal of Sports Medicine* 26: 276–280.

James, J.E. (2004) Critical review of dietary caffeine and blood pressure: A relationship that should be taken more seriously. *Psychosomatic Medicine* 66: 63–71.

James, J.E. (2012) Death by caffeine: How many caffeine-related fatalities and near misses must there be before we regulate? *Journal of Caffeine Research* 2(4): 149–152.

Jee, S.H., He, J., Whelton, P.K. et al. (1999) The effect of chronic coffee drinking on blood pressure: A meta-analysis of controlled clinical trials. *Hypertension* 33: 647–652.

Kalmar, J.M. and Cafarelli, E. (1999) Effects of caffeine on neuromuscular function. *Journal of Applied Physiology* 87: 801–808.

Kamimori, G.H., Karyekar, C.S., Otterstetter, R. et al. (2002) The rate of absorption and relative bio-availability of caffeine administered in chewing gum versus capsules to normal healthy volunteers. *International Journal of Pharmaceutics* 234: 159–167.

Kang, H., Kim, H. and Kim, B. (1998) Acute effects of caffeine intake on maximal anaerobic power during the 30s Wingate cycling test. *Journal of Exercise Physiology Online* 1.

Knutti, R., Rothweiler, H. and Schlatter, C. (1981) Effect of pregnancy on the pharmacokinetics of caffeine. *European Journal of Clinical Pharmacology* 21: 121–126.

Kovacs, E.M.R., Stegen, J.H.C.H. and Brouns, F. (1998) Effects of caffeinated drinks on substrate metabolism, caffeine excretion and performance. *Journal of Applied Physiology* 85: 709–715.

Laska E.M., Sunshine, A., Mueller, F. et al. (1984) Caffeine as an analgesic adjuvant. *Journal of the American Medical Association* 251: 1,711–1,718.

Laurence, G, Wallman, K. and Guelfi, K. (2012) Effects of caffeine on time trial performance in sedentary men. *Journal of Sport Sciences* 30(12): 1,235–1,240.

Lelo, A., Birkett, D.J., Robson, R.A. et al. (1986a) Comparative pharmacokinetics of caffeine and its primary demethylated metabolites paraxanthine, theobromine and theophylline in man. *British Journal of Clinical Pharmacology* 22: 177–182.

Lelo, A., Miners, J.O, Robson, R.A. et al. (1986b) Quantitative assessment of caffeine partial clearances in man. *British Journal of Clinical Pharmacology* 22: 183–186.

Lieberman, H.R., Tharion, W.J., Shukitt-Hale, B. et al. (2002) Effects of caffeine, sleep loss and stress on cognitive performance and mood during US Navy SEAL training. *Psychopharmacology* 164: 250–261.

Lieberman, H.R., Wurtman, R.J., Emde, R.J. et al. (1987) The effects of low doses of caffeine on human performance and mood. *Psychopharmacology* 92: 308–312.

Lindinger, M.I., Graham, T.E. and Spriet, L.L. (1993) Caffeine attenuates the exercise-induced increase in plasma $[K^+]$ in humans. *Journal of Applied Physiology* 74: 1,149–1,155.

Lindinger, M.I., Willmets, R.G. and Hawke, T.J. (1996) Stimulation of Na+, K+-pump activity in skeletal muscle by methylxanthines: Evidence and proposed mechanisms. *Acta Physiologica Scandinavica* 156: 347–353.

MacIntosh, B.R. and Wright, B.M. (1995) Caffeine ingestion and performance of a 1,500-metre swim. *Canadian Journal of Applied Physiology* 20: 168–177.

Malinauskas, B.M., Aeby, V.G., Overton, R.F. et al. (2007) A survey of energy drink consumption patterns amongst college students. *Nutrition Journal* 6: 35.

Meyers, B.M. and Cafarelli, E. (2005) Caffeine increases time to fatigue by maintaining force and not by altering firing rates during submaximal isometric contractions. *Journal of Applied Physiology* 99: 1,056–1,063.

Mintel (2017) Grande growth: UK coffee shop sales enjoy a growth high. Available at: http://www. mintel.com/press-centre/food-and-drink/uk-coffee-shop-sales-enjoy-a-growth-high (Accessed on 25 July 2017).

Mohr, M., Nielsen, J.J. and Bangsbo, J. (2011) Caffeine improves intermittent exercise performance and reduces muscle interstitial potassium accumulation. *Journal of Applied Physiology* 111(5): 1,372–1,379.

Morck, T.A., Lynch, S.R. and Cook, J.D. (1983) Inhibition of food iron absorption by coffee. *American Journal of Clinical Nutrition* 37: 416–420.

Morton, A.R., Scott, C.A. and Fitch, K.D. (1989) The effects of theophylline on the physical performance and work capacity of well-trained athletes. *Journal of Allergy and Clinical Immunology* 83: 55–60.

Nehlig, A. and Debry, G. (1994) Caffeine and sports activity: A review. *International Journal of Sports Medicine* 15: 215–223.

Pasman, W.J., van Baak, M.A., Jeukendrup, A.E. et al. (1995) The effect of different dosages of caffeine on endurance performance time. *International Journal of Sports Medicine* 16: 225–230.

Paton, C.D., Hopkins, W.G. and Vollerbregt, L. (2001) Little effect of caffeine ingestion on repeated sprints in team-sport athletes. *Medicine and Science in Sports and Exercise* 33: 822–825.

Paton, C.D., Lowe, T. and Irvine, A. (2010) Caffeinated chewing gum increases repeated sprint performance and augments increases in testosterone in competitive cyclists. *European Journal of Applied Physiology* 110: 1,243–1,250.

Pedersen, D.J., Lessard, S.J., Coffey, V.G. et al. (2008) High rates of muscle glycogen resynthesis after exhaustive exercise when carbohydrate is coingested with caffeine. *Journal of Applied Physiology* 105: 7–13.

Penetar, D., McCann, U., Thorne, D. et al. (1993) Caffeine reversal of sleep deprivation effects on alertness and mood. *Psychopharmacology* 112: 359–365.

Plaskett, C.J. and Cafarelli, E. (2001) Caffeine increases endurance and attenuates force sensation during submaximal isometric contractions. *Journal of Applied Physiology* 91: 1,535–1,544.

Reeves, R.R., Struve, F.A. and Patrick, G. (1997) Somatic dysfunction increase during caffeine withdrawal. *Journal of the American Osteopathic Association* 97: 454–456.

Riesselmann, B., Rosenbaum, F., Roscher, S. et al. (1999) Fatal caffeine intoxication. *Forensic Science International* 103: S49–S52.

Rosenberg, L., Palmer, J.R., Kelly, J.P. et al. (1988) Coffee drinking and nonfatal myocardial infarction in men under 55 years of age. *American Journal of Epidemiology* 128: 570–578.

Sawynok, J. and Yaksh, T.L. (1993) Caffeine as an analgesic adjuvant: A review of pharmacology and mechanisms of action. *Pharmacological Reviews* 45: 43–85.

Shimada, J. and Suzuki, F. (2000) Medicinal chemistry of adenosine receptors in brain and periphery. In Kase et al. (eds) *Adenosine Receptors and Parkinson's Disease*. Oxford, Elsevier, 31–48.

Silverman, K., Evans, S.M., Strain, E.C. et al. (1992) Withdrawal syndrome after the double-blind cessation of caffeine consumption. *New England Journal of Medicine* 327: 1,109–1,114.

Schneiker, K.T., Bishop, D., Dawson, B. et al. (2006) Effects of caffeine on prolonged intermittent-sprint ability in team-sport athletes. *Medicine and Science in Sports and Exercise* 38: 578–585.

Smit, H.J. and Rogers, P.J. (2000) Effects of low doses of caffeine on cognitive performance, mood and thirst in low and higher caffeine consumers. *Psychopharmacology* 152: 167–173.

Spriet, L.L. (2002) Caffeine. In M.S. Bahrke, C.E. Yesalis (eds) *Performance-Enhancing Substances in Sport and Exercise*. Champaign, IL, Human Kinetics, 267–278.

Spriet, L.L. (2014) Exercise and sport performance with low doses of caffeine. *Sports Medicine* 44(Suppl 2): S175–S184.

Stuart, G.R., Hopkins, W.G., Cook, C. et al. (2005) Multiple effects of caffeine on simulated high-intensity team sport performance. *Medicine and Science in Sports and Exercise* 37: 1,998–2,005.

Tarnopolsky, M. (2008) Effect of caffeine on the neuromuscular system: Potential as an ergogenic aid. *Applied Physiology Nutrition and Metabolism* 33: 1,284–1,289.

Tarnopolsky, M. and Cupido, C. (2000) Caffeine potentiates low frequency skeletal muscle force in habitual and nonhabitual caffeine consumers. *Journal of Applied Physiology* 89: 1,719–1,724.

Undem, B.J. and Lichtenstein, L.M. (2001) Drugs used in the treatment of asthma. In J.G. Hardman, L.E. Limbird and A.G. Gilman (eds) *Goodman and Gilman's The Pharmacological Basis of Therapeutics*, 10th edition, New York, McGraw-Hill, 733–754.

Van Duinen, H., Lorist, M.M. and Zijdewind, I. (2005) The effect of caffeine on cognitive task performance and motor fatigue. *Psychopharmacology* 180: 539–547.

Van Thuyne, W. and Delbeke, F.T. (2006) Distribution of caffeine levels in urine in different sports in relation to doping control before and after the removal of caffeine from the WADA Doping List. *International Journal of Sports Medicine* 27: 745–750.

WADA (2003) Play true magazine: Policy into practice. Available at: https://www.wada-ama.org/sites/default/files/resources/files/PlayTrue_2003_3_Policy_Into_Practice_EN.pdf (Accessed on 25 July 2017).

WADA (2015) World Anti-Doping Code. Available at: https://www.wada-ama.org/sites/default/files/resources/files/wada-2015-world-anti-doping-code.pdf (Available on 25 July 2017).

Weatherby, R.P. and Rogerson, S. (2002) Caffeine potentiation of the performance enhancing effects of pseudoephedrine. *Medicine and Science in Sports and Exercise* 35: 110.

Wemple, R.D., Lamb, D.R. and McKeever, K.H. (1997) Caffeine vs caffeine-free sports drinks: Effects on urine production at rest and during prolonged exercise. *International Journal of Sports Medicine* 18: 40–46.

Wiles, J.D., Bird, S.R., Hopkins, J. and Riley, M. (1992) Effect of caffeinated coffee on running speed, respiratory factors, blood lactate and perceived exertion during 1500-m treadmill running. *British Journal of Sports Medicine* 26: 116–120.

Zhang, Y., Coca, A., Casa, D.J. et al. (2015) Caffeine and diuresis during rest and exercise: A meta-analysis. *Journal of Science and Medicine in Sport* 18: 569–574.

Zhang W.Y. and Li Wan Po, A.(1996) Analgesic efficacy of paracetamol and its combination with codeine and caffeine in surgical pain--a meta-analysis. *Journal of Clinical Pharmacy and Therapeutics* 21: 261–282.

Zhang W.Y. and Li Wan Po, A. (1997) Do codeine and caffeine enhance the analgesic effect of aspirin? A systematic overview. *Journal of Clinical Pharmacy and Therapeutics* 22: 79–97.

Section 4

Evolving issues concerning drug use in sport

Chapter 26

Drug use in society and the impact on the anti-doping movement

Neil Chester and Jim McVeigh

26.1 Introduction

Whilst the focus of this book is to examine the use of drugs within sport, particularly amongst those involved in competitive sport, there is a need to cast the net a little further. The prevalence and issues surrounding non-therapeutic drug use outside of organised sport has been widely documented for decades. Indeed, the use of illicit recreational drugs within society is a serious problem involving organised crime and with wide-reaching effects, having significant economic and social impact. The social and economic cost of drug supply in England and Wales is estimated to be £10.7 billion a year (Mills et al., 2013). Similarly, the use of performance- and image-enhancing drugs (PIED) is no longer simply the domain of serious body builders or high performance athletes, but is much more widespread amongst recreational athletes and those looking to enhance their body image. This is a global issue (Sagoe et al., 2014) with growing evidence from the UK (McVeigh and Begley, 2017), USA (Kanayama and Pope, 2012), Australia (Iverson et al., 2013) and Scandinavia (Bojsen-Møller and Christiansen, 2010). Indeed the growth in enhancement technologies within society signals an acceptance of advancement either to restore impaired function or to extend function beyond (perceived) normal limits. The ethical issues surrounding such developments are particularly important and warrant continual examination. A particular concern is the impact of the growing acceptance of enhancement technologies and the normalisation of societal drug use on sport and anti-doping.

26.2 Recreational psychoactive drug use

The addictive nature of many psychoactive drugs, coupled with their serious adverse health effects, has meant that many are classified as illicit under state law. Such classification is an attempt to control their use and thus limit their negative impact on health. Nevertheless, the continual development of new, designer drugs (e.g. variants of amphetamine and cannabis) makes law enforcement challenging. The effect of criminalisation on drug use and the reported harms are important questions that need to be resolved to ensure effective harm minimisation.

The non-medical use of psychoactive drugs has been regarded as a serious public health issue for some time. Whilst evidence of psychoactive drug use dates back to some of the earliest human records (Crocq, 2007), widespread non-medical use of psychoactive drugs has increased markedly throughout the twentieth century (Pickering and Stimson, 1994). Determining the scale of the problem of illicit drug use is particularly difficult due to the illegality and the stigmatisation of use. In the review by Degenhardt and Hall (2012) an estimated 149–271 million individuals worldwide used an illicit drug in 2009 of which 125–203 million were cannabis users and 15–39 million used opioids, amphetamines and cocaine. In developed countries, it was estimated that one in twenty individuals between 15 and 64 years had used illicit drugs in the last year (Degenhardt and Hall, 2012). In the UK, according to the Health and Social Care Information Centre (HSCIC, 2016), one in twelve adults (between 16 and 59 years) reported the use of illicit drugs in the previous year (2015/16). Despite such widespread use, there is evidence that overall use of illicit psychoactive drugs is declining (HSCIC, 2016), with the latest estimates of the number of people using drugs considered the most dangerous (i.e. opioids and crack cocaine) being 293,879 in the UK (Hay et al., 2014).

Recently the use of novel psychoactive substances has received notable attention not least due to the growth in their use and their purported negative effects on health. However, while the prevalence remains relatively low, approximately 100 new substances are being identified and monitored in Europe each year (European Monitoring Centre for Drugs and Drug Addiction, 2016). Often referred to as 'legal highs' such a term may be considered a misnomer, not least since this might suggest a level of safety, thus adding to their attraction but also due to recent changes to legislation in the UK (and elsewhere) that have meant it is now illegal to manufacture and supply such drugs under the Psychoactive Substances Act (2016). However, the chemicals contained in such products are generally unknown and there is a lack of toxicology data. Furthermore, a lack of quality assurance in their manufacture makes contamination of such products extremely likely (Gilani, 2016) – a public health issue they have in common with the PIED market (Chatwin et al., 2017). The intention of legislation is to reduce the prevalence of psychoactive substance use by limiting the production and supply. Whilst such legislation excludes substances such as nicotine, caffeine and alcohol, there appears to be some ambiguity with regards prohibited and exempt substances. Although food or drinks are typically considered exempt they may be considered a novel psychoactive substance if they contain an ingredient that is psychoactive – in such cases cocoa and nutmeg may be exempt. Nitrous oxide, used as a propellant in whipped cream, would be exempt from the Act unless it were to be sold for its psychoactive effect. There is concern as to the definition of the term psychoactive substances and whether it might be considered too broad. This concern highlights an important issue in terms of the blurring of boundaries between legal and illegal substances and what is considered acceptable and unacceptable drug use.

Despite the focus on illicit drugs, it is important to consider the many psychoactive drugs that are more socially accepted within many societies. Alcohol consumption and tobacco smoking is particularly common and legal amongst adults in many nations. Age restrictions are typically placed on their use and regulated through taxation. Nevertheless, it is pertinent to highlight the considerable harmful effects of widespread use of such psychoactive drugs. Nutt et al. (2010) considered a range of recreational drugs commonly used in the UK and concluded that both alcohol and nicotine had significant adverse effects and were particularly burdensome from a health perspective, in line with illicit drug use. In recent years, tobacco use has declined in the UK (Office for National Statistics, 2017a) and this trend is mirrored globally, particularly in high-income nations (WHO, 2015). Whilst alcohol consumption has declined marginally, it remains high in the UK (Office for National Statistics, 2017b)

As in the wider society, athletes are also susceptible to the use of illicit recreational drugs. Whilst many do not confer any ergogenic advantage, they are present on the

World Anti-Doping Agency Prohibited List since they pose a health risk to the athlete and their use would be considered against the spirit of sport. A recent example includes the British tennis player Dan Evans, who tested positive for cocaine at the Barcelona Open in April 2017. Although there is typically no intention to enhance performance athletes are generally held in high esteem and as role models, thus the use of recreational drugs is deemed unacceptable.

26.3 Performance- and image-enhancing drug use

Outside of sport, the use of many performance and image-enhancing drugs (PIED; e.g. anabolic androgenic steroids) is permitted in many nations other than Australia, the USA and parts of the European Union. Many state laws allow possession for personal use but prohibit trafficking. Nevertheless, a negative public perception around such drug use means that their use continues to be underground. This has implications on the accurate determination of the prevalence and characteristics of use of such drugs and on the extent to which such drugs have a negative impact on health. Indeed accessing such individuals for harm reduction purposes and wider health-related interventions can be extremely difficult.

For decades, the use of such drugs has centred on the bodybuilding community and, in a more covert manner, amongst elite athletes. More recently, PIED use has extended into the wider gym culture and has been embraced by adolescents and young men simply to improve their body image and wellbeing (Christiansen et al., 2016; McVeigh et al., 2012). Middle-aged and older men are also attracted to the use of PIEDs for the purpose of counteracting the effects of ageing. Historically, whilst there is a predominance of males using anabolic agents, drugs targeting weight loss are particularly attractive to females. This includes products that have been banned due to health concerns such as sibutramine and rimonabant and those classed as a metabolic poison such as dinitrophenol (DNP) (Evans-Brown et al., 2012)

The extent of image-enhancing drug use has risen dramatically over recent years. Evidence to support this rise has come from several sources, including UK official drug statistics (Lader, 2016). In the UK this rise has been acknowledged by the Advisory Council on the Misuse of Drugs (ACMD, 2010) and the National Institute for Health and Clinical Excellence harm minimisation schemes (NICE, 2014). These schemes were established in the UK in the 1980s to reduce the adverse effects of psychoactive drug use, in particular the prevention of HIV transmission (Stimson and O'Hare, 2010) and have been made accessible to those using drugs for image enhancement purposes such as anabolic androgenic steroids (AAS). The numbers of AAS users accessing syringe exchange clinics in the UK has increased dramatically (McVeigh and Begley, 2017).

Despite the significant increase in AAS use and widening use throughout society, particularly amongst adolescents there appears to be a reticence towards support aimed at reducing use and minimising harm. Such reticence might be based on the perceived impact of such drug use on public health. A priority within the UK has been to avoid driving the use of such drugs further underground, away from help and support and in avoiding the criminalisation of large numbers of young men, and the inherent risks attached to this. This is an ongoing strategy since AAS were first controlled under the Misuse of Drugs Act in 1996 (ACMD, 2010).

In a study by Nutt et al. (2010) AAS use was deemed to be a low risk drug of abuse when compared with illicit psychoactive drug use (e.g. cocaine, amphetamine and cannabis) as well as more socially acceptable drugs such as nicotine (tobacco) and alcohol. Whilst this might be the case there is growing evidence that anabolic agents have significant side effects and as the prevalence of use grows, particularly amongst younger generations, so does the impact on public health.

According to the Partnership for a Drug Free Kids survey, lifetime prevalence of AAS and human growth hormone misuse amongst US adolescents was found to be 7 per cent and 11 per cent, respectively (Partnership for Drug-Free Kids, 2013). Whilst adolescents constitute a minority in terms of the users of PIEDs they are a particularly important group as a consequence of their vulnerability with respect to the adverse side-effects.

Muscle dysmorphia is a condition whereby individuals have a negative perception of themselves in terms of their body image and musculature. Those with muscle dysmorphia perceive themselves to be unattractive and to be dissatisfied with their body composition. The use of AAS is believed to be a perpetuating factor in the development of muscle dysmorphia (Rohman, 2009). Pope et al. (1997) proposed the following diagnostic criteria for muscle dysmorphia:

- An individual with a preoccupation with their body composition and an opinion that their body is not sufficiently lean or muscular.
- The preoccupation causes significant distress relating to at least two of the following criteria:
  - A need to maintain training and diet at the expense of important social, occupational or recreational activities;
  - Avoidance of situations that involve exposure of their body to others or endure such situation with significant distress;
  - The preoccupation of the inadequacy of their body size causes clinical distress or impairment of functioning in social and occupational areas of their life;
  - Continuation of their training and dietary programme (and use of PIEDs) despite the awareness of the physical and psychological impact.

- The primary concern for the individual is their size and muscularity rather than body fat (as in anorexia nervosa).

While the potential for AAS dependence was first raised many years ago (Wright, 1980) there is now a growing concern regarding the development of AAS dependence syndrome amongst some AAS users. Kanayama et al. (2009) describe a form of dependence of the use of AAS that is coupled with prominent adverse psychological effects (Pope et al., 2017). Whilst muscle dysmorphia may be a predisposing factor for initiating AAS use for some, it may also play a part in the continuation of use and possible AAS dependence. Other proposed mechanisms include the withdrawal effects associated with AAS abstinence and classical rewarding or hedonic effects associated with AAS-induced positive psychological effects (Kanayama et al., 2010). Further research is warranted to further the understanding of the aetiology of AAS dependence together with risk and resilience factors.

The use of PIEDs has also been attributed to occupational motives amongst individuals occupying positions in the military, police force, prison and security services, the entertainment industry, and the sex industry. Whilst substances used to enhance lean body mass might be desirable to those roles that are physically demanding and require a physical presence, with the 'drive for muscularity' playing a significant role (McCreary and Sasse, 2000), the use of cognitive enhancers (smart drugs) may be attractive to those employed in a number of roles, for example in academia. However, the evidence surrounding the use of cognitive enhancers is weak, predominantly based on personal anecdotes and small-scale niche surveys (Lennard, 2009; Maher, 2008).

A particular issue of note amongst such drug users is the practice of polypharmacy. Competitive bodybuilders might focus their drug use specifically on PIEDs and possibly ancillary drugs to counteract any drug-related side effects that they may be experiencing. However, the gym user may be less discerning and combine PIEDs with recreational psychoactive drugs. Such polypharmacy is particularly concerning since there is limited information regarding the safety of such practices (Dodge and Hoagland, 2011; Sagoe et al., 2015).

The source of most PIEDs and psychoactive drugs is the illicit market. The internet is particularly important in serving this market, enabling access to a wide range of restricted drugs. Evidence indicates that the majority of available PIEDs have been manufactured illicitly without safeguards (Evans-Brown et al., 2012), with products untested, often contaminated with impurities and adulterated with additional active ingredients (Evans-Brown et al., 2009; Graham et al., 2009; MHRA, 2007; Stensballe et al., 2015). The unscrupulous marketing of illicit, contaminated products is also a significant factor in the high levels of localised infections (Hope et al., 2015).

26.4 Performance-enhancing drug use in recreational/non-elite athletic groups

Recent evidence suggests an increasing number of positive drug tests amongst those competing at lower competitive levels. According to the Rugby Football Union (RFU: Governing body for rugby Union in the UK) annual report (2015–2016) all players currently sanctioned for an anti-doping rule violation were those competing in what is considered amateur rugby (RFU, 2017). Whilst the data set is not large, in light of the fact that most drug testing occurs at the highest level of sports competition, it does suggest a possible shift in culture. Clearly it is difficult to ascertain the reasons for the use of PIEDs within this group; however, it is likely that not only might individuals be attracted to the increased performance capabilities ascribed to such use but also the concomitant improvements in body image that they enjoy/benefit from. A study by Frenger et al. (2015) examined data from a large-scale online survey (n = 13,910) targeting amateur athletes in Germany and the USA as well as university students in four European countries. The results from the survey showed that 5 per cent of respondents took prohibited substances with the intention of enhancing their sporting performance.

Currently anti-doping measures are centred almost entirely on elite competitors at senior or junior levels. Any deterrent acting on non-elite/amateur athletes is likely to be one that the individual athletes place on themselves. Indeed, Henning (2014) highlights how self-surveillance occurs at a non-elite level in road runners, through their interpretation of the anti-doping rules via media reports relating to elite athletes. Self-surveillance is clearly reliant on the knowledge of the athlete regarding anti-doping rules and their own integrity. In many respects, such athletes are most likely to be influenced by changes in societal norms and opinion regarding drug use and enhancement since they are not confined by the constant surveillance that their elite counterparts are exposed to and might not consider the anti-doping rules to be directly applicable or relevant to them.

26.5 Human enhancement technology

Human enhancement technology is a broad term, which incorporates a wide range of bio-technological advances designed to enhance human function and appearance. The interest in human enhancement technology has traditionally focused on health requirements and the restoration of function or appearance to a desired norm. However, in recent years there has been growth in the interest in lifestyle requirements and enhancement beyond normal capacity. Human performance is an important target for those looking to develop or embrace human enhancement technology.

Human enhancement can be categorised into the following:

1   Life extension;
2   Physical and image enhancement;
3   Mood and personality enhancement; and
4   Cognitive enhancement.

On the surface, it might be difficult to appreciate the negative implications of human enhancement technology; however, it raises important ethical questions which need addressing. For example:

1   Which types of human enhancement should we accept and which should we discourage?
2   Who should benefit or access human enhancement technology?
3   What boundaries, if any should we put in place to protect individuals and society against human enhancement?
4   In what arenas or environments will society permit enhancement and where would it be considered deviant?

The acceptance of human enhancement is clearly not a simple argument. Whilst the technology and the skills tend to be already available, comprehensive debate is necessary in an attempt to provide some answers to the key questions and thus protect those tempted to embrace such enhancement.

Enhancement technologies may be categorised in the following way:

1)   Pharmaceutical enhancement: a wide range of substances, both licit and illicit are used with the aim of improving performance of a particular task or activity, enhancing body image (Table 26.1) or improving health;
2)   Medical/surgical enhancement: numerous interventions with the intention of improving quality of life, health and saving life are available, including organ replacement, sensory implants (e.g. cochlear implants used to restore hearing), cosmetic surgery, prosthetics;
3)   Genetic enhancement: the transfer of genetic material with the intention of modifying human traits. Whilst genetic enhancement is often attributed to doping it may also include gene therapy used to improve health;
4)   Mechanical and computer technological enhancement: a wide range of technological advances have helped to enhance health, sports performance and lifestyle across all spheres. Examples might include medical imaging techniques (e.g. magnetic resonance imaging), mobile phones and computers.

Table 26.1 Examples of pharmacological agents used to enhance performance and image
(Evans-Brown et al., 2012)

Pharmacological agent	Reasons for use	Legal status in UK
Anabolic androgenic steroids	Stimulates muscle growth	POM; controlled drug
Human growth hormone	Stimulates muscle growth	POM; controlled drug
IGF-1	Stimulates muscle growth, mediates the action of GH	POM
Insulin	Enhance muscle mass and endurance	POM
Aromatase inhibitors	Limits conversion of testosterone to oestrogen	POM
Anti-oestrogens (e.g. Tamoxifen)	Blocks the action of oestrogen	POM
Human chorionic gonadotropin (HCG)	Stimulates testosterone production	POM; controlled drug
Selective androgen receptor modulators (SARMs)	Enhance muscle mass	Untested
Clenbuterol	Enhance muscle mass	Not licenced in UK; controlled drug
Sibutramine	Supresses appetite	Banned
Orlistat	Reduces dietary fat absorption	POM
Thyroid hormone (T3; T4)	Increases metabolic rate	POM; Not licenced for weight loss
Ephedrine	Increases metabolic rate	POM; Not licenced for weight loss
Dinitrophenol (DNP)	Increases metabolic rate	Untested
Melanotan II	Increases melanin production in skin; darkens skin colour	Untested
Finasteride	Increases hair growth on scalp	POM
Botulinum toxin	Muscle relaxant to reduce wrinkles	POM
Isotretinoin	Reduces sebum secretion/acne	POM
Sildenafil (i.e. Viagra)	Increases sexual function; increases blood flow to the penis	POM
Modafinil	Promotes wakefulness/ alertness; dopamine reuptake inhibitor	POM
Methylphenidate (i.e. Ritalin)	Stimulant; dopamine reuptake inhibitor	POM; controlled drug
Fluoxetine (i.e. Prozac)	Selective serotonin reuptake inhibitor; enhances mood	POM
Diazepam	Reduces anxiety	POM

POM – prescription only medicine

Enhancement technology is typically embraced for self-improvement and in many cases offers corrective measures to various disabilities including long or short sightedness, poor hearing and ambulation. Nevertheless, it is difficult to ascertain or define disability. A disability might be considered a physical or mental impairment that affects an individual to the extent that they are unable to perform particular activities required within daily living.

26.6 The normalisation of drug use in society and the impact on the anti-doping movement

A developing threat to the anti-doping movement is considered to be the normalisation of drug use within society. The growing trend towards the use and acceptance of enhancement technologies is likely to have a detrimental effect on anti-doping. As society continues to embrace the 'body beautiful' ideal and continues the quest for the ultimate anti-ageing elixir so too does drug-free sport become an ideal within a sub-section of society that is effectively dissociated and eroded.

The normalisation of adolescent recreational drug use is a well-known concept that has been described by several researchers including Measham et al. (1994) and Parker et al. (1998). It refers to the acceptance or justification of what is essentially deviant behaviour by both those that participate in the activity and society at large, to the extent that it enters mainstream culture.

The process by which such behaviour has become normalised may be under discussion; however, it is likely to become so, in part as a consequence of increased imagery relating to drugs and drug use particularly by major companies to market their products in a positive light (Blackman, 2010). The advent of the internet has clearly been a significant landmark in the legitimisation and normalisation of non-therapeutic drug use. For the first time, individuals across a wider sector of society have been introduced to and bombarded with images relating to drug use, and their availability has rocketed. The internet also provided a platform for information and misinformation relating to drug use (Evans-Brown et al., 2012).

There is a danger that the use of PIEDs, which is currently viewed as risky behaviour, will become normalised and therefore accepted behaviour within society. Indeed, subliminal messages from advertising are considered to play their part in normalising drug use. For example, the portrayal of male physiques with heavy musculature and the use of the term 'steroids' in a positive light to describe power and muscular bulk all help to change the perception of PIED use within society to one that is more acceptable. Clearly such a change in perception creates a contradiction in terms of the legislation of PIEDs in sport. The perceived ineffectiveness of doping control is further amplified by the normalisation of PIEDs within society.

However, the interaction between PIED use, sport and the wider society is multidirectional. Indeed, the high sense of morals and ethics in the protection of sport from doping may have an influence on the legislation and control of substance use beyond the realms of sport (Kayser et al., 2007; Kayser and Smith, 2008).

There is evidence of a growing acceptance of PIED use as an inevitable part of competitive sport. According to findings from interviews with athletes who had used PIEDs, doping was considered an established and essential behaviour in competitive sport and none viewed their activity as abnormal (Pappa and Kennedy, 2013). It is this acceptance of PIED drug use in competitive sport that enables athletes to legitimise their behaviour. Clearly, this ability to rationalise is deemed to have a direct impact on the prevalence of PIED use amongst athletes. Nevertheless, since the anti-doping rules set out in the World Anti-Doping Code establish a framework for the welfare and safety of athletes and attempt to ensure fair play, such normalisation of doping from an athlete's perspective might be disregarded. However, it might be argued that the normalisation of non-therapeutic drug use within the wider society could have a greater effect on PIED use in sport as a consequence of the impact on the anti-doping movement. Of course without an effective anti-doping programme PIED use in sport will inevitably mushroom.

Within the wider society the following factors are thought to undermine the anti-doping movement:

1   Widespread use of recreational, illicit drugs across all classes and ages (although generally centred on the young);
2   Increased use of image-enhancing and anti-ageing drugs/products across a wide spectrum of society in response to media-driven images and expectations;
3   Use of cognitive-enhancing drugs amongst students and the workforce alike to maintain or increase productivity; and
4   The increased entertainment value of sport for the general public and the audience attitudes towards doping, such as the ambivalence towards athletes who are caught and their enjoyment of watching high-level performance however it may be achieved.

As these factors, as well as others become more accepted or central in daily living it is likely that the zero tolerance approach to PIED use in sport will appear ever more alien. Whilst sport may always be able to justify its position as a 'rule-based' institution it may become more difficult to justify and indeed legislate against something that is becoming increasingly acceptable elsewhere in society.

26.7 Summary

The reasons behind drug use are multi-factorial and whilst anti-doping is focused largely on substances (and methods) for the purpose of performance enhancement, athletes and the wider society may use drugs for a wide variety of non-therapeutic reasons, including for both recreation and enhancement purposes. Furthermore, these drugs may not only be legal but also heavily advertised and promoted within certain environments (e.g. alcohol being one of the most prevalent enhancement drugs). Enhancement incorporates numerous technologies that serve to augment all aspects of human function and activities. The development of enhancement technologies is testament to the general acceptance of self-improvement, empowerment and a medicalised society. The continually shifting societal values towards youthfulness and immediate gratification further amplifies the demand for and acceptance of enhancement technologies.

It is essential that the anti-doping movement continues to debate the issues relating to PIED use within the context of societal drug use. Whilst the focus of anti-doping will remain on competitive sport, the wider issues relating to health and welfare of all those engaged in sport and exercise must be considered. The wider debate around enhancement technologies must also be brought to the fore to establish clear guidance with respect to acceptable behaviour. The acceptance of technology to enhance capabilities beyond what are deemed to be 'normal' must be questioned; so too must the issues around individual human rights. For example, is it acceptable for an individual to choose whether to employ enhancement technology to develop physical and cognitive characteristics with the aim of excelling in their chosen activity, yet for it to be forbidden in sport? Also, why is society more tolerant of the artist, poet or musician who may stimulate their imagination through substance use compared to the athlete? No artist has been stripped of their achievements or banned from engaging in their work as a consequence of substance use. The issue of doping and drug use in general highlights complex societal issues which cannot be examined in isolation.

The public perception and opinion of enhancement technology and non-therapeutic drug use, particularly with respect to sport, is an essential issue to consider by sports and anti-doping organisations. Public opinion is central to the anti-doping movement and is likely to have particular influence in terms of the success of future control strategies.

26.8 References

ACMD (2010) *Advisory Council on the Misuse of Drugs, Consideration of the Anabolic Steroids*. London: Home Office.

Blackman, S. (2010) Youth subcultures, normalization and drug prohibition: The politics of contemporary crisis and change? *British Politics* 5: 337–366.

Bojsen-Møller, J. and Christiansen, A.V. (2010) Use of performance-and image-enhancing substances among recreational athletes: A quantitative analysis of inquiries submitted to the Danish anti-doping authorities. *Scandinavian Journal of Medicine and Science in Sports* 20: 861–867.

Chatwin, C., Measham, F., O'Brien, K. and Sumnall, H. (2017) New drugs, new directions? Research priorities for new psychoactive substances and human enhancement drugs. *International Journal of Drug Policy* 40: 1–5.

Christiansen, A.V., Vinther, A.S. and Liokaftos, D. (2016) Outline of a typology of men's use of anabolic androgenic steroids in fitness and strength training environments. *Drug Education, Prevention and Policy* 24: 3.

Crocq, M.A. (2007) Historical and cultural aspects of man's relationship with addictive drugs. *Dialogues Clinical Neuroscience* 9(4): 355–361.

Degenhardt, L. and Hall, W. (2012) Extent of illicit drug use and dependence and their contribution to the global burden of disease. *Lancet* 379: 55–70.

Dodge, T. and Hoagland, M.F. (2011) The use of anabolic androgenic steroids and polypharmacy: A review of the literature. *Drug and Alcohol Dependence* 114(2-3): 100–109.

European Monitoring Centre for Drugs and Drug Addiction (2016) European Drug Report 2016: Trends and developments. Available at: http://www.emcdda.europa.eu/publications/edr/trends-developments/2016 (Accessed on 31 July 2017).

Evans-Brown, M., Kimergard, A., and McVeigh, J. (2009). Elephant in the room? The methodological implications for public health research of performance-enhancing drugs derived from the illicit market. *Drug Testing and Analysis* 1: 323–326.

Evans-Brown, M., McVeigh, J., Perkins, C. and Bellis, M.A. (2012) *Human Enhancement Drugs: The Emerging Challenges to Public health*. North West Public Health Observatory, Liverpool. Available at: http://www.cph.org.uk/wp-content/uploads/2012/08/human-enhancement-drugs---the-emerging-challenges-to-public-health---4.pdf (Accessed on 31 July 2017).

Frenger, M., Pitsch W. and Emrich, E. (2015) Doping in mass sport: An inexplicable problem? *Performance Enhancement and Health* 3(2): 116.

Gilani, F. (2016) Novel psychoactive substances: The rising wave of 'legal highs' *British Journal of General Practice* 66(642): 8–9.

Graham, M.R., Ryan, P., Baker, J.S., Davies, B. et al. (2009) Counterfeiting in performance- and image-enhancing drugs. *Drug Testing and Analysis* 1: 135–142.

Hay, G., Rael dos Santos, A., and Worsley, J. (2014). Estimates of the Prevalence of Opiate Use and/or Crack Cocaine Use, 2011/12: Sweep 8 Report. Available at: http://www.nta.nhs.uk/uploads/estimates-of-the-prevalence-of-opiate-use-and-or-crack-cocaine-use-2011-12.pdf (Accessed on 31 July 2017).

Henning, A. (2014) (Self-) surveillance, anti-doping and health in non-elite road running. *Surveillance and Society* 11(4): 494–507.

Hope, V.D., McVeigh, J., Marongiu, A. et al. (2015). Injection site infections and injuries in men who inject image- and performance-enhancing drugs: Prevalence, risks factors, and healthcare seeking. *Epidemiology and Infection* 143: 132–140.

HSCIC (2016) Statistics on drug misuse. Available at: http://content.digital.nhs.uk/catalogue/PUB21159 (Accessed on 31 July 2017).

Iversen J., Topp L., Wand H., Maher L. (2013). Are people who inject performance and image-enhancing drugs an increasing population of Needle and Syringe Program attendees? *Drug and Alcohol Review* 32: 205–207.

Kanayama, G., Brower, K.J., Wood R.I. et al. (2009) Anabolic-androgenic steroid dependence: An emerging disorder. *Addiction* 104: 1,966–1,978.

Kanayama, G., Brower, K.J., Wood R.I. et al. (2010) Treatment of anabolic-androgenic steroid dependence: Emerging evidence and its implications. *Drug and Alcohol Dependence* 109: 6–13.

Kanayama G., Pope H. G. (2012). Misconceptions about anabolic-androgenic steroid abuse. *Psychiatric Annals* 42: 371–375.

Kayser, B, Mauron, A. and Miah, A. (2007) Current anti-doping policy: A critical appraisal. *BMC Medical Ethics* 8: 2.

Kayser, B. and Smith. A.C. (2008) Globalisation of anti-doping: The reverse side of the medal. *British Medical Journal* 337: a584.

Lader, D. (2016) Drug misuse: Findings from the 2015/16 Crime Survey for England and Wales. Available at: https://www.gov.uk/government/collections/drug-misuse-declared (Accessed on 24 July 2017).

Lennard, N. (2009) One in ten takes drugs to study. *Varsity* 6 March 1: 5.

Maher, B. (2008) Poll results: Look who's doping. *Nature*. 452: 674–675.

McCreary, D.R., and Sasse, D.K. (2000). An exploration of the drive for muscularity in adolescent boys and girls. *Journal of American College Health* 48(6): 297–304.

McVeigh, J. and Begley, (2017) Anabolic steroids in the UK: An increasing issue for public health. *Drugs Education Prevention and Policy* 24(3): 278–285.

McVeigh, J., Evans-Brown, M., and Bellis, M.A. (2012) Human enhancement drugs and the pursuit of perfection. *Adicciones* 24(3): 185–190.

Measham, F., Newcombe, R. and Parker, H. (1994) The normalization of recreational drug use amongst young people in North-West England. *British Journal of Sociology* 45(2): 287–312.

MHRA (2007) *Rules and Guidance for Pharmaceutical Manufacturers and Distributors*. London, Pharmaceutical Press.

Mills, H., Skodbo, S. and Blyth, P. (2013). *Understanding organised crime: Estimating the scale and the social and economic costs*. Home Office Research Report 73. London: Home Office. Available at: https://www.gov.uk/government/publications/understanding-organised-crime-estimating-the-scale-and-the-social-and-economic-costs (Accessed on 21 July 2017).

NICE (2014) Needle and syringe programmes. Available at: https://www.nice.org.uk/guidance/ph52/chapter/What-is-this-guidance-about (Accessed on 31 July 2017).

Nutt, D.J., King, L.A. and Phillips, L.D. (2010) Drug harms in the UK: A multicriteria decision analysis. *Lancet* 376: 1,558–1,565.

Office for National Statistics (2017a) Adult smoking habits in the UK: 2016. Available at: https://www.ons.gov.uk/peoplepopulationandcommunity/healthandsocialcare/healthandlifeexpectancies/bulletins/adultsmokinghabitsingreatbritain/2016 (Accessed on 8 July 2017).

Office for National Statistics (2017b) Adult drinking habits in Great Britain: 2005 to 2016. Available at: https://www.ons.gov.uk/releases/adultdrinkinghabitsingreatbritain2015 (Accessed on 8 July 2017).

Pappa, E. and Kennedy, E. (2013) 'It was my thought . . . he made it a reality': Normalization and responsibility in athletes' accounts of performance-enhancing drug use. *International Review for the Sociology of Sport* 48(3): 277–294.

Parker, H., Measham, F. and Aldridge, J. (1998) *Illegal Leisure: The Normalization of Adolescent Drug Use.* London, Routledge.

Partnership for Drug-Free Kids (2013) The partnership attitude tracking study. Available at: https://drugfree.org/wp-content/uploads/2014/07/PATS-2013-FULL-REPORT.pdf (Accessed on 31 July 2017).

Pickering, H. and Stimson, G.V. (1994) Prevalence and demographic factors of stimulant use. *Addiction* 89: 1,385–1,389.

Pope, H.G., Khalsa, J.H. and Bhasin, S. (2017) Body image disorders and abuse of anabolic-androgenic steroids among men. *Journal of the American Medical Association* 317(1): 23–24.

Pope, H.G., Gruber, A.J., Choi, P., Olivardia, R. and Phillips, K.A. (1997) Muscle dysmorphia: An unrecognised form of body dysmorphic disorder. *Psychosomatics* 38: 548–557.

Psychoactive Substances Act (2016) Explanatory notes. Available at: http://www.legislation.gov.uk/ukpga/2016/2/notes/division/1/index.htm (Accessed on 8 July 2017).

RFU (2017) Anti-Doping Programme 2015–16 Annual Report. Available at: http://www.england rugby.com/mm/Document/General/General/01/32/25/82/RFU_Anti-DopingReport2015_16_Version4_English.pdf (Accessed on 31 July 2017).

Rohman, L. (2009) The relationship between anabolic androgenic steroids and muscle dysmorphia: A review. *Eating Disorders* 17:187–199.

Sagoe, D., McVeigh, J., Bjornebekk, A. et al. (2015) Polypharmacy among anabolic-androgenic steroid users: A descriptive metasynthesis. *Substance Abuse Treatment Prevention and Policy* 15(10): 12.

Sagoe D., Molde H., Andreassen C. S. et al. (2014). The global epidemiology of anabolic-androgenic steroid use: A meta-analysis and meta-regression analysis. *Annals of Epidemiology* 24: 383–398.

Stensballe, A., McVeigh, J., Breindahl, T., and Kimergard, A. (2015). Synthetic growth hormone releasers detected in seized drugs: New trends in the use of drugs for performance enhancement. *Addiction* 110: 368–369.

Stimson, G.V. and O'Hare, P. (2010) Harm reduction: Moving through the third decade. *International Journal of Drug Policy* 21: 91–93.

WHO (2015) WHO report on the global tobacco epidemic, 2015. Available at: http://apps.who.int/iris/bitstream/10665/178574/1/9789240694606_eng.pdf?ua=1&ua=1 (Accessed on 9 July 2017).

Wright, J.E. (1980) Anabolic steroids and athletics. *Exercises and Sports Science Review* 8: 149–202.

Chapter 27

Governance and corruption in sport with respect to doping

Neil King

27.1 Introduction

The issue of doping is central to understanding the governance of sport. Since the 1960s, high profile doping 'scandals' involving elite athletes, international governing bodies and state agencies have raised public awareness of corruption, bribery and mismanagement in sport (Numerato, Baglioni and Persson, 2013). Subsequently, governing bodies of sport have been subject to increased scrutiny and intervention by government agencies in a context of relatively weak regulatory oversight and increasing commercialisation (Houlihan, 2003). In an effort to coordinate anti-doping measures across sports and nation states, a World Anti-Doping Agency (WADA) was founded in 1999. Today, the anti-doping governance infrastructure is a global labyrinth of organisations, legislation, regulation, policies and interventions funded by both governing bodies and governments. The scale of doping in sport however remains unquantified and given the recent investigation of doping in Russia (McLaren, 2016a, 2016b) it is clear that the anti-doping coalition face significant challenges if doping-free sport is ever to be realised.

For an analysis of sport governance and policy in respect of doping, this chapter draws on a growing body of research, most notably by Houlihan (1999a, 1999b, 2002a, 2002b, 2003, 2007, 2014) but also by David (2008), Kayser, Mauron and Miah (2007), and Reid and Kitchen (2013), and the broader sport governance literature (Hoye and Cuskelly, 2007; King, 2016) where the key themes are:

- Legal and regulatory change (Gardiner, 2009; Parrish, 2003; Reilly, 2012);
- Stakeholding (Casini, 2009; Houlihan, 2013; Thibault et al., 2010);
- Organisational performance (Robinson, 2012; Winand, 2011);
- Accountability, transparency and ethical practice (Bovens, 2007; Henry and Lee, 2004; Pound, 2011); and
- Compliance (Green and Houlihan, 2006; Houlihan, 2002b; Pieth, 2010; Tallberg, 2002).

In terms of structure, this chapter is divided into four sections. First, an overview of anti-doping policy traces key developments in doping policy and governance from the 1960s to the current date. Second, the extensive worldwide governance infrastructure to challenge doping in sport is mapped in order to foreground the expanding role of government (and more broadly, state) agencies in doping. However, despite an extensive anti-doping infrastructure with a remit to eradicate or diminish the use of drugs that may enhance athlete performance, the size of the challenge facing governing bodies remains large, as illustrated by a case study of doping in Russia in the third section. The fourth section assesses the prospects for the effective governance of drugs in sport. The chapter concludes with a brief discussion that pinpoints doping as a 'test case' for governing bodies of sport. A bullet point summary and list of sources completes the chapter.

27.2 The evolution of anti-doping policy: an overview

Today's extensive global governance infrastructure to tackle doping in sport emerged from government, media and public concerns dating back to the 1960s (Houlihan, 2002a). In a volatile political and ideological context in the 'cold war' era, sporting competition between capitalist and communist states enabled a doping culture to become embedded in some sports where athlete doping was effectively ignored or encouraged by agencies of the state (Hoberman, 1984). Arguably, the International Olympic Committee (IOC) did not thoroughly investigate doping allegations due to concerns regarding the image of sport, notwithstanding the likely costs and complexity associated with an investigation (Houlihan, 2003). Although difficult to prove beyond a reasonable doubt, it can be concluded on a balance of probabilities that coaches, athletes and government departments colluded in the use of performance-enhancing drugs in the former Soviet states as noted in trials related to doping programmes in the former East Germany (Franke and Brendonk, 1997).

However, outside of state-controlled doping regimes, a culture of doping was also detected in the Australian Institute of Sport, resulting in a high-profile government investigation (Australian Government, 1989). Where commercial sector interests drive sport, the Bay Area Laboratory Collective (BALCO) supplied athletes with drugs initially unbeknown to the US Anti-Doping Agency until whistleblowing occurred (Holt et al., 2009; Reid and Kitchen, 2013). These examples serve to highlight that doping is a feature of elite sport both where the state effectively steers the governance of sport and where the state has limited oversight for sport. However, it may be more deeply embedded where sport is under state control as the McLaren (2016a and 2016b) reports highlight.

Sport governance in respect of doping has in part been driven by a series of doping scandals such as the Ben Johnson affair in 1988 (Dubin, 1990). This in turn led to calls for more effective interventions by governing bodies and pressure from government agencies concerned with sport policy, investment, legislation and regulation. Policy harmonisation across sports, between sports organisations and across nation states was proving to be challenging (Houlihan, 1999a). A tipping point was reached at the 1998 Tour de France when the extent of doping was uncovered by French police and customs authorities (Houlihan, 2003). It is noteworthy that the governance of the doping issue became no longer solely the remit of sports bodies and government agencies with oversight for sport policy as doping became an issue meriting criminal investigations. The apparatus of the state began to mobilise around the doping issue and this trend has continued, as is discussed in the following section. Given the increasing commercialisation of professional sport, powerful sports organisations such as the IOC were no longer exempt from a tightening legislative and compliance framework.

The 1960s to late 1990s can be characterised as an era when government powers increased in respect of the governance of doping and the autonomy of international and national governing bodies for sport diminished, apart from the larger international organisations such as the IOC thanks to its relative wealth and influence. For most sports bodies, however, given their limited resources and dependency on external sources of funding, government now plays a key role in sport governance. In part, the role of government expanded as a result of sports bodies avoiding or evading the significant challenge presented by doping. More specifically, the reputational and commercial damage of governing bodies finding evidence of doping in their sport prohibited or constrained effective intervention, as did the legal costs of accusing athletes of using performance-enhancing drugs. Moreover, costly mistakes could be made by governing bodies such as by the former British Athletic Federation (BAF) who took action against the athlete Diane Modahl based on testing errors (Hartley, 2013). As a result, doping infringements in some sports remained unchallenged and doping became normalised over time. Further, over this timespan, a variety of approaches to doping were applied by different governing bodies across different sports and nations that in turn led to inconsistencies in policy and practice, interoperability issues, a lack of transparency, stakeholder disengagement, limited compliance with regulation and litigation by athletes accused of doping (for more detailed accounts see Holt et al., 2009; Houlihan, 2002a and 2003).

Subsequently, the founding of WADA in 1999 was an attempt to find a consensus regarding definitions of doping, the classification of prohibited substances, procedures for testing, sanctions, appeals, and educational interventions (David, 2008). More recently, the latest World Anti-Doping Code (WADA, 2015a) has been signed by 660 stakeholders in the sport sector including major governing bodies for sport and public authorities across many nation states, resulting, to an extent, in a harmonisation of rules and regulations. However, the implementation and evaluation of anti-doping interventions since the creation of WADA has proven to be more problematic, as will be discussed in Sections 27.4 and 27.5. First, however, the core components of the contemporary anti-doping infrastructure are detailed.

27.3 The anti-doping governance infrastructure

An extensive organisational and regulatory infrastructure exists today to challenge doping in sport. It is part state funded where government departments and agencies have intervened in sports governance and part funded by the IOC for those sports that have Olympic status. Of note is that a narrative of governance reform or 'modernisation' (Green and Houlihan, 2006), steered by government agencies with significant financial and political resources, has replaced a narrative of self-governance by governing bodies. The dominant governance narrative today is underpinned by a layered framework of compliance (Houlihan, 2002b, 2014) consisting of legal, regulatory and policy components, including a layer of scrutiny and surveillance in order to monitor and evaluate the effectiveness of interventions.

The main components of an evolving anti-doping infrastructure include:

- A World Anti-Doping Agency (WADA);
- A World Anti-Doping Code (2015a) and a code compliance monitoring programme;
- Funding from government targeted at doping. WADA receives 50 per cent of its funding from the IOC and 50 per cent from a number of governments;
- Multi-national treaties and agreements such as the International Convention Against Doping in Sport (UNESCO, 2012) that is ratified by 183 nation states;
- An International Anti-Doping Arrangement;
- The Council of Europe (COE) Monitoring Group and the European Committee for WADA;
- National anti-doping agencies such as the US Anti-Doping Agency (USADA) and UK Anti-Doping (UKAD);

- Partnerships and collaborative bodies across nation states formed to increase interoperability including the Institute of National Anti-Doping Organisations (iNADO);
- Legislative bodies to deal with specific cases such as the Anti-Doping Division within the Court of Arbitration for Sport (CAS);
- An expanding list of banned substances and agreed upon athlete suspensions, fines and bans;
- Accredited laboratories to test for banned substances;
- Athlete surveillance mechanisms to monitor doping;
- Investigatory panels or committees within sports governing bodies at the international and national levels;
- A plethora of strategies, codes of practice and educational initiatives drawn-up by the numerous organisations responsible for sport governance, including the IOC and the International Association of Athletic Federations (IAAF);
- Forums and conferences that bring together sports federations, governing bodies, National Anti-Doping Organisations (NADOs), professional athletes, sponsors, lawyers, academics, scientists and consultants;
- Taskforces such as the IAAF taskforce that investigated the Russian Athletics Federation (RAF) (see Section 27.4);
- Elements of the criminal justice system such as the police and customs authorities employed in the investigation into the Tour de France;
- Components of the 'deep state', including Intelligence agencies and INTERPOL who work with the IOC and COE;
- Government bills in respect of good governance (e.g. UK Parliament, 2015); and
- Good governance guides and codes of practice (e.g. UK Sport, 2004).

This extensive and complex infrastructure with a remit to detect, deter and prevent doping has emerged from a loose affiliation of organisations, pressure groups and individuals advocating governance change that has become an epistemic community consisting of advocates who share values and ideas, pool resources and seek policy change, or more broadly, governance change (Haas, 1990; Houlihan, 1999b). This community has acquired a level of political support, pooled expertise and established an evidence base to make the case for investment in an anti-doping governance infrastructure. However, the current level of efficacy of the community is questionable given the unknown extent of doping in sport. Nonetheless, the patchwork approach to doping prior to the establishment of WADA has been replaced with one that is more coherent and better resourced.

The period since WADA was founded until 2016 could be considered as almost two decades of 'progress' in tackling doping in sport, with a level of policy harmonisation acquired across states and across sports; the closure of organisations supplying drugs such as BALCO; successful prosecutions of high-profile athletes; and the rectification of the image and integrity of sport to some extent. However, the WADA-led investigation undertaken by McLaren (2016a and 2016b) demonstrates clearly that doping in sport has not been addressed in at least one nation state, namely Russia. Moreover, it is unlikely that Russia is unique in this regard. This chapter will turn next to the damning conclusions of the two McLaren reports.

27.4 Case study: doping in Russia and the McLaren reports

The three key findings of the first McLaren report (2016a: 1), commissioned by WADA are unequivocal:

- The Ministry of Sport in Russia directed, controlled and oversaw the manipulation of athlete's analytical results or sample swapping, with the active participation and assistance of the lead intelligence agency and both the Moscow and Sochi laboratories.
- The Moscow laboratory operated, for the protection of doped Russian athletes, within a state-dictated failsafe system, described in the report as the 'Disappearing Positive Methodology'.
- The Sochi laboratory operated a unique sample swapping methodology to enable doped Russian athletes to compete at the (Olympic) Games.

The second report (McLaren, 2016b: 1-3) is more comprehensive, adding significant detail to the earlier report. Nonetheless, the assertion that elements of the Russian state intentionally doped athletes remains the core finding. The key points of the report in brief are:

- An institutional conspiracy existed across summer and winter sports athletes involving Russian officials within the Ministry of Sport and its infrastructure. In other words, athletes were not acting alone.
- The manipulation of the doping control process occurred over a timespan that included the London 2012 Summer Games and the Winter Games in Sochi in 2014.
- The evolution of the doping infrastructure was in response to WADA regulatory changes and out-of-competition testing.
- Over 1,000 Russian athletes competing in summer, winter and Paralympic sports can be identified as being involved in or benefiting from manipulations to conceal positive doping tests.

It can be concluded that Russian athletes benefitted from a centralised and systematic approach to doping involving components of the state. Subsequent to the first report, Russia was suspended from the 2016 Olympic and Paralympic Games in Rio de Janeiro. However, a generic ban was not agreed by the IOC and a reduced squad of Russian athletes competed. Around 100 athletes were barred, however. After the second report, the IOC appointed two commissions to investigate McLaren's findings and opened disciplinary proceedings against specific Russian athletes who competed in 2014 at the Sochi Winter Olympics. Critically, this action was not taken on the basis of AAFs (adverse analytical findings) pertaining to failed doping tests but on the basis of the manipulation of samples, which is indicative of a proactive approach to doping violations rather than a reliance on 'proof'. The Sochi games were targeted as Russia hosted the event and was therefore in a position to manipulate a favourable outcome. Given that investigatory bodies in Russia are directed by the state, the opportunities to introduce a doping programme funded and managed by state agencies were enhanced.

The IAAF has noted a lack of reform in the governance of Russian athletics. The Russian Athletics Federation (RAF) had been barred from international competition (prior to the reports) and has not submitted athlete biological passport samples to the IAAF for independent testing. Moreover, athlete whereabouts for out-of-competition testing is unknown in some cases. Following the McLaren reports, the Russian Anti-Doping Agency was viewed as non-compliant with the World Anti-Doping Code and Russia's drug-testing operations have been decertified. However, to date the Russian Olympic Committee (ROC) has not been suspended following the McLaren reports. Given the number of organisations responsible for governing sport in Russia (as elsewhere) and the number of unknown and perhaps unquantifiable aspects of doping, it has proved to be problematic for the IOC and WADA to guarantee anti-doping measures are having an impact.

In conclusion, the extent of doping in Russia appears to be extensive and intentional. In this context, at the time of writing, whether Russian athletes can compete in the 2018 Winter Olympics in PyeongChang, South Korea is undetermined. The state-funded systemic use of drugs for acquiring political if not ideological advantage clearly remains a key motive for some nation states, undermining the integrity of sport in the international arena. On the other hand, banning all Russian athletes from competing can be viewed as arbitrary and capricious, if not a 'political decision' in the wider political context. Critically, it is problematic for 'clean' Russian athletes to prove their innocence. Nonetheless, many Russian athletes competed at the 2016 Olympic Games under a neutral flag which in itself draws attention to the limitations of anti-doping investigations. Despite the McLaren reports, harmonising anti-doping policy and practice across nation states remains an aspiration rather than a reality. The final section of this chapter assesses the prospects for the effective governance of drugs in sport.

27.5 Building an effective governance infrastructure and anti-doping policy

Creating effective governance including anti-doping policy and practices would require political support within governing bodies for sport and within government agencies, coupled with a regulatory and legislative framework that would enable action to be taken against individuals and organisations facilitating the use of performance enhancing drugs or obfuscating drug-use. Effective governance also requires the organisational capacity to address doping including adequate financial resources to implement and assess interventions. An effective form of governance also requires public support, media responsibility, a voice for athletes, cooperation between agencies and accountability. This section identifies and analyses components of effective governance and highlights a number of constraints to effective anti-doping interventions.

Political leadership

The governing bodies for sport with a responsibility for tackling doping, such as the IAAF, were cited by the second WADA-commissioned McLaren report (2016b) as lacking political leadership in tackling doping. The report cites corruption, nepotism and abuse of power, including an undermining of the anti-doping structure itself and even a 'cover up' of athlete doping (Play the Game, 2016). Subsequently, the IAAF (2016) and other bodies have sought reform leading to a more robust approach to doping within athletics. The evidence and intelligence cited in the McLaren reports is also being used to embed World Anti-Doping Code compliance at sports events and among individual athletes. As noted, governing bodies have historically sought to evade reputational and financial damage, from sponsors withdrawing support for example, should doping cases come to light. As a result, recommendations cited in reports, following reviews of governance, have typically included: revisions to governance structures and principles, a separation of anti-doping work from the political work, the establishment of an independent compliance committee and safeguards for whistle-blowers. Clearly, building effective anti-doping measures requires strong political leadership by governing bodies with oversight for doping.

Financial resources to address doping

As noted, WADA receives 50 per cent of its funding from the IOC and 50 per cent from a number of governments. Almost half of the government contribution derives from Europe (via the Council of Europe), with almost an equivalent contribution made by Asia and the Americas (mainly sourced from the USA and Canada). In respect of the government contribution, in 2003, 193 governments signed the Copenhagen Declaration on Anti-Doping in Sport, demonstrating a commitment to tackle doping. In practice, however, securing funding for WADA operations has been problematic. Currently, the IOC is required to match-fund the contribution by governments. Therefore, WADA requires governments to increase their funding in order to access a greater share of IOC funds. Unfortunately, government commitment has been inconsistent in practice despite policy statements and rhetoric. It can also be noted that the IOC generates significant and increasing levels of income as broadcasting revenue increases and it could therefore increase its contribution. Despite this, real term cuts to WADA's budget may compromise its goals. Moreover, investigations into doping are resource intensive, with the McLaren reports (2016a, and 2016b) costing 12.5 per cent of WADA's annual budget (Association internationale de la presse sportive, 2017). It can be argued that without sufficient financial resources, coupled with the effective use of these resources, securing impactful and sustainable measures to challenge doping lacks feasibility.

Compliance with the World Anti-Doping Code

Assuming a level of political will to tackle doping is manifest in both public authorities and sports governing bodies, and financial resources are adequate to tackle doping, effective anti-doping measures also require the compliance of organisations to deliver practices aligned with the World Anti-Doping Code. It can be noted, however, that actions such as signing the Code, writing policy statements, formulating sport-specific codes of practice, establishing an ethics committee to investigate doping, and so on, are more readily achievable than the more difficult challenges associated with implementation and evaluation.

It was the case that some sports initially resisted signing or implementing the Code but as of mid-2017, a broad consensus is established. This is in part due to increasing government (or more broadly, state) intervention resulting in governing bodies administering a level of self-governance in order to retain semi-autonomous status. For example, the Olympic Charter was amended in 2003 to state that the World Anti-Doping Code is mandatory for the whole Olympic Movement. Currently, sports governing bodies and athletes must seek to be fully compliant with the Code in three stages: acceptance, implementation, and enforcement (Houlihan, 2014). Government agencies have concluded that where there is an embedded culture of weak governance in respect of doping, inducements or penalties such as sanctions for non-compliance, at least in the short term, are justifiable. However, there are limitations to enforcement as a compliance strategy. Research suggests that 'non-compliance is best addressed through a problem-solving strategy of capacity building, rule interpretation, and transparency, rather than through coercive enforcement' (Tallberg, 2002: 613). In practice, it cannot be claimed that governing bodies are wholly compliant with the Code in respect of doping, as it is 'work in progress'. Nonetheless, the Code has had an impact on sport governance.

To what extent WADA is an independent global regulator with powers to enforce compliance is debatable given its resource dependency on external funding, most notably from the IOC, and a lack of sanctioning powers. In other words, compliance with the World Anti-Doping Code is diminished by the regulator's resources and scope for influence. The McLaren reports serve to highlight not only the extent of doping in specific states but also issues of governing body compliance with WADA. Currently, WADA can recommend specific actions are undertaken by sports governing bodies but recommendations are not conditions that require action and audit. Nonetheless, the IOC has accepted the thrust of the McLaren reports and has agreed to retest all Russian athlete samples from London 2012 and Sochi 2014. The outstanding issue across different nations and sports bodies is finding consensus regarding WADA's remit and jurisdiction. Moreover, WADA and national anti-doping agencies have limited control if the state apparatus for sport effectively condones or promotes athlete use of drugs. In sum, it can be claimed that WADA's prospects for success in meeting its goals have improved since its foundation (Houlihan, 2000). However, there remain significant obstacles to effective anti-doping policy.

Legal and regulatory robustness

A substantive regulatory infrastructure exists today for sport, including legislative components. Given the potential for litigation by wealthy elite athletes, for example, with serious financial and reputational consequences for sports organisations, disputes can be resolved in the Court of Arbitration for Sport (CAS) and all International Federations have recognised the jurisdiction of CAS for anti-doping rule violations. Governing bodies, such as the IAAF, have also adopted a strict liability definition where 'a doping offence is deemed to have been committed if a prohibited substance is present in an athlete's urine sample, irrespective of whether the drug was taken knowingly or whether the drug was capable of enhancing performance' (Houlihan, 2003: 223). However, there can be medical exemptions, which in itself raises questions about defining what constitutes performance enhancement.

In the last decade, an incremental shift towards the criminalisation of doping has occurred in Italy and Spain and Kenya, for example. Germany has gone further in criminalising athlete support workers such as coaches and managers for doping infractions. Treating doping as a criminal offence creates a parallel approach with recreational drug-use legislation and regulation that has resulted in a 'war on drugs' in sport (Kayser, Mauron and Miah, 2007). The criminalisation of athletes is not the preferred position of WADA but governments taking action against the distribution and trafficking of banned substances is encouraged (WADA, 2015b). This is in part a response to criminal operations becoming associated with professional sport.

It is debatable whether there are sufficient ethical grounds for an anti-doping policy situated within a model of prohibition (Kirkwood, 2012). Instead, governing bodies could focus on harm-reduction through education programmes and imposing penalties that pertain only to sport. Currently, under the World Anti-Doping Code (2015a) a first offence for doping carries a four-year ban, where it was two years previously, and a second offence equates to a lifetime ban. Further, those found guilty of doping can be banned for at least one Olympic Games cycle. Despite this robust stance, however, since 2015, the UK government has considered making doping a criminal offence (Brown, 2015). Criminalisation aside, an expanded culture of surveillance has emerged to monitor and detect athlete doping via a 'whereabouts' rule, which in itself is contentious (Moller, 2011). Further, a role for

INTERPOL in investigating doping demonstrates that it is no longer only government agencies with a sport-related remit that oversee professional commercialised sport. As a response, sports organisations are seeking to retain legitimacy for those that govern sport by adopting the World Anti-Doping Code, albeit with varying levels of commitment in practice.

Interoperability, collaboration and trust

The relationship between governing bodies for sport and government agencies is pivotal for anti-doping policy and governance practices to be effective. As noted, this relationship has been complicated by an increasing level of commercialisation in professional sport, changes in the legal and regulatory environment, and a growing media spotlight on sport.

Houlihan (1999a, 1999b and 2003) analyses the development of international cooperation that emerged in response to problems of disjointed and uncoordinated anti-doping efforts, including, among others: a high degree of mutual suspicion, a scarcity and splintering of resources required to conduct research and testing, a lack of knowledge about specific substances and procedures being used and to what degree, an inconsistent approach to sanctions for those athletes found guilty of doping, and other interoperability issues. However, despite the emergence of an epistemic community centred on reducing doping and securing the integrity and authenticity of sport, significant interoperability issues remain in a fluid policy environment vulnerable to crisis and distrust between sports bodies operating at different levels of governance, between government agencies and departments, and not least between government and governing bodies for sport. As a hybrid public-private body, WADA is nested within this complex governance super-structure and multifaceted policy environment (Casini, 2009). It can be argued that the effective governance of doping requires more extensive cooperation and coordination than is currently the case.

Extended stakeholding

Hierarchic governance has proven to be a major source of conflict in sport, since those that are excluded from the decision-making process may want to challenge regulations and decisions but have limited scope to do so (García, 2007). However, due to the traditional hierarchic governance of sport, policy and governance has rarely been stakeholder-driven (Henry and Lee, 2004). Moreover, a failure to consult stakeholders increases the potential for unproductive levels of conflict in sport governance. Athletes acquiring a voice in organisational decision-making processes and structures can take the form of athlete representation on committees with a focus on doping, within a wider process of democratisation (Houlihan, 2013). Of course, for effective anti-doping measures to become the norm, the case for extending athlete representation is strengthened where athletes themselves comply with best practice in respect of doping.

Where athletes have a legitimate concern regarding doping, sports bodies must have an effective whistleblowing policy (Thibault, Kihl and Babiak, 2010). However, in such cases, particularly given that doping cases can bring reputational and financial damage to a governing body, whistleblowers can be marginalised, especially as the economic and communications 'fire power' rests within the organisation on which the individual has informed. It can be noted that the evidence underpinning the McLaren investigation into doping in Russia was supplied by a whistleblower, without which the investigation may never have taken place. The key point here is that it is problematic for 'good governance' to emerge when the fullest extent of the problem is unquantified. In order to more accurately quantify the extent of doping, governing bodies require athlete and support worker participation in the policy process. Given that accountability is a core component of corporate governance (Low and Cowton, 2004) and powerful sports organisations are in effect corporate bodies, albeit in the non-profit sector, doping can no longer be treated purely as a matter for administrators to address. Instead, extending stakeholder engagement and participation in sport governance can be one component of a strategy to address doping.

Managing the media, doping 'scandals' and public perceptions

Public perceptions are critical for anti-doping measures to take effect (Houlihan, 2003). However, the mainstream media portrays sport governance as being in a permanent state of 'crisis' with few if any solutions. Research conducted by UK Anti-Doping (UKAD) in 2017 found that almost half of adults in the sample believed that doping is widespread based on media reports (UKAD, 2017). Stamm et al. (2008) observed an increased public awareness of doping from research in Switzerland and research findings from a poll in the USA suggest a declining public trust in doping-free sport (Longman and Connolly, 2003). It may be the case that frequent 'scandals' as defined by media organisations have, over time, shaped public perception. Perhaps more concerning for WADA and the coalition working against doping is the findings of research by Vangrunderbeek and Tolleneer (2010), who observed that between 1998 and 2006 student attitudes to doping had shifted from one of zero tolerance towards a more diffuse ethical attitude. These findings raise concerns over the efficacy of educational programmes targeted at doping in sport if societal attitudes are changing.

In response to media and public perceptions, governing bodies have sometimes responded positively and pro-actively (MacAloona, 2011) whilst others have denied that there is a 'crisis' until a tipping point was reached, for example in the Lance Armstrong case (Dimeo, 2014). Governance by reaction to crisis is clearly insufficient as a tactic to address doping, and the media, by focusing on 'scandals', exacerbate the tendency of governing bodies to react defensively. Facilitating informed debate and conducting an internal investigation of doping within sports, led by governing bodies, is necessary if public perceptions are to be modified. A lack of honesty, transparency and accountability in respect of the doping issue in sport has arguably undermined public trust in sport.

Embedding good governance practices

In recent years, cases of corruption in the corporate sector have led to calls for 'good governance' (Transparency International, 2009a, 2009b) and as sports bodies have adopted corporate governance practices (King, 2016), a similar narrative has emerged where weak governance is cited. As a result, sports governing bodies, such as for tennis (Miller, 2011), have responded by taking actions to introduce good governance practices. The IOC (2008) has introduced a focus on good governance along with other governing bodies who have adopted the principles cited by the Council of Europe (2005). The COE define 'good governance' in terms of a complex network of policy measures and private regulations to promote the core values of sport such as democratic, ethical, efficient and accountable sports activities. Further, the International Sport and Culture Association (2005) notes that good governance is a prerequisite for the legitimacy, autonomy and survival of sports organisations. Introducing a set of rules and regulations does not ensure good governance, however. Fully addressing doping may require a 'democratic environment' to emerge over time and this requires the application of principles pertaining to accountability and transparency.

Fundamentally, accountability entails identifying who is accountable, for what, how, to whom and with what outcome (Bovens, 2007; Mulgan, 2000). Houlihan (2013) adds that accountability also relates to: efficiency in the pursuit of organisational objectives; a culture of trust, honesty and professionalism; and organisational resilience. A distinction can also be made between accountability (providing an answer) and responsibility (liability). Accountability clearly involves a relationship between those who call for modifications to existing practices such as WADA and those with oversight for existing practices (governing bodies) who are in effect 'held to account'. Transparency can be conceived as an intrinsic component of democratic, accountable organisations, and a safeguard against corruption (Hood and Heald, 2006).

As debates around good governance are bound-up with issues of autonomy and regulation (Geeraert, Alm and Groll, 2013), accountability is important to provide a democratic means to monitor and control conduct ('the democratic perspective'); for preventing the development of concentrations of power ('the constitutional perspective'); and to enhance the learning capacity and effectiveness of an administration ('the learning perspective'). Unfortunately, as Pound (2011) observes, sports organisations have been deficient with regard to accountability and many have resisted any suggestion that its governance should be transparent. A challenge to operationalising transparency is how to make information available regarding doping. Governing bodies can adopt a model of 'real time transparency' (where there is continuous athlete surveillance for example) or a model of 'retrospective transparency' (where information is released in a reporting cycle). Another form of retrospective transparency was recently proposed by the European Athletics Federation (EAF) that would make null and void all world records set in athletics prior to 2005 when more sophisticated drug screening was introduced (BBC, 2017). Clearly this mitigates against 'clean' athletes who competed fairly and has understandably met with athlete objection.

Extending accountability and transparency is arguably compromised by the more powerful international sports organisations choosing to be based in an optimal regulatory context for their semi-autonomous operations. In Switzerland, the IOC, for example, is embedded into a legal system that gives them a level of protection against internal and external examination. Bringing the operation of powerful sports organisations into a legal and regulatory framework applied to less powerful sports bodies may result in stronger governance regarding the doping issue. The less powerful and resource dependent governing bodies by contrast find themselves subject to ever-expanding state powers in the sport sector.

In respect of organisations with oversight for doping, it cannot be claimed that good governance is currently a norm, despite policy rhetoric. This suggests a more robust and longer-term strategy to tackle doping is required, especially given the governance challenges identified in this chapter. WADA does offer some flexibility for how organisations implement good governance within the Code, given the differing resources for sports bodies. However, government agencies require short-term solutions and the push towards criminalisation of doping is indicative of the urgency with which the doping issue is being treated. The catalyst for this sense of urgency has to some extent been as a result of the damning conclusions of the McLaren reports.

27.6 Discussion: at a crossroads – doping as a test case for sport governance

The anti-doping policy community has grown in influence, particularly since the creation of WADA. However, many governing bodies for sport face significant challenges in building the optimal capacity to be effective in meeting the challenges posed by doping infringements and doping cultures. In a context of limited resources, competing organisational agendas, variable political will across states and sports, resource dependencies that compromise WADA's aspirations, and state or governing body collusion in obfuscating the true extent of doping in sport in some cases, the policy environment is both complex and, following the damning McLaren reports, toxic. On the other hand, the McLaren reports may prove to be a catalyst for fundamental change in the sector, although 'tipping points' have been identified before without fundamental changes to governance practices, such as after the Ben Johnson affair.

Ostensibly, for doping in sport to be addressed, organisations are required to investigate themselves, ensure safeguards for whistleblowers, provide a more robust voice for athletes as key stakeholders, and develop a culture of trust and information-sharing. Further, governing bodies would have to address problematic relationships with the media, government and regulatory agencies to ensure a negotiated level of scrutiny and compliance. In some cases, this requires a cultural shift in sports with a history of normalising doping such as professional cycling. Effective action, however defined, is compromised further where the extent of doping is simply not known and there is little incentive to uncover what may prove to be a much larger issue than sport bodies and government agencies would want to admit.

It can be argued that the dominant elite sport paradigm, located within economic, political and socio-cultural forms of neo-liberalism, results in doping cultures that shape the decisions of some athletes, support workers, administrators and those leading governing bodies. In neo-liberal societies where personal and organisational success in terms of medals and the associated financial and reputational rewards can compromise athlete welfare, a percentage of athletes, support workers and in some cases state agencies will, for personal, financial and ideological reasons, seek to obfuscate the extent of doping in a bid to profit from 'unfair advantage'. In this context, athletes face a number of inter-related pressures that may enable doping, including changing attitudes to drug use in society, peer pressure within a sport that has an embedded doping culture, and not least the financial and reputational rewards of winning 'at all costs'.

Looking to the future, further state-led intervention in sport governance is likely, resulting in further legislation, regulation and criminalisation, but a 'war on drugs' is highly unlikely to be successful. As the anti-doping infrastructure expands, so too does its commitment to resource anti-doping, eventually resulting in the overload and potential breakdown of this infrastructure into competing factions. Sports organisations and government must weigh-up the value of national and athlete success in international competition against the values of participation, fairness, democratic processes and the integrity of sport. This requires sports organisations to normalise, embed, deliver, evaluate and share 'good governance' in respect of doping. Tackling a doping culture in sport requires those in positions of authority and influence to demonstrate leadership, build organisational capacity and enact changes with limited resources. More fundamentally, it requires a paradigm shift in sport governance and the dominant narratives that drive it.

Doping is arguably the 'test case' for the government bodies of sport and government agencies investing in anti-doping measures. This chapter highlights the nature of the challenge and the significance of doping for the future of sport governance.

27.7 Summary

- The issue of doping is central to understanding the governance of sport.
- Sport governance in respect of doping has in part been driven by a series of 'scandals'.
- An extensive organisational and regulatory infrastructure exists today to challenge doping in sport.
- The founding of WADA was an attempt to find a consensus in anti-doping policy.
- Securing adequate funding for WADA operations has been problematic.
- Harmonising anti-doping policy and practice across nation states remains an aspiration rather than a reality.
- The effective governance of doping requires more extensive cooperation and coordination.
- An expanded culture of surveillance has emerged to monitor and detect athlete doping.
- There has been an incremental shift towards the criminalisation of doping as government expands its influence in sport governance.
- Doping is deeply embedded in sport governance where it is under state control.
- It is problematic for 'good governance' to emerge when the fullest extent of the problem is unquantified.
- A declining public trust in doping free sport threatens the effective governance of doping.
- Governing body accountability is critical for successful anti-doping interventions to take effect.
- Doping is a 'test case' for the government bodies of sport and government agencies investing in anti-doping measures.

27.8 References

Association internationale de la presse sportive (2017) *Anti-Doping Reality: We All Get What We Pay For*. Available at: http://www.aipsmedia.com/2017/02/11/20322/anti-doping-wada-funding-mclaren-report-alan-abrahamson (Accessed on 11 February 2017).

Australian Government (1989) *Drugs in Sport*. Interim report of the Senate Standing Committee on the Environment, Recreation and the Arts. Canberra, Australian Government Publishing Service.

BBC (2017) *Doping: European Athletics to Examine Credibility of All Records*. Available at: http://www.bbc.co.uk/sport/athletics/38765253 (Accessed on 26 January 2017).

Bovens, M. (2007) Analysing and assessing accountability: A conceptual framework. *European Law Journal* 13(4): 447–468.

Brown, A. (2015) *UK Government to Consider the Criminalisation of Doping*. The Sports Integrity Initiative. Available at: http://www.sportsintegrityinitiative.com/uk-government-to-consider-criminalisation-of-doping/ (Accessed on 30 October 2017).

Casini, L. (2009) *Global hybrid public-private bodies: The World Anti-Doping Agency (WADA)*. Draft paper for the Global Administrative Law Conference on 'Practical Legal Problems of International Organizations', Geneva, 20–21 March 2009, 4.

Copenhagen Declaration on Anti-Doping in Sport (2003) Available at: http://www.wadaama.org/Documents/World_Antidoping_Program/Governments/WADA_Copenhagen_Declaration_EN.pdf (Accessed on 30 October 2017).

Council of Europe (2005) *Recommendation Rec (2005)8 of the Committee of Ministers to Member States on the Principles of Good Governance in Sport*. Available at: https://wcd.coe.int/ViewDoc.jsp?id=850189&Site=CM (Accessed on 30 October 2017).

David, P. (2008) *A Guide to the World Anti-Doping Code: A Fight for the Spirit of Sport*. Cambridge University Press, Cambridge.

Dimeo, P. (2014) Why Lance Armstrong? Historical context and key turning points in the 'cleaning up' of professional cycling. *The International Journal of the History of Sport* 31(8): 951–968.

Dubin, C.L. (1990) *Commission of Inquiry into the Use of Drugs and Banned Practices Intended to Increase Athletic Performance*. Ottawa, Canadian Government Publishing Centre.

Franke, W.W. and Berendonk, B. (1997) Hormonal doping and androgenisation of athletes: A secret program of the German Democratic Republic. *Clinical Chemistry* 43(7): 1,262–1,279.

García, B. (2007) From regulation to governance and representation: Agenda-setting and the EU's involvement in sport. *Entertainment and Sports Law Journal* 5(1): 1–13.

Gardiner, S. (2009) Sport and the law. In K. Bill (ed.) *Sport Management*. Exeter, Learning Matters, chapter 14.

Geeraert, A., Alm, J. and Groll, M. (2013) Good governance in international sport organizations: An analysis of the 35 Olympic sport governing bodies. *International Journal of Sport Policy and Politics* 6(3): 281–306.

Green, M. and Houlihan, B. (2006) Governmentality, modernization and the 'disciplining' of national sporting Organisations: Athletics in Australia and the United Kingdom. *Sociology of Sport Journal* 23(1): 47–71.

Haas, E.B. (1990) *When Knowledge is Power: Three Models of Change in International Organisations*. Berkeley and Los Angeles, University of California Press.

Hartley, H. (2013) Modahl V British Athletic Federation (1994-2001) in Anderson, J. (eds.) *Leading Cases in Sports Law*. ASSER International Sports Law Series. The Hague, T.M.C. Asser Press.

Henry, I.P. and Lee, P.C. (2004) Governance and ethics in sport. In S. Chadwick and J. Beech (eds) *The Business of Sport Management*. Harlow, Pearson Education, 25–42.

Hoberman, J. (1984) *Sport and Political Ideology*. Austin, The University of Texas Press.

Holt, R.I.G., Erotokritou-Mulligan, I. and Sonksen, P.H. (2009) The history of doping and growth hormone abuse in sport. *Growth Hormone and IVF Research* 19(4): 320–326.

Hood, C. and Heald, D. (2006). *Transparency: The Key to Better Governance?* Oxford, Oxford University Press.

Houlihan, B. (1999a) Policy harmonization: The example of global anti-doping policy. *Journal of Sport Management* 13(3): 197–215.

Houlihan, B. (1999b) Anti-doping policy in sport: The politics of international policy co-ordination, *Public Administration* 77: 311–334.

Houlihan, B. (2000) The World Anti-Doping Agency: Prospects for Success. In J. O'Leary (ed.) *Drugs and Doping in Sport*. Cavendish, London, 125.

Houlihan, B. (2002a) *Dying to Win*, 2nd edition. Strasbourg, Council of Europe.

Houlihan, B. (2002b) Managing compliance in international anti-doping policy: The world anti-doping code. *European Sport Management Quarterly* 2(3): 188–208

Houlihan, B. (2003) Doping and sport: More problems than solutions? In B. Houlihan (ed.) *Sport and Society: A Student Introduction*. London, Sage, 218–234.

Houlihan, B. (2007) The politics of sports policy in Britain: The example of drug abuse. In A. Tomlinson (ed.) *The Sport Studies Reader*. London, Routledge, 157–164.

Houlihan, B. (2013) Stakeholders, stakeholding and good governance in international sport federations. In J. Elm (ed.) *Action for Good Governance in International Sports Organisations*. Copenhagen, Danish Institute for Sports Studies, 185–189.

Houlihan, B. (2014) Achieving compliance in international anti-doping policy: An analysis of the 2009 World Anti-Doping Code. *Sport Management Review* 17(3): 265–276.

Hoye, R. and Cuskelly, G. (2007) *Sport Governance*. Oxford, Elsevier Butterworth-Heinemann.

IAAF (2016) *Reform of the IAAF: A New Era*. Monaco, IAAF.

International Olympic Committee (2008) *Basic Universal Principles of Good Governance of the Olympic and Sports Movement*. IOC, Lausanne. Available at: 2016.http://www.olympic.org/Documents/Conferences_Forums_and_Events/2008_seminar_autonomy/Basic_Universal_Principles_of_Good_Governance.pdf (Accessed on 19 August 2016).

International Sport and Culture Association (2005) *Good governance: A Code for the Voluntary and Community Sector*. Available at: http://www.governancecode.org/wp-content/uploads/2012/06/Code-of-Governance-Full1.pdf (Accessed on 30 October 2017).

Kayser, B., Mauron, A. and Miah, A. (2007) Current anti-doping policy: A critical appraisal. *Medical Ethics* 8(2): 1–10.

King, N. (2016) *Sport Governance: An Introduction*. London, Routledge.

Kirkwood, K. (2009) Considering harm reduction as the future of anti-doping policy in international sport. *Quest* 61(2): 180–190.

Longman, J. and Connolly, M. (2003) Americans suspect steroid use in sport is common, poll finds. *New York Times*, 16 December.

Low, C. and Cowton, C. (2004) Beyond stakeholder engagement: The challenges of stakeholder participation in corporate governance. *International Journal of Business Governance and Ethics* 1(1): 45–55.

MacAloona, J.J. (2011) Scandal and governance: Inside and outside the IOC 2000 Commission. *Sport in Society: Cultures, Commerce, Media, Politics* 14(3): 292–308.

McLaren, R.H. (2016a) *WADA Investigation of Sochi Allegations: The Independent Person Report*. Lausanne, WADA.

McLaren, R.H. (2016b) *WADA Investigation of Sochi Allegations: The Independent Person 2nd Report*. Lausanne, WADA.

Miller, S. (2011) Good governance and anti-doping policy: An international federation view. *International Journal of Sport Policy and Politics* 3(2): 279–288.

Moller, V. (2011) One step too far: About WADA's whereabouts rule. *International Journal of Sports Policy and Politics* 3(2): 177–190.

Mulgan, R. (2000) 'Accountability': An ever-expanding concept? *Public Administration* 78(3): 555–573.

Numerato, D. Baglioni, S. and Persson, H.T.R. (2013) The dark sides of sport governance. In D. Hassan and J. Lusted (eds) *Managing Sport: Social and Cultural Perspectives*. London, Routledge, 284–300.

Parrish, R. (2003) The politics of sports regulation in the EU. *Journal of European public policy*, 10(2), 246–262.

Pieth, M. (2010) *Harmonising Anti-Corruption Compliance*. Zurich, OECD Good Practice Guidance.

Play the Game (2016) *Corruption 'Embedded' in the IAAF: Second WADA Report*. Available at: http://www.playthegame.org/news/news-articles/2016/0140_corruption-embedded-in-the-iaaf-second-wada-report/ (Accessed on 30 October 2017).

Pound, R. (2011) *Responses to Corruption in Sport*. Presentation to Play the Game Conference, 3 October 2011.

Reid, D. and Kitchin, P. (2013) The management of anti-doping: An ongoing challenge for sport. In D. Hassan and J. Lusted (eds.) *Managing Sport: Social and Cultural Perspectives*. Oxford: Routledge, 34–50.

Reilly, L. (2012) Introduction to the Court of Arbitration for Sport (CAS) and the role of national courts in international sports disputes. *Journal of Dispute Resolution* 1: 63–80.

Robinson, L. (2012) Contemporary issues in the performance of sports organisations. In L. Robinson, P. Chelladurai, G. Bodet and P. Downward (eds) *Routledge Handbook of Sport Management*. New York, Routledge, 3–6.

Stamm, H., Lamprecht, M., Kamber, M., Mart, B. and Mahler, N. (2008) The public perception of doping in sport in Switzerland, 1995–2004. *Journal of Sport Sciences* 26: 235–242.

Tallberg, J. (2002) Paths to compliance: Enforcement, management, and the European Union. *International Organization* 56(3): 609–643.

Thibault, L., Kihl, L. and Babiak, K. (2010) Democratization and governance in international sport: Addressing issues with athlete involvement in organizational policy. *International Journal of Sport Policy and Politics* 2(3): 275–302.

Transparency International (2009a) *Business Principles for Countering Bribery: A Multi-Stakeholder Initiative Led by Transparency International*. Berlin, Transparency International.

Transparency International (2009b) *Corruption and Sport: Building Integrity and Preventing Abuses (TI Working Paper # 03/2009)*. Berlin, Transparency International.

UNESCO (2012) *International Convention against Doping in Sport*. Available at: http://www.unesco.org/eri/la/convention.asp?KO=31037&language=E&order=alpha (Accessed on 30 October 2017).

UK Anti-Doping (UKAD) (2017) *UKAD Issues Urgent Wake-up Call as Doping Stories Hit Public Trust in the Integrity of Sport*. Available at: http://ukad.org.uk/news/article/ukad-issues-urgent-wake-up-call-as-doping-stories-hit-public-trust-in-the-i/ (Accessed on 30 October 2017).

UK Sport (2004) *Good Governance: A Guide for National Governing Bodies of Sport*, London, Institute of Chartered Secretaries and Administrators.

UK Parliament (2015) *Governance of Sport Bill*. Available at: http://www.publications.parliament.uk/pa/bills/lbill/2014-2015/0020/15020.pdf (Accessed on 30 October 2017).

Vangrunderbeek, H. and Tolleneer, J. (2010) Student attitudes towards doping in sport: Shifting from repression to tolerance? *International Review for the Sociology of Sport* 46(3): 346–357.

Winand, M., Rihoux, B. and Qualizza, D. (2011) Combinations of key determinants of performance in sport governing bodies. *Sport, Business and Management: An International Journal* 1(3): 234–251.

World Anti-Doping Agency (WADA) (2015a) *World Anti-doping Code*. Lausanne, WADA. Available at: https://www.wada-ama.org/en/what-we-do/the-code (Accessed on 30 October 2017).

World Anti-Doping Agency (WADA) (2015b) WADA statement on the criminalization of doping in sport. https://www.wada-ama.org/en/media/news/2015-10/wada-statement-on-the-criminalization-of-doping-in-sport (Accessed on 30 October 2017).

Index

Page numbers in **bold refer to Tables**. *Page numbers in italics refer to Figures.*

CPSIA information can be obtained
at www.ICGtesting.com
Printed in the USA
LVHW06s1831210518
577950LV00014B/250/P

9 780415 789417